Veterinary Notes for Dog Owners

Veterinary Notes for Dog Owners

Edited by
Trevor Turner BVet Med, MRCVS, FRSH

Popular Dogs
London Sydney Auckland Johannesburg

Popular Dogs Publishing Co. Ltd

An imprint of the Random Century Group
20 Vauxhall Bridge Road, London SW1V 2SA

Random Century Australia (Pty) Ltd
20 Alfred Street, Milsons Point, Sydney, NSW 2061

Random Century New Zealand Limited
PO Box 40–086, Glenfield, Auckland 10

Century Hutchinson South Africa (Pty) Ltd
PO Box 337, Bergvlei 2012, South Africa

First published 1990

Set in Linotron Sabon by 🅰 Tek Art Ltd, Addiscombe, Croydon, Surrey

Photographic origination by Thomas Campone, Southampton

Printed and bound in Great Britain by Butler & Tanner

British Library Cataloguing in Publication Data
Veterinary Notes for dog owners
1. Livestock: Dogs. Veterinary care
I. Turner, B. Trevor
636.7089

ISBN   0 09 174374 5 (cased)
        0 09 173817 2 (paper)

ACKNOWLEDGEMENT OF ILLUSTRATIONS

The majority of the photographs were provided by Trevor Turner and the authors. In addition the publishers would like to thank the following for allowing reproduction of photographs as indicated:

Dr Peter Emily DDS, Diplomate ACVS Plates 16, 17, 20, 21, 27, 28; *Dr M.T. Fox BVet Med, PhD, MRCVS* Figs 176, 178; *Professor Colin E. Harvey BVSc, MRCVS, Diplomate ACVS* Plate 26; *Marc Henri ASC/Dr Roger Mugford BSc, PhD* Figs 36a, 36b, 36c, 37a, 37b, 37c, 38a, 38b, 38c, 38d, 39, 40; *J.G. Lane BVet Med, FRCVS* Plate 22; *Cooper Pitman-Moore* Plate 6; *The Royal Veterinary College* Plates 2, 4; *Sally Anne Thompson* Figs 1, 2, 3, 4, 5, 6, 8, 10, 14, 17, 22, 23, 24, 30; *R.T. Willbie* Fig 21

Thanks are also due to Dr Peter Emily for providing the illustrations for Figs 199, 200, 204 and 205.

CONTENTS

Infectious Diseases

Medical and Surgical

Miscellaneous

ABOUT THE AUTHORS

Dr W.E. ALLEN, MVB, PhD, FRCVS
Ed Allen qualified in Dublin in 1968. After 18 months in general practice he joined the Department of Surgery and Obstetrics at the Royal Veterinary College to study reproductive problems. He was awarded a PhD in 1973 and Fellowship of the Royal College of Veterinary Surgeons in 1983. He is now Senior Lecturer in Animal Reproduction at the College, and his main professional interests centre on reproductive problems in the dog and horse.

Dr P.G.C. BEDFORD, BVet Med, PhD, FRCVS, DVOphtal
Peter Bedford qualified from the Royal Veterinary College London in 1967. He is currently University Reader in Veterinary Ophthalmology at the College. In 1974 he gained his PhD for work on canine glaucoma and in 1977 Fellowship of the Royal College of Veterinary Surgeons. In 1982 he was made a Foundation Diplomate in Veterinary Ophthalmology. His interests include all aspects of veterinary and comparative ophthalmology and upper respiratory tract disease. Current research includes new techniques for the relief of glaucoma and the aetiology of retinal pigment epithelial dystrophy (central progressive retinal atrophy) in the dog.

Dr W.P. BERESFORD-JONES, MA, PhD, MRCVS
Peter Beresford-Jones read agriculture at the University of Cambridge and graduated with a BA degree and a certificate of proficiency. Vacations spent on Shropshire farms led to his interest in farm animal disease and as a result he entered Glasgow Veterinary School in 1939, having converted his BA degree to an MA. During the war he served in the Territorials but returned to Glasgow after demobilisation. He transferred to the Royal Veterinary College London in order to complete his studies for the MRCVS diploma, graduating in December 1949. He spent some time in practice and was then appointed as an assistant lecturer in Veterinary Parasitology at the Royal Veterinary College. Rising to Head of Department, during his 27 years in the division he reorganised the syllabus in order to emphasise its veterinary importance. He was awarded his PhD in 1964 for work in parasitology and has published papers on both endo and ecto parasites, many of which refer to those found in the dog, cat and fox. Together with Professor D.E. Jacobs he contributed to the chapter on endoparasites published in *Canine Medicine and Therapeutics*, now entering its third edition and regarded as the authoritative textbook on the subject. Peter Beresford-Jones also examined veterinary students on the subject of parasitology. Now retired, he regularly lectures to veterinary undergraduates at the Royal Veterinary College.

PATSY BLOOM, Company Director, Associate Member BSAVA
Patsy Bloom had a successful career in advertising and marketing when she founded PetPlan, a company specialising in pet health insurance in 1977. The company very soon established itself as a market leader in its field. Patsy was a finalist in the 1988 Veuve Clicquot Business Woman of the Year competition and is an admitted insurance broker under the Institute of Registered Insurance

Brokers. In recognition of her association with the veterinary profession she was made an associate member of the British Small Animal Veterinary Association. A workaholic, she lives in Central London with her Yorkshire Terrier 'Champers'.

Dr B.M. BUSH, BVSc, PhD, FRCVS
Barry Bush qualified from the University of Bristol in 1961 and worked in small animal practice before moving to the Royal Veterinary College where he is now Senior Lecturer in Small Animal Medicine. In addition to teaching commitments he acts as a consultant in the referral hospitals of the Royal Veterinary College. His main interests are internal medicine laboratory medicine and first aid for dogs and cats. He has published several books and was responsible for establishing the first organised courses for the education of veterinary nurses and continues to be associated with their training and examination.

J.E.F. HOULTON, MA, Vet MB, MRCVS, DVR
John Houlton qualified from the University of Cambridge Veterinary School in 1970 and subsequently spent six years in practice before returning to Cambridge as assistant University surgeon. In 1982 he gained the Diploma in Veterinary Radiology from the Royal College of Veterinary Surgeons. Now University Surgeon at the Veterinary School he is responsible for the small animal orthopaedic lecture course and orthopaedic cases. A Freeman of the City of London, in 1985 he was awarded the British Small Animal Veterinary Association 'Simon' Award for outstanding contributions to Veterinary Surgery. His main professional interests include orthopaedic surgery, trauma and radiology.

Dr IAN S. MASON, B Vet Med, PhD, MRCVS
Ian Mason qualified from the Royal Veterinary College London in 1981. After three years in practice he returned to the College as a research fellow and in 1987 became clinical resident in Dermatology at the Queen Mother Hospital of the Royal Veterinary College. Awarded a PhD in 1990 he currently provides a referral service in veterinary dermatology.

SUSAN E. MATIC MA, BVSc, MRCVS, DVC, DVR
Sue Matic emigrated to South Africa with her parents in the early 1960s and qualified there as a veterinary surgeon in 1974. Following brief but varied experiences in mixed practice she returned to Britain and spent six years in small animal practice during which time she gained a Certificate in Veterinary Radiology. She spent a year in the radiology department at Cambridge veterinary school gaining the Diploma in Veterinary Radiology in 1983, then joined the staff at the Cambridge veterinary school teaching small animal medicine. During this time she developed an interest in cardiology and to further this interest visited several centres in the USA and gained the Diploma in Veterinary Cardiology in 1989. Recently Sue left teaching and is involved at present in animal welfare and employed by the Government.

Dr I.A.P. McCANDLISH BVMS, PhD, MRCVS
Irene McCandlish qualified from Glasgow University Veterinary School in 1973. She returned to Glasgow to investigate kennel cough in dogs, was awarded her

PhD in 1977 and is currently Senior Lecturer in Veterinary Pathology and a member of the Canine Infectious Disease research unit there. This unit achieved world wide recognition following work on canine parvovirus infection and Dr McCandlish, together with Dr Hal Thompson received the prestigious Blaine award of the British Small Animal Veterinary Association in recognition of this work. Dr McCandlish has also been awarded the G. Norman Hall medal of the Royal College of Veterinary Surgeons for research into animal diseases and the Argus medal of the National Canine Defence League for outstanding services to canine welfare. In her spare time Dr McCandlish is a devotee of Rough Collies except, she says, when sodden and muddy but still intent on sitting on her knee.

PROFESSOR DAVID B. MORTON, BVSc, PhD, MRCVS

David Morton qualified as a veterinary surgeon from the University of Bristol in 1965 and subsequently studied for his PhD at Liverpool Veterinary School. This was followed by a research fellowship at Cambridge. He then moved to the University of Leicester Medical School to teach human anatomy where he became Director of the Unit of Biomedical Services. Currently he is Professor of Biomedical Science and Ethics at the University of Birmingham. At Leicester he collaborated with Professor Alan Jeffreys, pioneer in the field of genetic fingerprinting, resulting in the technique being developed to determine uncertain canine paternity. Recently the Canine Molecular Genetics Laboratory has been set up at the University of Leicester where techniques are presently being developed to detect inherited disease in dogs.

Dr ROGER A. MUGFORD, BSc, PhD

Roger Mugford graduated in Zoology and Psychology from the University of Hull and was subsequently awarded a PhD. In 1970 he joined the new Animal Behaviour section of the Animal Studies Centre at Pedigree Petfoods. In 1979 he started a referral practice dealing with behavioural problems in domestic animals, mainly dogs and cats. The practice is now the world's largest centre committed to the treatment of animal behavioural problems, employing two veterinary surgeons, two PhDs and two other graduates. Roger contributes regularly to radio and TV and is the author of many articles on the subject of animal behavioural therapy.

Dr ANDREW S. NASH, BVMS, PhD, MRCVS

Andrew Nash qualified from Glasgow Veterinary School in 1967. He spent five years in general practice before returning to Glasgow in 1973 as House Physician. In 1975 he became a lecturer in small animal medicine at Glasgow and is now Senior Lecturer at the Veterinary School. He was awarded his PhD for work on renal biopsies in dogs and cats in 1984. Always interested in kidney disease, since 1985 he has taken a special interest in juvenile nephropathies in dogs. Other interests include anaemia in dogs and cats, endocrine diseases and infectious diseases of cats. More recently he has turned his attention to the problems associated with obesity and hyperlipidaemia in dogs. He has published widely on many aspects of small animal internal medicine and is a regular speaker at professional and lay meetings at home and abroad.

Dr LARRY N. OWEN MA, DVSc, FRCPath, FRCVS

Larry Owen has just celebrated 40 years as a veterinary surgeon, qualifying from Liverpool Veterinary School in 1950. He spent some time in general practice and then returned to Liverpool as a lecturer in Veterinary Pharmacology. He worked in the Bahamas for three years and it was there that he developed an interest in oncology. Upon his return to England in 1958 he joined the staff of Cambridge University Veterinary School specialising in oncology. For several years he was actively involved in work for the World Health Organisation as well as being leader of a very successful research group in Cambridge. He retired from Cambridge University in 1982 and has run a veterinary cancer consultation service at the Animal Health Trust for the last eight years. Larry has contributed over 100 articles to veterinary or cancer journals and is an advocate of using methods developed for treating human cancer to which many 'hopeless' cases in animals are found to respond. Since his return to England in 1958 he estimates he has seen more than 10,000 dogs with cancer.

SUSANNA PENMAN, BVSc, MRCVS

Sue Penman qualified from the University of Bristol Veterinary School in 1980. For the next six years she worked mainly in small animal practice and then spent a year travelling around the world. While in Denver, Colorado in 1987 she was privileged to work with some of the leaders in the field of veterinary dentistry. She returned to the United Kingdom and further developed her interest in the subject and now runs a dental referral practice in addition to lecturing and writing on the subject. She is currently president of the British Veterinary Dental Association.

G.C. SKERRITT, BVSc, FRCVS

Geoff Skerritt qualified from the University of Liverpool Veterinary School in 1971. He spent a short time in small animal practice and then joined the veterinary faculty in Liverpool as a member of the academic staff. Originally appointed as a lecturer in veterinary anatomy he now teaches and practises veterinary neurology. He gained fellowship of the Royal College of Veterinary Surgeons in 1985 for a thesis concerned with neurological disease. Geoff Skerritt has lectured widely throughout Europe and North and South America and has acted as external examiner in five out of the six United Kingdom veterinary schools. Currently he is chairman of the Neurological Study Group of the British Small Animal Veterinary Association and council member of the European Society of Veterinary Neurologists. He has published extensively, both at home and abroad, on veterinary anatomy and neurology and is co-author of a popular veterinary textbook. He has also contributed to a number of other textbooks and pet care books and is translator of a French veterinary textbook into English. He has been interviewed several times on radio and television news programmes in the United Kingdom and South America. His current interests include clinical neurological disease in domestic animals, especially canine epilepsy.

M.J.R. STOCKMAN, MRCVS

Mike Stockman qualified from the Royal Veterinary College London over 40 years ago. Associated with dogs all his life he showed his first dog, a Golden Retriever, in 1942. He has had first hand experience with many breeds, buying his first Keeshond in 1947. He bred his first litter in 1962 and has campaigned three home-bred champions. A member of the Kennel Club since 1967, he chaired the Breeds Standards Committee for six years and is now chairman of Crufts committee. He is qualified to award Challenge Certificates in eleven breeds. Married to a Veterinary Surgeon with two sons and a daughter Mike has recently retired after 34 years in practice. In recent years he has engaged in purely canine practice. He writes irregularly for the veterinary and canine press and co-presents Crufts TV programmes with Angela Rippon and Peter Purves.

JEAN TURNER, VN
Jean Turner qualified originally as a secretary and worked for many years in a large organisation as PA to the Managing Director. Married to Trevor Turner she became involved in running a busy small animal practice and as soon as her responsibilities as a mother would allow, studied to qualify as a veterinary nurse in 1971. A member of Council of the British Veterinary Nursing Association she is presently Public Relations Officer for the association. An examiner in Veterinary Nursing for the Royal College of Veterinary Surgeons, she regularly lectures and writes on nursing topics both in the veterinary and dog and cat press. Working full time as hospital secretary her current interests include all aspects of veterinary nursing in addition to promoting the professional image of the veterinary nurse. Sharing a home with dogs, cats and other small animals, appearances in the exhibition ring are infrequent but nonetheless enjoyed.

TREVOR TURNER, BVet Med, MRCVS, FRSH
Trevor Turner qualified from the Royal Veterinary College in 1958. Brought up with dogs all his life he immediately entered the small animal field and within a few months established his own practice. From the same, but somewhat enlarged premises, he now runs a veterinary hospital employing over 30 people. A supporter of the veterinary nursing scheme from its inception he is past president and an honorary member of the British Veterinary Nursing Association. He speaks widely on veterinary and canine related topics and has twice been honoured by the British Small Animal Veterinary Association as the recipient of the prestigious 'Melton' award, latterly for his contributions towards forging links between the veterinary profession, breeders and members of the pet owning public. At present he and Jean share their home with three dogs and four cats.

D.J. WATSON, BVet Med, MRCVS
David Watson qualified from the Royal Veterinary College London in 1972 and spent seven years in predominantly small animal practice before entering commerce. Presently he is manager of the veterinary services division of Pedigree Petfoods. This work demands a detailed working knowledge of pet nutrition and a close understanding of the bond between owners and their pets.

Dr SUSAN P. YEO, BVet Med, PhD, MRCVS
Sue Yeo qualified from the Royal Veterinary College in 1981 and spent a couple of years in practice. She then joined Bristol University School as large animal house physician. In 1984 she became a veterinary research fellow at Bristol sponsored by the Agriculture and Food Research Council which led to the award of a PhD in 1988 for work in the field of Immunology. She is presently engaged in general practice.

INTRODUCTION

Veterinary Notes for Horse Owners was first published in 1877 at a time when the horse reigned supreme. It has gone through seventeen editions, three major revisions and countless reprints and is still extremely popular. Today the dog has replaced the horse as the major companion animal and far more practising veterinary surgeons are concerned with the welfare of dogs than with horses or farm livestock. This was the reasoning that led to the idea of this book late in 1987. The enthusiasm and excitement surrounding it did not wane throughout the many months of gestation.

Canine medicine and surgery, like many other branches of veterinary science, have progressed over the last few years. Successful treatment depends upon precise diagnosis and in this area the canine speciality is no laggard.

Owners' attitudes have also changed radically. The modern dog owner is informed, understanding and with or without the help of pet health insurance, prepared to invest heavily in the wellbeing of the family pet.

Veterinary Notes for Dog Owners is not intended as a do-it-yourself manual, nor is it to be regarded as a canine encyclopaedia. It is precisely as the title suggests, a collection of veterinary notes intended to inform, guide and assist all those involved with the welfare of dogs. With this object we have been particularly fortunate in managing to secure the enthusiastic cooperation and support of twenty-one authors, all experts in their fields. The thirty-six chapters are intended to present in an intelligible fashion up-to-the-minute facts relating to dogs and their management. Obviously some subjects are more complicated than others and while every effort has been made to ensure that explanations are kept as simple as possible, the temptations to distort by over-simplification or to assume that all readers are dog owning technocrats have been resisted.

The opening chapters on the responsibilities of dog owning, the breeds and genetics hopefully set the scene. This is not intended to be a heavy-going textbook but a readable account of all that is best in relation to dogs.

Breeds are described but not individually; such information may be obtained from a myriad of available texts today. Not so, however, information on canine immunology or on genetic fingerprinting, both fields in which far-reaching strides will be made in the next few years. In consequence these subjects are considered in depth.

Dog care does not depend solely upon advances in nutrition or cardiology, a knowledge of the endocrine system or elucidation of the complexities of infectious disease. From humble beginnings nearly thirty years ago veterinary nurses now play an indispensable support role in modern veterinary practice. In consequence veterinary nursing and the nurses' training and responsibilities are discussed in depth, followed by a chapter on nursing the sick dog.

The book is divided into specific sections. It opens with a section on the new owner which discusses the responsibilities of owning a dog as well as a general outline of the breeds. Genetics, breeding and the problems of inherited disease form a separate section, as does general management which encompasses the fast growing field of behavioural problems.

The various organs of the body are dealt with separately as are infectious diseases, including parasites. Canine dentistry is a rapidly expanding field and is covered in detail, sharing a section with chapters on subjects as diverse as cancer in the dog, poisoning and first aid and it is in this latter chapter, incidentally, together with the chapter on nursing the sick dog that comprehensive do-it-yourself advice is offered. Throughout the rest of the book the emphasis concentrates on information and explanation.

Kennels and kennel management is a separate chapter, not only to guide in selecting kennels but also to advise should you need to build a kennel in the garden or decide to open a boarding kennels.

The rest of the final miscellanous section encompasses topics as wide ranging as showing your dog, veterinary certification, the complexities of veterinary medicines, client/professional relationships and not least, pet health insurance and its growing importance in the UK.

The book is not intended to be comprehensive, omissions I am sure will come to light. I will be glad to learn of them and do my best to rectify faults in the future. Repetition will be apparent in some areas and this has been entirely deliberate. I hope the book will be of value and interest to the dog owner, professional breeder and pet owner alike, not to mention those veterinary surgeons and veterinary nurses looking for authoritative, easily understood, up-to-the-minute explanations of sometimes complex issues. I am grateful to my co-authors for making it possible.

Trevor Turner
Mandeville Veterinary Hospital, 1990

The New Owner

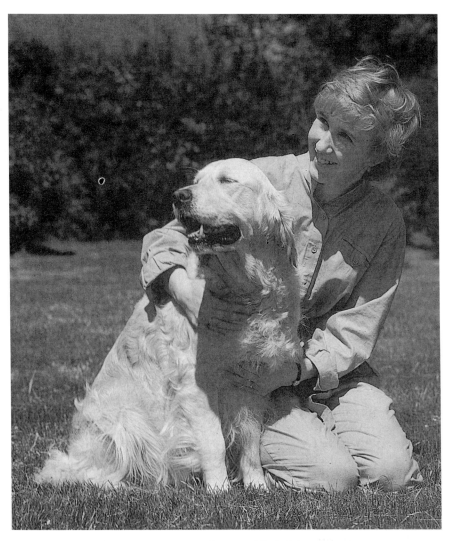

Figure 1   Owning a dog is a delightful experience

1

THE NEW OWNER

Owning a dog is one of the truly delightful experiences of life. It gives us companionship, which is good for us all whether we live alone or in a large household; it gives us exercise, or should do, because every dog needs exercise irrespective of age. It also gives us responsibility and for many that can be the one thing that forces the unhappy person to go on with living rather than give in to the 'miseries'. Above all it gives us love, a love which is not dependent on wealth, position, temperament or looks. That's what you and I can get out of owning a dog.

We have to make sure that the dog isn't the one who does all the giving, receiving little or nothing in return. It is not sufficient to feed the dog, water him, groom him and give him the canine equivalent of a roof over his head. You will notice that I say 'him' and 'his'. That doesn't mean I am only concerned with the male, but if we are going to have to say 'him or her' every time we come to it, it will become tedious in the extreme.

All these basic needs are essential to any dog, he cannot get along without them, but the one thing that to him means more than a full stomach, a clean coat and a dry bed, is TLC, or Tender Loving Care. He needs to be let out to relieve himself regularly, he needs his meals to be provided on a similar basis and he loves the sound of his collar and lead being taken down off that hook behind the back door. Dogs are social animals and therefore the best sound of the lot is to be told that he is a silly old so-and-so in a friendly voice, to feel that hand caress him round the back of his ears.

You may say that is sentimental nonsense from someone whose dogs are nothing more than pampered pets. However, I have seen shooting men, whose dogs seemed to mean nothing more than a means of fetching and finding, stifle a tear, unable to speak when the end of the road had come for some faithful old favourite.

If you haven't the time or the inclination to give back to your dog something of that which he will give you unstintingly each and every day

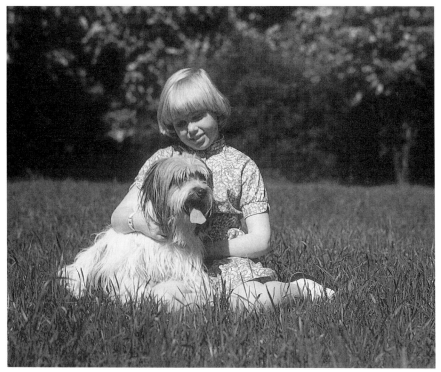

Figure 2   TLC – Tender Loving Care

for anything up to and beyond 15 years, then change your mind and buy a goldfish! That is not to say that goldfish do not need to be properly looked after, but they won't bring you a lead on a cold winter's night with the snow six inches deep outside.

If you want to own a dog you will have to cope with all the responsibility and be prepared to give of your time and effort. Every year thousands of dogs of all shapes and sizes are discarded by owners who thought they wanted a dog and then found that the commitment was too great when it came to proper caring.

That's the sermon over! Let us assume that you have made up your mind that a dog is for you and you are right for a dog. That is undoubtedly the biggest decision, but there are a whole lot more decisions which will need to be made.

Are you going to look for a pedigree dog or would you rather have a crossbred? This is a dog whose parents were both purebred but who were not of the same breed. What about a mongrel? This is one whose parents were possibly mixtures themselves and perhaps Mum didn't even remember who Dad was!

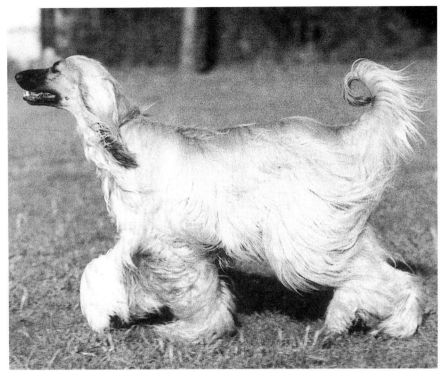

Figure 3 The hairy Afghan

Now the sexual decisions – a male or a female?

Are you going to have a baby puppy around the 8–10 weeks old mark or will you see if you can find a young adult who needs a change of home for perfectly good reasons?

Now size, large or small? Dogs come in all sizes from less than 20 cm (9 in.) at the shoulder to over 1m (3 ft). They can weigh anything from 1 kg (2½ lb) to 100 kg (200 lb).

Hairy like a sleek Afghan, indecipherable like an Old English Sheepdog, short coated like a Boxer or even naked like a Chinese Crested dog?

Athletic like a Border Collie? Dignified like an Irish Wolfhound? Slightly ponderous like a St. Bernard or delightfully extrovert like a Dalmatian?

Is it to be a guarding type like a Rottweiler, or a one-track-minded puller like a Siberian Husky, an easy going multi-purpose dog like a Golden Retriever or just a pure companion like a Cavalier King Charles Spaniel, although even those smashing little so-called Toys are capable of reverting to their origins and doing a bit of retrieving given the chance.

It's decisions all the way! It is important that you get it right because you may be living with the final answer for a decade and a half. You may

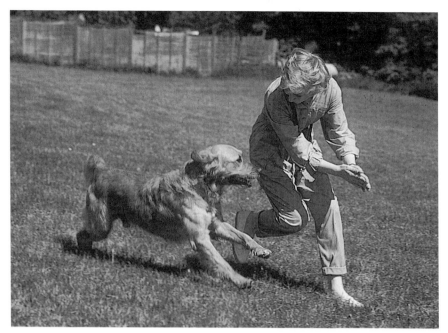

Figure 4   Golden Retriever, 'the easy-going multi-dog'

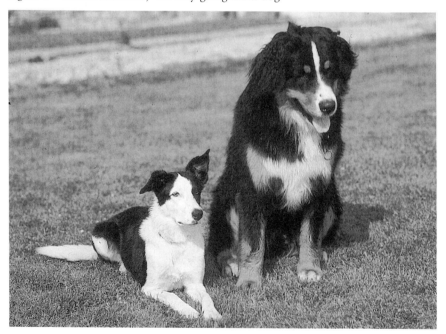

Figure 5   Bernese Mountain Dog and 'friend'. Do you have a pedigree or a mongrel . . . decisions, decisions!

take on the babe as a 55-year-old and still be getting the signals for a walk on a foggy night when you have reached your three score years and ten.

To try to help, let us look at all those alternatives in order.

PEDIGREE OR MONGREL

Whether to have a pedigree or mongrel is an age-old argument. Everybody will tell you their particular view. Experts abound in the dog world as they do in every field. If they don't know by direct experience of their own they will start the Gospel according to St Soapbox with those famous words, 'My grandfather, who bred Miniature Heelbiters in North Wales for 50 years and Knew All There Was to Know About Dogs, always used to say . . .' Then you will be told, 'Mongrels are much more intelligent than pedigrees,' or 'You can't trust pedigree dogs, they're all so highly bred that they have had all the brains bred out of them.'

The fact is that there is something to be said for both sides and the truth may be somewhere in the middle.

Mongrels are just that – mongrels. The word covers every sort of combination. There are those who are only just slightly more of a mix than the result of mating two purebred animals of different breeds. There are also mongrels, who are the results of canine free love, where every roving Romeo has paid court to any attractive lady whose owners just happened to leave the back door open during the period when little 'Bonnie' was actively thinking about the birds and the bees. That scene has been repeated time and time again as the generations rolled by with the Romeo/Bonnie offspring meeting up with other similarly 'doubtful' characters, until the end product is of the proverbial 'Heinz 57' variety.

When we get to the chapter on basic genetics we will see just how much influence, say, great-grandparents have on a particular descendant, but for the moment let us just accept that each illicit relationship is responsible for a little bit of the final furry bundle. That means that we have precious little guarantee that just because Mum was grey, short coated and shaped like a Greyhound and Dad was black, hairy and fat, that the progeny will be a halfway house. Dad's parents may have been nothing like him to look at and Mum's Mum would say it happened on a dark night and she couldn't give a description of Mum's Dad if she was asked.

As a veterinary surgeon practising for several decades I was always amazed at how many mongrels were reported by their fond owners to be part Labrador simply because they were black! I am willing to accept that the Labrador can be as randy as the next chap, but I can't quite see how it comes about that he always seemed to be about whenever that back door came to be left open! The very fact of the puppy being a mongrel means that there is no pedigree to prophesy what the puppy will look like or, for that matter, behave like when it grows up. It's all a little bit of chance; all in the lap of the Gods! There is some basic logic in the oft repeated statement that 'mongrels are healthier than purebreds'. The fact is that when a litter of mongrels is conceived it is almost always an accident and the result is not enthusiastically greeted by the bitch's owners. If there are a lot of pups there is often a decision to keep only a few and the ones which are kept are very often the biggest and strongest. This does not happen with pedigree litters unless the particular breed concerned is one which has big litters which are not easily sold even though they are pedigree. Breeders of pedigree litters are not going to 'put down' puppies just because they are not all that big or less than robust at birth, if by rearing them with care they can be sold for a reasonable sum of money.

I am not referring to the true 'runts' here, just to the smallest in a litter, which might be the one to go if demand were not as good as supply, or if those pedigree puppies had just happened to be mongrels.

If the pregnancy was unintended and the bitch a mongrel, the experience of rearing pups may be wanting. These puppies then have to fight their way to success rather than be 'coddled'. This means in some cases what Darwin called the 'survival of the fittest' or, in other words, nature's natural selection.

A lot of pedigree puppies are overfed during weaning. A little 'healthy neglect', provided it isn't sheer malnutrition, may slow the growth rate down in the early stages so the mongrel may, after all, not lose out on the score of its owner's less than professional ideas on rearing. Anyway, the mongrel is a bit like the kid from the 'wrong side of the tracks', he had to get there the hard way so perhaps he has to be just that bit tougher.

It is said that mongrels are more resistant to disease, sometimes as an excuse for owners not spending money on vaccination or annual boosters. This is just rubbish. The diseases that occur in dogs such as distemper, parvovirus and the rest couldn't care less what went to make up the genetic bundle and will attack the mongrel just as much as the pedigree.

Mongrels are, of course, likely to cost less to buy in the first place. There are breeds of dog where a large purse is needed to obtain a puppy, but in most of the popular breeds the initial outlay should not be more than £250–300, since in Britain, even compared with the rest of Europe, prices of pedigree puppies compare very favourably. There are some that would even call them cheap in the UK. But if the price is a stumbling block in the first place it may be worthwhile considering whether a dog is really within the scope of the family budget.

A year's feeding and maintenance, including veterinary attention, can quite easily come to that sort of sum without there being any catastrophe of illness or injury. At least we are lucky in the UK that such catastrophes can today be effectively covered by pet health insurance, which at least takes away the worry of the unexpected expense. Nevertheless the protection has to be paid for and one has to budget for the premium.

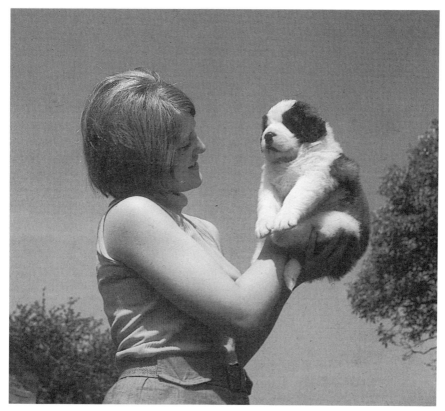

Figure 6 St Bernard puppy. Many pedigree puppies are overfed during weaning

The pedigree dog, on the other hand, is very much more predictable in practically every respect – its size, its coat length, its energy, its enthusiasm, its intelligence and to a certain extent its temperament.

DOG OR BITCH?

Which sex? This is always a difficult question to answer. The male in most breeds is usually larger. He is also likely to be rougher and tougher.

His attitude to the opposite sex varies from a constant mild interest to a downright tendency to be randy. He may not pick the fights, but few of the boys can resist an obvious challenge. He will not, of course, come into season, so he doesn't have to spend regular periods either shut away in kennels or being carefully guarded when he leaves the safe confines of the house.

The bitch tends to be more of a home-loving companion, but I have to admit that my current male dog is every bit as loving as the gang of girls with whom he consorts. Hairy bitches usually cast their coats extremely thoroughly twice a year and take perhaps a bit more grooming than the male counterpart. Do remember that the dear little bitch who never allows any freshness on the part of the lads most of the year can turn into a right little flirt when she gets the urge, and 'heat' or season happens usually twice a year!

PUPPY OR ADULT?

Most people prefer to take on a real youngster so that it grows up with the family household from a very early age. Any faults are hopefully eradicated before they become a problem. Taking on an adult usually means that the vital element of housetraining has already been organised. For the elderly, the youngish adult may be the answer because there is less likelihood of the dog getting under feet and causing a painful accident to dog and owner.

However, do remember when you take over an adult animal, a 'second-hand' dog, there may be undisclosed reasons why the dog is homeseeking. It may be dirty in the house. It may bite children because it has been teased rotten. It may become deaf to all entreaties when it sees a passing bicycle, squirrel or car. It may have had absolutely no training. All this can apply whether the dog comes from an animal welfare society, a breed rescue scheme or just from the family next door, who seem so nice and are emigrating.

This does not mean that the dog should not be given a second chance, but do try to discover the hidden problems and decide dispassionately whether or not you can cope with the foibles, otherwise you may have provided just another temporary home for yet another difficult dog. Remember most dogs are made difficult by people's mistakes and I do not think that dogs are really meant to be recycled.

SIZE

The range is vast, from the Chihuahua and the Yorkshire Terrier, through the Fox Terriers and the smaller Spaniels, to the mediums such as the Labrador and the German Shepherd. At the top end of the scale are the Irish Wolfhounds and the Mastiffs. It is an unfortunate fact that most of the truly giant breeds have relatively short lifespans (10 years or less). Compare this with the West Highland White Terriers, Cairns and Jack Russells, which go on for 15 years or more! One point to remember is that if the unfortunate moment arrives when massive Mastiff is unlucky enough to walk across a road in the path of a car or because of old age becomes partially paralysed and cannot walk up and down the front steps, it is not going to be easy to pick him up to rush him to the vet or even to get him

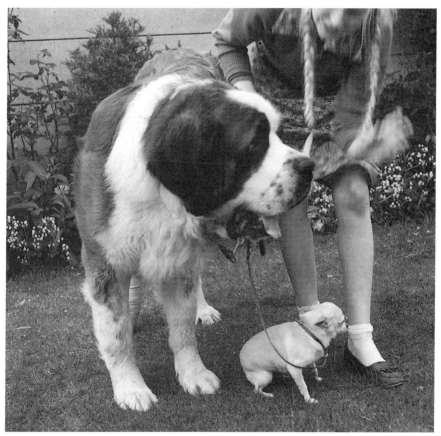

Figure 7 Chihuahua and St Bernard. Dogs come in all proportions

in from the garden through the back door. Big dogs tend to produce big problems, which include even larger veterinary bills. The dose rate of expensive drugs is considerably greater for a Rottweiler than a Pekingese!

HAIR COAT

The range of coats is quite staggering. There are breeds whose outer hairs measure in feet rather than inches. There are some whose jackets are so harsh that they feel like sandpaper; others have neat, short hair all over their bodies, while there are some who are to all intents and purposes naked, with only an odd tuft on the extremities to remind their owners which way they are going! Each type of coat needs grooming in a particular fashion. With some it is absolutely essential that they are given a 'going over' with a brush and comb every day, others will last for two weeks or more without becoming like a matted hearthrug. There are even those who require a rub over with a chamois leather and nothing more. Remember there are also those which do not moult at all and therefore need frequent and regular trimming. This can be an expensive item on the annual budget!

WHAT TO DO?

Before deciding on a breed it is as well to talk to breed enthusiasts and see just what is involved in keeping Fido fit and fashionable and avoiding Tim from becoming terribly tatty. If the hairy sort is the choice, there should be close liaison with the breeder in the first few months to make sure that regular maintenance is being properly carried out. A scruffy, filthy dog is not just an eyesore, it is also quite likely to be an animal suffering unnecessarily.

ACTIVE OR PASSIVE?

All dogs need exercise. That is a fundamental factor in keeping any dog healthy. 'We don't need to give Johnny walks because we have a large garden' is heard in veterinary consulting rooms the length and breadth of the country every day of the year. Rubbish! Johnny gets let out of the back door, frightens the living daylights out of the neighbour's cat, sundry squirrels and possibly the postman, cocks his leg on all his favourite aiming posts and then saunters back up to the same back door and lies on the step until he is let back in three hours later. This does quite a lot for his ego in the first ten minutes but precisely nothing for the length of his nails, because they never touch a hard surface in his entire exercise period. It also leaves him flabby and plump, because the only form of exercise he has had was a mad rush, rather like an overweight person running up the street to catch the bus which turned up for once a minute before it was expected! A period of controlled exercise, either on a lead or under total control off one, with some exercise on a hard surface, every day, will do wonders for a dog's muscles and his nails, not to mention the owner's coronary arteries!

The amount of exercise required varies enormously. The hounds and the gundogs, the workers and the terriers, the utility jobs and the toys, all have their different demands. Some will accompany their fit/ambitious owners doing the Pennine Way from end to end and then look round for more, others will enjoy a polite stroll round the park with 'Nanny and Master Arbuthnot' feeding the ducks and chatting to the park-keepers. The majority of breeds will be delighted to follow the family for a mile, or 20, across the road to the pub, or up and down Skiddaw or Cairngorm, without ever seeming to notice the difference. It is the owners who will notice it the next day with a vengeance!

Decide on your requirements and pick a dog to suit them. If the requirement is for a quiet, steady companion, there are plenty of breeds from Bichons to Bulldogs. If fizz is your fancy, what better than a Border Terrier or the Finnish Spitz. If jogging is your joy, the Dalmatian may be the dog for you. On the other hand, if you are happiest in the great outdoors then a middling-sized gundog is for you.

Whatever the selection, remember that too much food and too little exercise has exactly the same effect on pooch or parson, mastiff or memsahib, obesity knows no bounds.

TEMPERAMENT

The word 'temperament' covers an enormous field. It means a lot more than the difference between the bred-in-the-bone guarding instinct of the Rottweiler and the friend-to-everyone approach of the Cavalier. There are those who think of the big aggressive male as giving a macho, streetwise image, but they are in the wrong scene from the start. You may buy the latest imported breed because it suddenly takes your fancy and then discover that it isn't used to living in tidy suburbia. Its ancestors may have roamed the pastures of Poland or the fields of France making sure that the marauding wolf kept a respectful distance from the flock of sheep. That sort of temperament will need time to adjust to Surbiton. In the canine world such a tremendous variety of types and temperaments exist so that anyone who cannot find a dog that is just right must indeed be hard to please.

The final message has, I am sure, been heard before but it bears repeating. BUY FROM A BREEDER. By doing so you will be able to go and see the breed at its worst as well as its best. You will be able to see at least one parent and sometimes both and thus be able to assess adult temperaments, size and coat. No disrespect to the petshop but all you see there is likely to be a pair of appealing eyes staring at you from a cuddly bundle of fur and you will have a devil of a job dragging the family away from the window. Picking out a ten to fifteen year companion and friend is far too important, not only for you but even more for the dog, to be a matter of impulse buying. Remember the National Canine Defence League's slogan – A Dog is for Life, Not Just For Christmas.

2

THE BREEDS

In the previous chapter we discussed the question of the choice between purebred and mongrel. Now we will examine the purebred dog in its amazing range of breeds. There are, as at September 1989, no fewer than 166 separate breeds or varieties for which the Kennel Club in Britain issues an individual standard. There is, in addition, an Imported Register and onto this go any breeds which are entirely new or have been here for many years but have not registered a single specimen in the past 10 years.

The Imported Register at present contains 23 and it will no doubt grow. As people travel abroad they see breeds that they have never seen before and decide to import one or more, despite the fact that it is expensive, since they have to go through quarantine. The importation of a breed will be referred to in Chapter 3 Breeding, Genetics and Inherited Disease, because it has considerable significance in relation to the numbers of each breed in this country. One wonders why folk need yet another breed with the incredible variety there is already available; however, that could have been said when the first Rottweiler was brought in by a returning British officer in the early 1950s. In 1989, the Kennel Club registered 10,341 individual Rottweilers.

For purposes of administration and classification, the Kennel Club, the registration authority for pedigree dogs in Britain, divides the breeds into two sub-divisions, *Sporting* and *Non-sporting*. The Sporting dogs are further split into three groups, *Hounds, Gundogs* and *Terriers*, while the Non-sporting are classed as *Utility, Working* and *Toys*.

With the exception of the Utility group, there is in each group a common factor or factors which is fairly obvious. That is not to say that all Hounds are identical, or for that matter all Toys, but it does mean that in the descriptions which follow, group by group, we can allow ourselves some generalisations and will not require to attempt the quite impossible task of describing each and every breed in detail. So let us start in the logical sequence with the first (from the Kennel Club viewpoint) group.

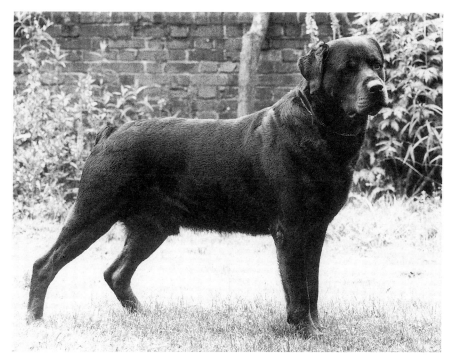

Figure 8   One of the first Rottweilers in the early 1950s

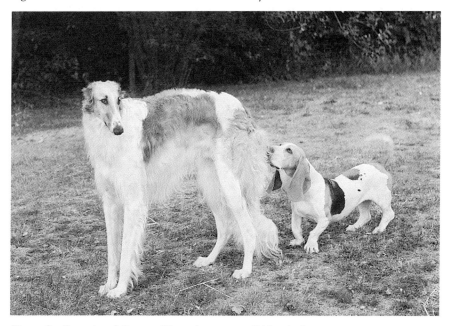

Figure 9   Borzoi and Basset. 'Hounds are not all identical'

The Hounds

By definition, hounds hunt. That means that they chase some form of quarry either by scent or sight or sometimes by hearing, or a combination of all three. Some do it in packs, others do it alone or with just one or two mates. Some gallop rapidly for short distances like a Greyhound after a hare, others cover vast distances like a Saluki after the gazelle. Others put their noses to the ground and proceed relatively slowly but with enormous stamina, like the Basset. There are others, such as the Dachshund, who spend a high percentage of their working day down a hole yelling at the badger or whoever happens to be at home at the time. There is even a vermin hound in the shape of the Basenji, or the fellow whose prey is the bird, the Finnish Spitz.

Because they all live to seek out and chase some form of prey they all have a common tendency to change from the faithful companion strolling round the park to a streak of greased lightning the second the bait appears. All you see is the rear end or, as it is known in the trade, the stern, disappearing into the middle distance at a rate of knots. If you could see them, the ears would be streaming out most picturesquely behind, but they will have become totally deaf to all entreaty from accompanying owner or,

Figure 10   Foxhounds. 'Some hounds do it in packs'

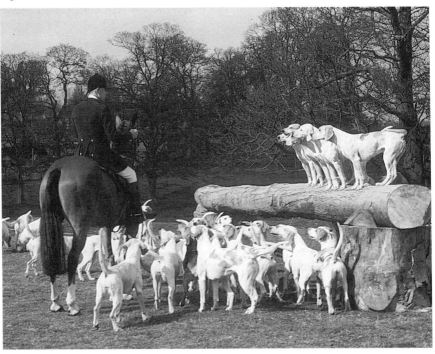

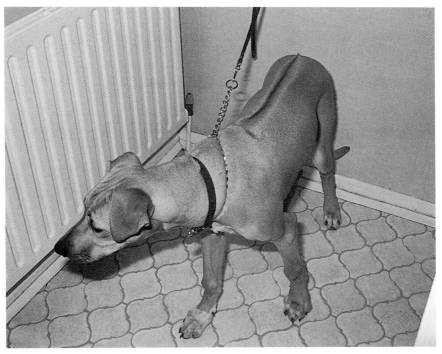

Figure 11 The powerfully built Rhodesian Ridgeback doesn't start out life as a manworker

unfortunately, to the sound of the large lorry with whom the hound is on a collision course.

The man you see walking around Clapham Common with a lead and no dog almost certainly owns a Beagle. The similarly outfitted lady in Mayfair has just been unwise enough to trust Caliph, her Afghan, when he said he needed to go behind that bush in Hyde Park to answer an urgent call of nature.

You need patience to master the art of living with a hound. They are not governed by modern sophistication, but by much more primitive instincts.

They have another general characteristic. Many of them not only chase their prey but also pull it down and possibly kill it. They are, however, super companions with very mild temperaments and with no great wish to hunt or hurt man. Even the Bloodhound selected with man in mind as his quarry does not seize the 'criminal' at the end of the trail. The powerfully built Rhodesian Ridgeback, trusted by his devotees in his country of origin to tackle a lion, doesn't start out in life as a 'man-worker', although he can be trained to be a very effective deterrent to the aggressor or the burglar if the need arises.

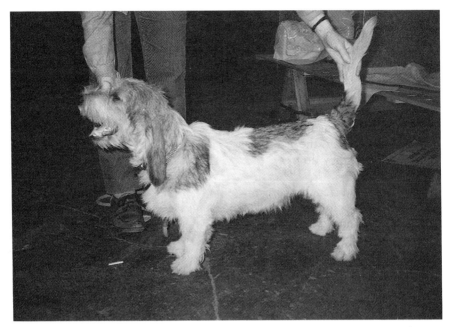

Figure 12 Petit Basset Griffon Vendeen. The rough and ready jacket is seen also on the Otterhound

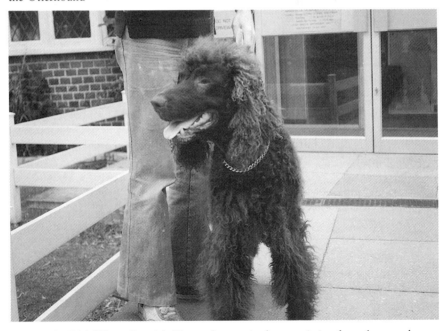

Figure 13 Irish Water Spaniel. The curly coat is characteristic of another gundog, the Curly Coated Retriever

Coat type varies in Hounds. There is the long haired elegance of the Afghan and the Saluki, the rough-and-ready jacket of the Otterhound or the Petit Basset Griffon Vendeen (who joined us recently from France), then there is the tight, shortish 'blazer' of the Elkhound and, finally, the smooth Mediterranean outfit of the Pharaoh and the Ibizan. A true spectrum of coats!

Show-wise the hounds are simply groomed, even if this may be a considerable task, as in the Afghan. They are not clipped or trimmed into a shape to satisfy the aesthetic imaginations of the breed standards aficionados, so they do not cost a great deal to keep wholesome, tidy and smart.

They are good trenchermen and the more actively they follow their basic function of pursuing the more fuel they will need. Conversely, as they are originally canine athletes they can run to fat when either they retire or perhaps if they never became active in the first place. The short-legged jobs such as the Dachshunds or the Bassets are particularly liable to become obese, so 'weight watchers' is one organisation which many have to join.

The Gundogs

It does not take a genius to find the common denominator in the gundog group. In one way or another they all work with the man carrying the gun, be he in search of feather or fur. The names of the types into which the group is further divided again gives an indication of particular roles played in the field. The Setters and Pointers show where game is concealed; the Retrievers retrieve. In addition there are many breeds which are multi-purpose; some of these such as the Hungarian Vizla, the German Pointer, with his two coat types, and the Weimaraner are actually referred to as HPRs, Hunt, Point and Retrieve dogs, while the various Spaniels tend to be pretty much jacks-of-all-trades but are by no means masters of none.

The coat is also characteristic in gundogs, whether it be short as in most of the HPR breeds, long and shiny as in the Setters, wavy as in some of the Retrievers and Spaniels or curly as in the Curly Coated Retriever and Irish Water Spaniel. Irrespective of the texture, all gundogs have a coat that is relatively easy to maintain and generally waterproof to keep their occupants ready and willing to stand up to the worst that British weather can offer.

The only oddity is the American Cocker Spaniel, which, although derived from English Cocker stock and intended to hunt and retrieve quail, has been developed until it has an exaggeratedly bushy coat on ears, chest, abdomen and legs. Indeed a show specimen trying to bustle its way through thorn and briar would soon find itself trapped by its hair.

The basic fact is that true gundogs are almost without exception good-natured. The odd one who transgresses sticks out like the proverbial sore

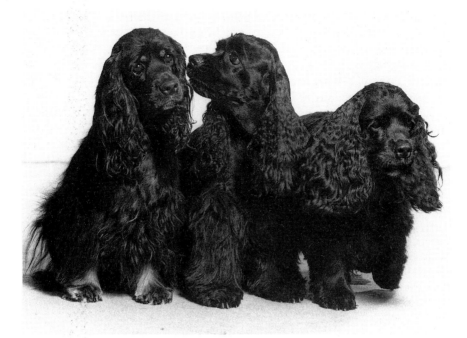

Figure 14   The American Cocker Spaniel. 'Has an exaggerated bushy coat for a gundog'

thumb. As a result they usually make wonderful household companions with good voices, but have no great yearning to accompany the bark with a bite. Some gundogs, like the Cocker Spaniel, have over the years become extremely popular as pets because of their ideal size and general characteristics but are presenting temperament problems today. These individuals, however, have usually been bred a long way from the original 'gun' stock.

Unfortunately, like the hounds their figures need watching, because most of them are pretty placid in nature, especially the retrievers and spaniels. They are also relative gluttons and, dare it be said, fairly adept as scavengers.

The Terriers

There is again a common denominator throughout the group – they are all effective 'pest control officers.' They may have different prey, but they are universally quick on the trigger. The possible exception is the Bull Terrier, whose name is in fact a misnomer. His origin is said to be from a judicious cross a long time back and he should have been referred to as the 'bull and terrier'! For all that, he has much of the temperament of the rest of the group, being on his toes at all times. He has something of a reputation as a fighter, and both the Bull Terrier and the Staffordshire Bull Terrier are not ones to back off if any other dog suggests a quick two or three rounds without much reference to the Queensberry rules. This goes for virtually all the terrier breeds, however, to some degree or another. It is as well to consider terriers as dogs that are not particularly amenable to discipline and not to take them round the local park off the lead. Remember the ranks of obedience champions do not number many terriers among their top echelons.

Nevertheless, they are terrific companions and super houseguards, ready to lay down their lives for their owners. They will accompany them over any terrain and for any distance. Temperamentally they are 'on-the-ball' at all times, never likely to be caught sleeping; none of them is enthusiastic over pain of any sort, so a visit to the vet is often an enlivening experience both for the owner and the other clients in the waiting room. The insertion of a thermometer in the rectum, accepted placidly by a retriever, is regarded as an insult by the average terrier and is considered a positive throwing down of the gauntlet by that more or less happy-go-lucky chap the Jack Russell Terrier.

Terriers last a long time and they are not tremendous eaters, so the whole gang has a great deal going for them. The Airedale is the tallest, while the West Highland White and his Scottish cousins the Cairn and the Scottie (all three are from a common ancestry) are the smallest. No, not the

Figure 15 The Skye Terrier. Less well known than some of his cousins, the Cairn, the Westie or the Scottie

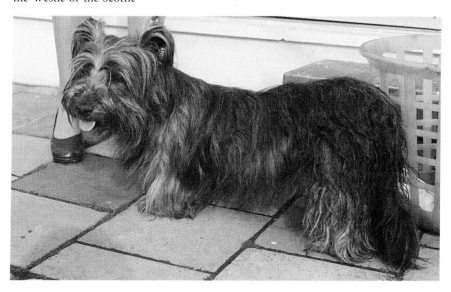

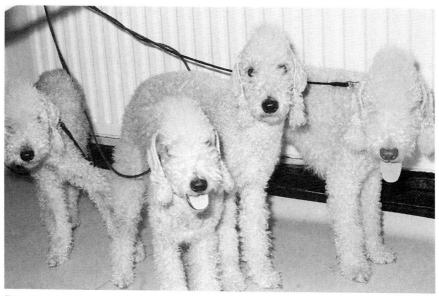

Figure 16 Bedlington Terriers. An unusual terrier coat

Yorkie, he is not a terrier at all but a Toy. In between there are all shapes and sizes; there are those which delight in their shagginess, those which are trimmed, those which have long coats and those which have very short ones. They mostly hail from individual geographic areas and are still to be found in numbers in their native localities.

There is such a variety that choice is hard, but a man must be hard to please if he can't find a terrier to suit him.

The Utility breeds

Originally the Utility and Working breeds were all one, but the group became too big for administrative purposes and they were split into two. It was relatively simple to find a common thread in the workers; they did a specific job such as guarding, herding or both at once. That left a whole lot of breeds which were 'non-sporting' but didn't truly have a specific role in life. Ever since the 'great divide' took place dog experts have been trying to express in easy terms what puts a breed into the Utility group. The best thing is to say that they are first and foremost companion dogs. The only other common factor which has been suggested is that they are all foreigners, but that isn't even 100 per cent true because they include the ever-so-British Bulldog.

Perhaps we had better settle for the fact that they constitute a sort of canine League of Nations. There are Yanks, Chinese, Japanese, Tibetans, and a whole host from the continent of Europe, so the true blue British

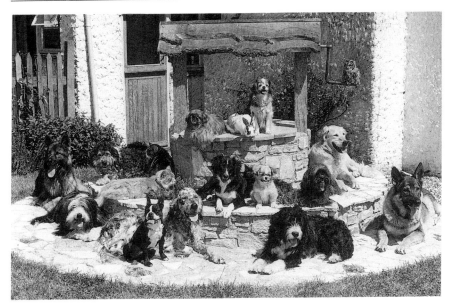

Figure 17 A Canine League of Nations

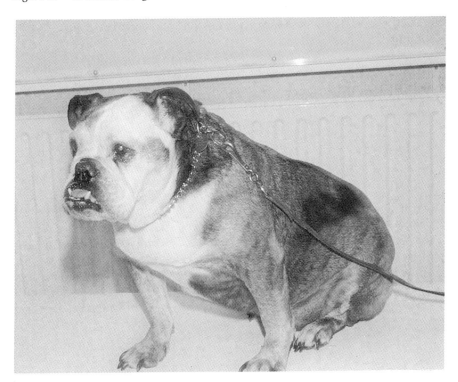

Figure 18 The Bulldog, a true blue Brit

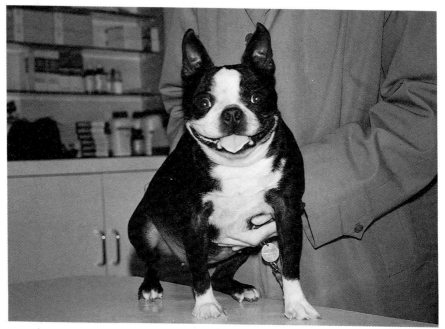

Figure 19   Boston Terrier. American answer to the British Bulldog?

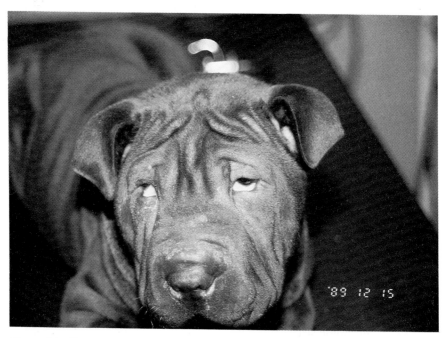

Figure 20   Shar Pei. A fairly illogical breed popular in spite of problems

Bulldog has a hard job to stand his corner against the myriad ethnic groups he meets in the group ring at the end of a multibreed show.

It is an interesting fact that with one or two exceptions the importation of these breeds into Britain has led to an improvement in quality overall. The country of origin often has to come to the UK now in order to buy really top-quality stock.

It would be a clever man who could find any physical similarity between the types. The four Tibetan breeds (Spaniel, Terrier, Lhasa Apso and Shih Tzu) are fairly similar in size and reasonably so in temperament. The Schnauzer and the Miniature Schnauzer are closer to the terriers than any other style. There are several Spitz types with prick ears and curly tail (Chow Chow, German Spitz, Japanese Akita, Japanese Spitz, Keeshond and the Schipperke), although this last doesn't customarily keep his tail even if born with one in the first place. The British Bulldog has his French counterpart as well as the American chap, the Boston Terrier. All have flattened or shortened noses. The Poodle in all three sizes is a highly intelligent fellow. The largest size will stand up to a day's shooting and the smaller versions will perform endless tricks with skill.

How the Dalmatian or the Leonberger got into the act is one of life's little mysteries. The Shar Pei is such a law unto itself that it is probably in the logical group just because it is a fairly illogical breed in the first place.

Temperamentally, size-wise coat-wise and even longevity-wise there is no thread running through the utility breeds. Frankly a visit to a major dog show on the day when the group is on exhibition is the only way that a prospective purchaser is to have any chance of finding the right breed if his intention is to own a Utility.

The Workers

We mentioned the split of the working breeds from the Utility breeds earlier. Even 30 years ago things were becoming busy on the working side of dogs. Since then some 28 new breeds have entered the country from Europe, the Arctic, Asia and Australia. In addition, the Lancashire Heeler, a small chap hailing from Ormskirk in Lancashire, has been 'rediscovered'. The choice is enormous and 'workers' from the Alaskan Malamute and the Neopolitan Mastiff down to the small Swedish Vallhund and the two sorts of Welsh Corgi, which are only slightly larger than the little Ormskirk fellow, are available in multiplicity. Some pull sledges and by and large practically pull their owners' arms out of their sockets, some herd sheep or cattle, while others guard against marauding wolves. Some are said to carry little barrels under their chins in case they bump into thirsty travellers in high places. Some scare the living daylights out of burglars, while others do the same to the police when they go to interview the burglars.

The Portuguese Water Dog earns its living taking messages from the captains of Portuguese fishing boats when they are going to be late home for supper, and presumably messages back saying the Portuguese equivalent of 'Your dinner's in the oven!'

Then there is the German Shepherd Dog, who is all things to all men and is the Alsatian to those of us old enough to remember! Finally there is the Boxer, who is dogdom's answer to Danny Kaye, a highly intelligent comedian.

All the working breeds had, and still largely have, the basic instincts which man appreciated when giving them roles to play. Those which were selected to haul man and his clobber across snowy wastes will do just that, whether man is sitting on a sledge or simply taking the family dog for a walk in the park. Those which will herd will do so unbidden just as readily as when they are doing it for the farmer for their keep. Those which make good police dogs are basically brainy. If the hand that feeds them doesn't teach them to be useful or competitive, they will think of ways in which to occupy their minds and their time. If they get bored, they may turn, like unsupervised children, to mischief or crime.

Those that have spent generations guarding animals (including humans) or property will not alter in temperament in a moment simply because they have become, as it were, 'domesticated'. They will continue to guard, and may well find it difficult to comprehend a law that says that if the owner leaves the front door unbolted in his absence, the dog is not entitled to do his job of keeping out even the nefarious intruder by sinking his teeth into some tender area.

It is doubtful whether the British penchant for foreign travel, coupled with a tendency to bring home yet another breed of dog from a different climate and a different culture, has always been in the dogs' best interests and never is this better illustrated than in this group.

If it's a worker you want, study them carefully before you buy. The large, fluffy bundle may become 200 lb of St Bernard; the handsome black and tan hunk may become a muscular macho Rottweiler; the Dulux puppy will bring an awful lot of the garden in with him when he's been playing in the rain. Have you the time or the commitment?

They're a fascinating bunch, but fascination is not enough. Understanding and discipline are even more necessary for your enjoyment and even more essential for the animal's well-being.

The Toys

There is an obvious theme running through the Toy group; they are all small. The largest, the Cavalier King Charles Spaniel, is limited by the breed standard to a maximum of 18 lb, even if in practice he tends to grow on a bit!

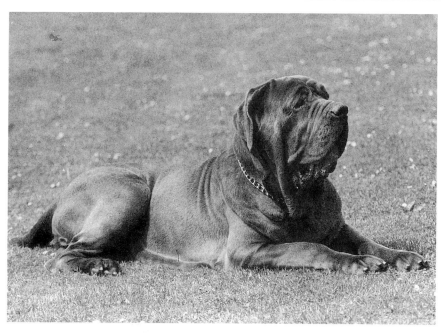

Figure 21   Neopolitan Mastiff. Working breeds are available in massive proportions

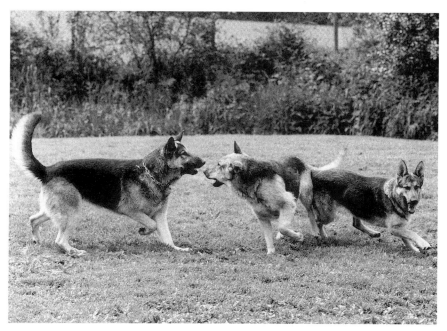

Figure 22   'Then there is the German Shepherd Dog . . . all things to all men'

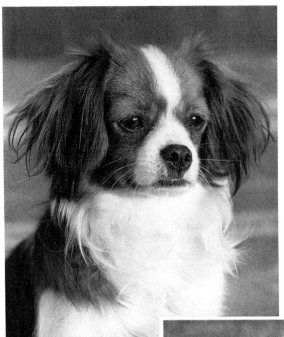

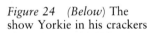
Figure 23 (Left) Cavalier King Charles Spaniel, the largest Toy

Figure 24 (Below) The show Yorkie in his crackers

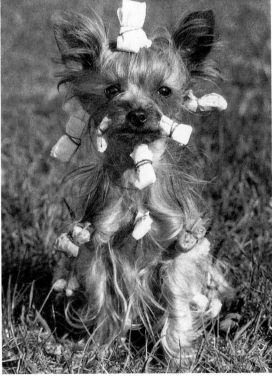

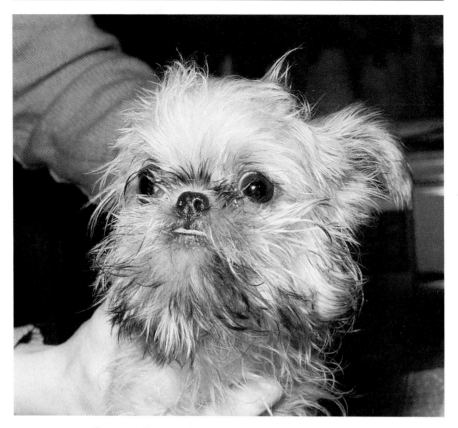

Figure 25   Griffon Bruxellois. Really a terrier trying to get out

While they are small in stature, they are not small in spirit. An offended Pekingese is an awesome sight and your average Chihuahua weighing at most 6 lb is quite happy to inform the neighbour's Irish Wolfhound that he is trespassing, even if the big fellow is only putting his head over the garden fence.

To be truthful, the Toy breeds are what their owners make them. The contrast in looks between the show Yorkie in his 'crackers' (curlers) and his rat-chasing cousin in the sticks is only that – a contrast in outward appearance. The ponderous, puffed-up Pekingese only got that way because his ancestors were supposed to spend their time sitting about, and modern man has bothered more about the dog's face and coat than about his health.

Some Toys are well known, others rarer. The Affenpinscher has a charm and mischief about him; the Griffon is really a terrier trying to get out. Even the Italian Greyhound is meant to have 'fine' bone, not 'delicate', a subtle difference indeed.

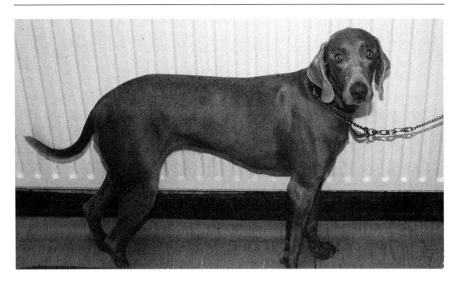

Figure 26   Weimeraner. Customarily docked, this one wasn't

If you are looking for a companion that will tell you when somebody sneaking about outside is there to no good purpose, but you need to be able to carry him upstairs on the bus to Clapham, then most of the Toys are for you.

They don't take a lot of food, though some of them will be faddy if they're allowed to get away with such behaviour by their nearest and dearest.

And even if they have, in some cases, got long silky coats there isn't so much hair in volume as on a Samoyed or a Briard, so the job should not take that long.

One last thought . . . some breeds have had various fractions of their tails amputated from time immemorial. The Poodles are seen with about half, the Cocker Spaniel with rather less, the Old English Sheepdog with nothing at all. They were almost all born with a perfectly normal length of tail and that is how they should have been left. The Kennel Club in all the relevant breed standards refers to them as 'customarily docked', but undocked they can be shown in competition with their mutilated mates. If you decide you want a 'customarily docked' breed, find a breeder and reserve an as yet unborn pup and say that you want its tail left as nature intended it. You will probably have to pay a deposit for the privilege, but you will be just one more person who has decided not to bow to what is purely fashion or 'custom' and your dog will be able to wag his tail, not just his stump. Furthermore have a go – show him with his customarily docked mates. They are sure to be envious and you may even win with him. More undocked animals are being shown each year.

General and Inherited Disease

3

BREEDING, GENETICS AND INHERITED DISEASE

It is all too easy for people who are interested in dogs, or, for that matter, any other kind of animal, to shudder when they hear the word genetics. I am sure that geneticists do not set out to blind their fellow mortals with science, but in genetics as in all scientific subjects there are new words to understand for the first time, and as a result the subject has a certain mystique about it. The word genetics simply means the study of heredity and variation in animals (and plants).

Heredity is the tendency of like to beget like; the property of organic beings by which offspring have the nature and characteristics of parents or ancestors.

These definitions are taken from the *Concise Oxford Dictionary of Current English* and are as simple and straightforward as anyone could ask.

Over the years there has been a great deal written and said about hereditary disease and quite naturally dog breeders have become somewhat nervous whenever the word heredity is used, especially when that word is used by either a veterinary surgeon or a geneticist! However, the aim of every dog breeder should be to produce pups which are capable of breathing easily, exercising freely, mating and whelping naturally, living to a reasonably ripe old age and, above all, fitting temperamentally into the modern society in which they will have to exist. That last sentence encapsulates what should be an ethical code for dog breeding. If it sounds a trifle pompous, so be it.

The point to grasp about inheritance is that it is inevitable, whether it refers to the purebred dog or the mongrel. The fact that when a breeder successfully mates a male Golden Retriever to a female Golden Retriever, the puppies are all Golden Retrievers, is a perfect example of inheritance. Similarly with any other coupling of dog and bitch of the same breed the outcome is predictable in that one can say that the pups will be like their parents. It is this point which distinguishes the purebred animal from its mongrel cousin. Purebred puppies will vary within certain very closely outlined limits, but they will all be basically recognisable. On the other hand the products of mating a male Corgi with a female Yorkshire Terrier will receive characteristics from their parents, but no two puppies will get exactly the same 'mix', so they will vary tremendously even in the first generation. In the same way other crossbreds from other breeds will be a bit on the unpredictable side and this is only the first generation.

Let us take this a little further. When we put a male 'Yorgi' (Corgi × Yorkie) in with a female 'Doodle' (Dachshund × Poodle) and the old urges are given free rein, the outcome is such as to defy prediction altogether! The pups may be quite delightful, may be healthy, may be the most perfect pets/companions/guards, etc., but one thing they will not be is predictable.

And predictability is the purpose of studying genetics as far as dog breeding is concerned.

We have no right as breeders to bring into the world dogs which have breathing problems as a result of the shape of their heads or the shortness of their noses. We have no right to breed dogs which we know to suffer from skeletal abnormalities of the joints. We have no right to breed from animals which will not mate naturally because of defects of the genitalia or lack of libido. We have no right to mate animals when we know that the chances of natural whelping are remote and the likelihood of surgical interference at parturition is excessive. Similarly, we should not continue breeding a strain of a particular breed which is known to die considerably younger than the average for that breed.

Finally, we should be breeding animals which are fitted to the purpose for which they are intended. If we are breeding working dogs they should be capable of carrying out that work. If we choose to breed dogs which are intended to be powerful, active guards with a 'short fuse', we should not be selling them into 'pet' households and then talk about unsuitable owners when accidents occur. The old adage of 'horses for courses' is as true of dog breeding as of any animal enterprise, and basic genetics are there to help.

In other words if you think you would like to breed dogs you should give the matter a great deal of thought. If you have any idea that there is money to be made out of breeding dogs, forget it. There are a few people who make a commercial success of the venture, but most of us breed a litter now and then in order to keep our own line going. We exhibit the ones we keep and this involves travelling all over the country. We pay stud fees, we feed the bitch and, hopefully, pups regardless of expense. We incur veterinary fees and we sell the pups we are not keeping at prices which seem far too cheap. We keep our bitches from the day they are born to the day they die and the average bitch is only producing puppies from the time she is two years old to the time she is seven or thereabouts. Most of them will not have more than two or three litters, so if you do your sums on those sort of figures you will soon see that financial gain is the last thing you can look forward to. If your motive is gain, you're in the wrong game!

Basic breeding

Once you are certain that you want to breed dogs you should start with a bitch. This may seem obvious, but it is surprising how many people feel that they will start with a dog. Keeping a stud dog is very easy, until you want to use him at stud! Although the average male dog demonstrates his sexual aspirations by chasing after and attempting to mate every female in sight, when he is actually presented with a bitch to be mated he frequently fails to perform appropriately. This may be easy enough for the experienced owner to put right, but can be extremely frustrating for the novice, both owner and dog.

The bitch you are going to start with is hopefully to be the foundation of your kennel, the first of a new 'line'. As such, therefore, she should be a good specimen of her breed without too many faults. You will be very fortunate indeed if you have bought a top-quality bitch as your first dog, but you should consult an established breeder of the same breed for an opinion of suitability for breeding. It is pointless commencing with a poor-quality animal and if the experts advise you to look for a better bitch, take their advice. You will then need to find an appropriate stud dog as a mate for your bitch. The mere fact that dog and bitch are of the same breed only ensures that the resultant puppies will be purebred; it does not guarantee that they will be good specimens. With luck you will have learned by observation and from conversation with experts in the breed any shortcomings of your bitch. All breeds have an official Kennel Club breed standard and you should compare your bitch against that standard.

If the standard says that the ears should be small, the neck of good length, the coat harsh, the hindlegs well angulated, and your bitch has large ears, a short neck, a soft coat and hindlegs without any angulation at all, you certainly don't want to breed her to a dog with the same faults. Select a dog who has as few faults as possible and definitely not one who is wrong in exactly the same areas. This is the practical application of genetics.

TERMS

There are various terms used when describing patterns of breeding:

'*In-breeding*' indicates that the type of mating has involved close relatives, such as grandfather to granddaughter, half brother to half sister. This system tends to 'fix' the good points quickly in the resultant offspring and their descendants, but it also tends to expose any major faults which the family is carrying. It is a system which many experienced breeders have used with great success, but experienced breeders are well aware of the possible dangers and will be prepared to stop whenever signs of problems arise. In-breeding should not be practised until one has experience.

'*Line-breeding*' involves using dogs and bitches with common ancestors in their pedigrees three or four generations back. It is used by the great majority of dog breeders. As a system it will usually help you to evolve the type of dog that you admire, but will 'fix' characterstics more slowly over a greater number of generations.

'*Outcrossing*' uses animals from totally different families. Such a system tends to produce pups which vary tremendously in type, and although it may throw up the occasional super dog, there will also be a great number of pretty nondescript ones. Judicious introduction of an 'outcross' into a line-bred strain will sometimes bring in a quality hitherto lacking, but it is not a form of breeding which should be consistently repeated at short intervals.

Thus, to recapitulate, you should start with as good a bitch as possible and select a dog as her mate on a combination of how his anatomical shape and his pedigree match with hers.

In the chapter on selecting a dog we discussed the influence which various ancestors have on their offspring. This is not an exact science, but one thing is certain, whatever the 'mix' between the parents they will each contribute 50 per cent to a puppy's make-up: in the same way grandparents will have a 25 per cent 'representation' and great-grandparents 12½ per cent, and by the fifth generation that one-off Champion in red on the pedigree which somebody will point to so proudly will only be able to lay claim to a mere 6¼ per cent contribution!

NEWLY IMPORTED BREEDS

When new breeds come into the UK from abroad, it is usual for an individual enthusiast to import perhaps a dog and two bitches, preferably from different lines. It costs a great deal of money to keep a dog in quarantine kennels for six months and it may be very difficult to persuade folk in other countries to part with their best stock in the first place. As a result the gene pool is not going to be large. If the new breed catches on, perhaps one or two other people will decide to bring in a couple of dogs, hopefully unrelated to any of the original lines.

If the breed becomes rapidly popular, there is all too likely to be a tendency for the importers to breed frequently from this small nucleus in order to recoup some of their considerable financial outlay. This means that the breed will have a large number of specimens all pretty closely related.

If the breed does not become popular quickly, there is no incentive for other imports and the result this time is a small number of specimens all closely related.

In either case, individual dogs and bitches may have an inordinate effect on the breed as a whole.

Basic genetics

We started by defining genetics as the study of heredity. Let us now have a look at all the factors which go to make up an individual and how they are passed on by the parents.

I have mentioned the 'jargon of genetics'. There are a few words with which we will need to be familiar if we are to understand genetics.

The basic unit of life is the cell. Within the cell there are structures called chromosomes. On the chromosomes there are a series of genes, and these have been defined as the units of inheritance. Chromosomes occur in pairs within each cell. Each species has a constant number of pairs: in the dog there are 39, of which 38 are identical pairs and are known as homologous chromosomes (autosomes); the 39th pair comprise the sex chromosomes, and here they are not identical. The female possesses two X chromosomes, the male has one X and one Y chromosome.

All the chromosomes other than the sex chromosomes are known as autosomes and thus a gene carried on an autosome is referred to as an autosomal gene, whereas those only carried on the sex chromosomes are sex-linked genes.

Each parent contributes one of each pair of chromosomes to the offspring and thus it is a matter of chance which one of each pair of chromosomes is transmitted. This is the basic reason why the individual members of a litter of puppies are not identical. As the chromosomes are paired, so are the genes which they carry. In some pairs of genes, one is capable of suppressing the effect of its opposite number in the pairing. The first gene is known as a dominant gene, while the other is the recessive gene. In the symbolic illustration of such a pairing the dominant is shown as 'A' and the recessive as 'a'. When a pair of genes influence the same trait or characteristic they are known as 'alleles'. When alleles combine they may do so in three ways, 'AA' or 'Aa' or 'aa'. These are known as genotypes. As 'A' is dominant to 'a' what we will actually see in the living animal will be the dominant appearance in 'AA' and 'Aa' and the recessive in 'aa'. Thus there are two phenotypes but three genotypes.

The genotype 'Aa' is therefore referred to as the carrier state for whatever factor the gene 'a' governs, since this is not apparent.

Let us now go on to the practical applications of genetics with particular regard to those defects in dogs which are either proven to be hereditary or have a high index of suspicion.

It is important as breeders that we try to avoid producing defective puppies at all costs. However, the matter must be viewed in perspective and we must acknowledge the fact that when we consider the whole miracle of mating, pregnancy and birth, nature does get it right most of the time. None the less many breeds of dogs have some problems in their genetic background. Some of these are well known, and genuinely committed breeders do their utmost to discover and eliminate such problems. Some of these problems are less well defined than others and are only recently being diagnosed as genetic in origin.

It is important to realise that there is no disgrace in producing a defective puppy for the first time. The disgrace lies in doing so and making no effort to establish the reasons, or even worse, trying to disguise the fact that a defect exists. Breeders who behave in this fashion are not observing the ethical codes of dog breeding.

Whatever breed you select you should study the breed standard. In some standards there are phrases which can be interpreted as advocating exaggeration of a particular feature. Recommendations that the nose should be as short as possible, that heads should be 'massive', that coats should be profuse, for example, all tend to invite breeders to select for shapes and types which may not be in the dog's best interests. Judges who are looking for these exaggerations and picking them out as highly desirable attributes at the expense of overall soundness and balance are often merely encouraging breeders to select for even more exaggeration.

Irrespective of the breed, discussion with knowledgeable breeders and interested veterinary surgeons will usually reveal if the breed is known to suffer from any hereditary defects. If you are lucky enough to have picked on a breed which genuinely has no obvious problems, be thankful, but don't just sit back and leave it at that; keep your eyes open for any sign that a problem is creeping into your favourite breed, for it can happen!

Inherited disease

Hip dysplasia is one of the commonest conditions causing anxiety among breeders as well as suffering for the dog. It affects the larger breeds more severely than the small ones. The hip joint in affected dogs is formed in such a way that it allows the top end of the thigh bone to sit in the cup of the joint somewhat loosely. As the dog grows there will be abnormally loose movement and a greater degree of wear than in a well-constructed hip. At its worst, hip dysplasia (HD) can be extremely painful and can render the dog permanently crippled (see Fig. 27).

There is an official scheme in Britain, run jointly by the British Veterinary Association and the Kennel Club, which assists and encourages breeders to control HD. Under this scheme the hip joints of a dog or bitch

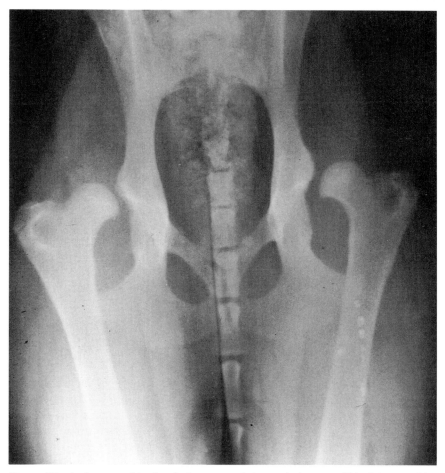

Figure 27 At its worst hip dysplasia can result in total absence of hip joints as this X-ray shows

from which it is intended to breed are X-rayed by the breeder's own veterinary surgeon and the X-rays are submitted for the opinion of acknowledged experts. A score is awarded and the advice of these experts taken in conjunction with discussion between the breeder and a practising veterinarian will assist in the decision regarding the suitability of the animal for breeding.

Many breeders of those breeds which are accepted as being afflicted with HD use the scheme to the advantage of both dog and owner. There are breeds which are of the size which might be expected to be affected with HD, but in fact are not, for example, the Siberian Husky, a breed which is growing rapidly in popularity here in the UK. Breeders of Huskies are understandably delighted at being in this situation, but are not sitting back and congratulating themselves on their good fortune. Most Huskies are X-rayed under the scheme before they are used for breeding simply because their owners do not want hip problems to creep in without their knowledge. HD is only one example of the action a breeder can take to maintain the high standard of his stock. It can be similarly repeated with other hereditary defects.

We discussed dominant and recessive genes earlier and we must now go back and look at them from a practical viewpoint. If a character is dominant, it is almost certainly going to be obviously so, not only in the genetic structure (genotype) but also in the visible creature itself (phenotype). So if you have a bitch with a silky coat when the standard calls for a harsh one, you go and look for a suitable dog whose coat is right and use him. With luck he will sire puppies which are correct in coat if the gene for quality of coat is dominant. A good example of dominance in gene pairing is black/brown coloration in many breeds. In general black is dominant over brown, so if you mate a pure black dog to a pure brown bitch all the pups will be black to look at, but they will all carry the recessive brown gene they got from Mum (Fig. 28):

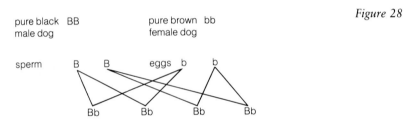

Figure 28

puppies all black in colour (phenotype) but they are all carriers for brown (genotype)

Now, if you mate two of these apparently black offspring together you will get (Fig. 29):

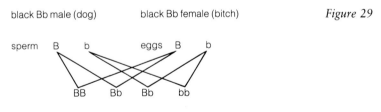

Figure 29

The BBs and the Bbs will all look black, and the bbs will all look brown and they won't carry any black at all. So if you mate two browns together you will get nothing but browns. As as rule, when you cross two 'carriers' you will get a ratio as above, where three out of four pups will be phenotypically black; two will be genotypically 'carriers' (Bb) and only one will be genotypically pure black (BB). The fourth will be genotypically and

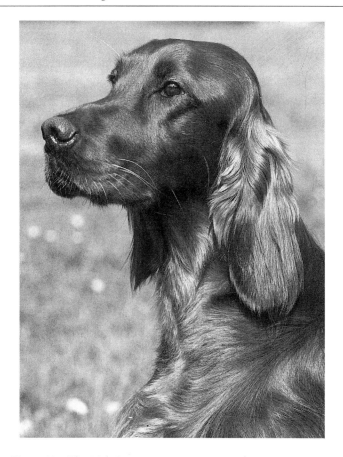

Figure 30 The Irish Setter. An autosomal recessive gene is involved in this breed when affected with PRA

phenotypically brown (bb). In nature it doesn't work out quite as neatly but over large numbers you will get a 1:2:1 ratio.

When we come to an inherited defect in which an autosomal recessive gene is involved as happens in the classic case of Progressive Retinal Atrophy (PRA) in the Irish Setter we find ourselves once again with three sorts of dog (see Fig. 30).

There are those which are totally free of the defect because they have only the dominant form of the gene (P), there are those which are carriers (Pp) and there are those which are affected with the defect whose sight will deteriorate as the cells of the retinae are gradually destroyed (pp). The PP and the Pp dogs will be normally sighted but while two PPs mated together will produce nothing but phenotypically and genotypically sighted pups, a Pp mated to a Pp will give us a ratio of pups of one PP, two Pps and one pp and this last will be potentially blind.

In order to decide whether a sighted dog or bitch is PP or Pp we have to carry out test-mating. We take an affected (pp) animal of the opposite sex to act as the mate. If the partner is a carrier we will get (Fig. 31):

Figure 31

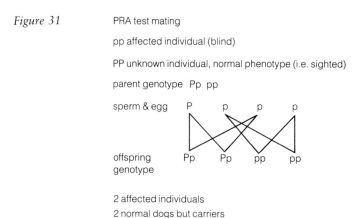

PRA test mating

pp affected individual (blind)

PP unknown individual, normal phenotype (i.e. sighted)

parent genotype Pp pp

sperm & egg

offspring
genotype

2 affected individuals
2 normal dogs but carriers

In other words two out of four puppies will be normally sighted but will be carriers while two will be affected. On the other hand if the mate is not a carrier (PP) we will get (Fig. 32):

Figure 32

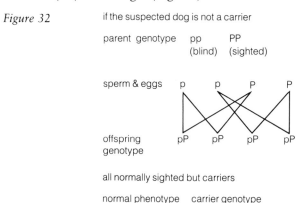

if the suspected dog is not a carrier

parent genotype   pp   PP
                   (blind)   (sighted)

sperm & eggs

offspring
genotype

all normally sighted but carriers

normal phenotype   carrier genotype

All the puppies will be normally sighted, but note that all will be carriers. Test-mating in this way over a sufficiently large number of puppies, usually at least 12 or more, is considered to establish whether an unknown dog is a carrier or not, since a clear dog, even though mated to an affected animal, will not produce a single affected offspring.

The snags to this approach are obvious:

(1) If the animal is a carrier, the tested condition has to be obviously diagnosable in an affected pup. In the case of PRA in the Irish Setter this is the case and fortunately at an early age. In the case of some other breeds

which suffer from PRA it may not be possible for an ophthalmologist to make a pronouncement until the animal is very mature. This means it would not be possible to 'clear' the tested parent until it was itself getting too old to breed from.

(2) In any test mating all the pups are going to be, at best, carriers. If the tested animal is itself a carrier, some of the pups from any mating are going to be blind. This means that the breeder, even with the best intentions in the world, will be risking producing blind animals which will have to be destroyed at an early age.

In practice, when an autosomal recessive gene is implicated the usual policy is to regard the affected animal as an indicator that *both* its parents are carriers and avoid using them further. Unfortunately this does not give the breeder any guidance on whether to use litter mates of the parents. Some of them, as we have seen, may be perfectly clear and to reject them might be the canine equivalent of throwing the baby out with the bath water!

This is not the place to explain all the subtleties of inherited defects in the dog. That is the realm of the individual book on the breed concerned or a book specifically on genetics. The whole subject is complicated and requires thorough and active investigation by individual breed clubs, utilising the information gleaned from the experience of all breeders. This information should be collated by the officials of the club and should be as factual as possible.

Veterinary diagnosis based on in-depth examination is essential. Rumour and innuendo have no place in any control scheme. The advice of geneticists is vital, as is the experience of other breeds which suffer from the same or similar problems.

We looked at an ethical code for dog breeders early on in this chapter; the study and control of hereditary defects forms a vital part of that code. Remember that there is no disgrace in producing a defective puppy the first time. The disgrace lies in producing a defective puppy and making no effort to discover the reasons or trying to disguise the fact that the defect exists.

Thus if you want to breed dogs, start with good stock, study the breed standard, go to shows, visit other breeders' kennels and see what the best dogs and bitches look like. Discover the problems in your breed and if possible where they occur in a pedigree.

Don't rush into that first mating just because you want to be able to call yourself a breeder. Remember that the people who appear to you to be the 'top breeders' in terms of successful production of high-quality stock only achieved this by experience and learning by mistakes. If you ask the really top ones they will, if they're honest, admit that they still get it wrong now and again. They still learn something new from every litter they breed!

Look carefully for the 'right' dog for your bitch. Don't use the latest champion or the dog who seems to be doing all the winning, unless he happens to have a pedigree compatible with your bitch and you are sure his characteristics will suitably complement those of your bitch.

If you intend to make a serious effort consider registering your own Kennel Club affix. Details can be obtained from the Kennel Club. This is your own breeding 'trademark' so that other breeders will recognize the name indicating that you were the breeder.

I have deliberately left the most important thing to the end because it has to stick in your mind . . . .

Never mate any dog to any bitch irrespective of the potential unless you have good reason to believe that you will be able to find good homes for every single puppy that your bitch produces. There are too many unwanted puppies and adult dogs about without you adding to their number. Remember your beloved 'Daisy' might well whelp eight pups even though the breed average is only four or five. Daisy may be the apple of your eye but there may not be eight people around who see her in the same light.

Dog breeding is a tremendous challenge; it can be enormously rewarding as a hobby.

But there is no place for the irresponsible . . . . Think before you mate . . . .

4

GENETIC FINGERPRINTING

'Genetic fingerprinting', sometimes known as 'DNA fingerprinting' is an exciting new discovery which makes it theoretically possible to identify every single person on this planet. It also enables us to make certain deductions about family relationships, for example to prove (or indeed disprove) who are our parents. This scientific discovery was made by Professor (then Dr) Alec Jeffreys at Leicester University during his research on the haemoglobin gene. Haemoglobin carries oxygen in the blood and some people have a genetic defect which reduces the blood's capacity to do this (sickle cell anaemia). Paradoxically, Professor Jeffreys was carrying out his work without any thought of an application to relationships, which serves to illustrate how basic or fundamental research can have an unpredictable, and sometimes far-reaching, impact on our lives. Jeffreys' discovery was published in the mid-1980s and since then many scientists have used his technique of genetic fingerprinting in various areas of research, such as looking at the fidelity of house sparrows, the conservation of rare species, and even to examine the evolution of animals.

Many of you will be familiar with its application for humans in forensic work and in immigration cases. Some of the crucial evidence against Colin Pitchfork, convicted of the infamous Enderby murders, was based on this technique, the first time such evidence had been used in English Courts. Thus the validity of the technique was accepted. The Home Office also accepted the technique to prove family relationships in immigration cases. ICI bought the patent for some of the chemicals used in the process and they now carry out the work commercially under the name of 'Cellmark' with their laboratories situated in Abingdon, Oxfordshire. So fast has the business expanded that they are already having to move laboratories in order to cope with the workload. However, it is expensive.

So how can it help the dog owner at present and in the future, and how does it work?

THE TECHNIQUE

DNA (or deoxyribonucleic acid) is the chemical name for the biological material that animals (including humans) inherit from their parents and it is this material that is responsible for how animals work and function – it controls in one way or another all the intricate processes that go on in our bodies. The DNA in an individual is also specific for how that animal looks, hence animal species look different, and even within a single species each individual is different. Thus we all look different, for example compare the shape of our noses, the colour of our eyes or skin, etc. The body is made up of many different organs (such as the heart and liver) and tissues (such as muscle and blood) and these in turn are made up of cells. Each cell has a nucleus which controls what that cell does (see Fig. 33). A muscle cell will contract, a cell on our head may produce a hair (if we're lucky!). The cell nucleus is made up of the DNA mentioned earlier and the DNA is organised in a highly specialised way so that segments of it carry specific information. Although all cells in the body have exactly the same amount of DNA, only some segments of the DNA – or genes as these segments are called – are switched on at any one time. Thus the muscle cell contracts and does not produce a hair as only the 'contraction gene' operates.

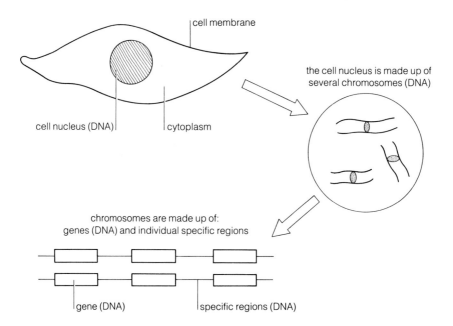

Figure 33 Diagrammatic representation of the cell, its nucleus and contained DNA

So how does this help us make a fingerprint? Nearly all tissues and secretions from the body contain cells and, therefore, contain the nuclear DNA, which, as mentioned above, not only controls what cells do but is also specific to that individual. Consequently, if we can obtain a blood sample we can then isolate the DNA and make a fingerprint – similarly, from a sample of semen, or from hair or indeed from any tissue or secretion which contains cellular material. Saliva cannot be used as it contains no cells. Recent technical developments indicate we shall soon be able to obtain a fingerprint from just a few cells in the near future – possibly even one. The sensitivity of this technique would then be quite remarkable and require simply a few hairs rather than a 5–10 ml blood sample, which is normally required at present.

WHERE DO WE GET OUR DNA?

We inherit our DNA directly from our parents, half coming from the mother and the other half from the father. Just as the DNA fingerprint of the parents is unique, so too is the fingerprint of the offspring. Thus brothers and sisters in a family look different, because the 50 per cent part of the DNA they inherit from each parent is different for each offspring. In fact we inherit our DNA at the time of fertilisation from the sperm (50 per cent paternal DNA) and the egg (50 per cent maternal DNA) giving 100 per cent unique offspring DNA. The only time when two fingerprints will be the same is when the DNA they inherit is the same, as in the case of identical twins, when during the early stages of development one fertilised egg-cell gives rise to two offspring.

Growth of this fertilised egg from just one cell into a full-term baby is by cell division, with the DNA reproducing itself exactly at each cell division. Subsequently, the number of cells increases dramatically and these eventually grow in an orderly manner to form organs, such as the liver, muscles, etc. These cells also differentiate so that only certain genes are switched on. The DNA in the cell nucleus is divided up into chromosomes and parts of these chromosomes are made up of precise sequences of DNA molecules, which are the blueprint for life (see Fig. 33). They carry the information for the cells in an animal's body for coat colour, or for a specified protein. These meaningful sequences of DNA are otherwise known as genes and sometimes we refer to this information as the animal's genotype (see Fig. 33). Interestingly, only some 3 per cent of the DNA seems to code for proteins such as muscle protein or blood albumin or immunoglobulins (antibodies), and the function of the other 97 per cent is not yet known. Some of it must control aspects such as shape (such as the shape of the liver or kidney, or a limb, or even a nose, etc.) and this organisation of cells we refer to as the animal's phenotype – it is what we can see and recognise. Other areas of non-shape DNA may well code for aspects such as predisposition to disease. What is of interest to our discussions on fingerprinting is that between these genes there are sequences of DNA which carry the blueprint for the identity of each individual, i.e., it is these DNA sequences that confer the uniqueness of an individual's fingerprint.

In order to obtain a fingerprint, a blood sample is normally taken and the DNA is extracted from the white blood cells. The DNA is then partly broken up by an enzyme in a similar way to that in which food is digested by chemical enzymes. The fragments are placed on a flat sheet of gel (literally like jelly) and an electric current applied across the gel. The DNA fragments then move towards one pole (i.e., towards the positive electrode) but at differing speeds, determined by the size of the fragment – smaller sizes move more rapidly. The current is then switched off, the gel 'fixed' so the DNA cannot move and it is then immersed in a solution containing special chemicals called DNA probes (the ones patented by ICI). These probes recognise and attach to sequences of DNA from the 'individual's

Figure 34　Genetic bar codes

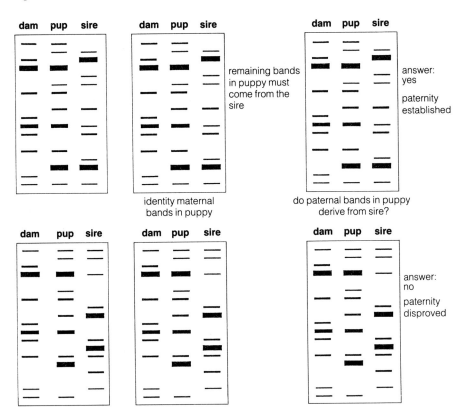

unique regions'. Some of the DNA fragments, in different positions on the gel, will contain these sequences and others will not, depending on the individual. The probes are labelled with a radioactive marker and in order to 'light up' where they have attached to pieces of DNA on the gel, the fixed gel is placed on to an X-ray film. The film is then developed to reveal a 'bar-code'-like pattern, very similar to that seen on the labels of goods in a shop (see Fig. 34). This then is the DNA fingerprint, unique to that individual, consisting of bands of different thicknesses and in different positions (both thickness and position are critically important when analysing fingerprints).

HOW ARE FAMILY RELATIONSHIPS SHOWN FROM A DNA FINGERPRINT?

As 50 per cent of the DNA comes from each parent, the offspring will inherit 50 per cent of its bands from its mother and 50 per cent from its father. Normally there is no dispute over the mother and an investigation of parentage, for example, more often than not involves proof of paternity rather than maternity. Fig. 34 shows two typical cases – one a positive match and the other a negative. In an analysis one first pairs off the bands that are common between the mother and child and any remaining (maternally unpaired) bands must then have come from the father; it is then a simple matter to check them off. Unlike other tests which can only rule out paternity, a complete match in a human DNA fingerprint is positive proof of paternity except, as mentioned earlier, in the case of identical twins.

HOW IS IT USED IN FORENSIC WORK?

Because each person has a unique DNA fingerprint and that fingerprint will be the same whether taken from blood, skin, semen, etc., a comparison of fingerprints from a suspect (based on a blood sample) and tissue taken from the scene of the crime (e.g., blood stain, seminal fluid from underpants) should help clarify the situation. The accuracy of this test is such that the odds of it being wrong are around a billion (10^9) to one in humans, providing it is carried out correctly.

HOW CAN IT BE USED IN THE CANINE WORLD?

We have shown that it is possible to make fingerprints from many species of animals, including dogs, cats, horses, sheep, rabbits, rats, mice, etc. However, from our investigations to date it is obvious that fingerprints between *unrelated* dogs do not show the same number of different bands as one would expect in humans. We think this is because dogs have been more closely bred throughout the centuries, and indeed have been line-bred and inbred to produce the breeds and lines that we can recognise today. Consequently, we cannot discriminate between individual animals with the same degree of certainty, i.e., the same odds as in humans. Nevertheless, some studies have shown that the odds may still be around 100,000:1, and in a paternity test this is still far better than any other existing method. What perhaps is important is that a negative match disproving parentage (rather than a positive proof of identifying the sire) has never been shown to be wrong in any species. Thus, so far as we can tell, based on all the evidence to date, a dog whose bands do not match up is extremely unlikely to be the true sire. However, it may not always prove possible to discriminate between two closely related dogs, although to date we have been able to do so. In practice, we need to see how much of a problem the close relationships in dogs proves to be – it may still be possible to discriminate between two potential sires, but with fewer bands being different than in humans the odds may not be as great. Nevertheless as there has been no recorded case of an animal with mismatched bands ever being related, a negative match will prove difficult to argue against!

In fact, the cases which have been investigated have been easily resolved. In one case of a double mating in a pack of Siberian Huskies one of the

Figure 35   Pack of Siberian Huskies

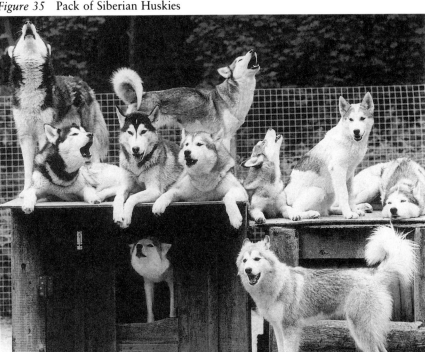

potential sires was ruled out (see Fig. 35). On another occasion a 'ringer' stud dog had been used and subsequent blood sampling of the dam, champion stud dog and pups showed that the offspring could not have come from the champion stud dog. The ringer was not to be found! One can appreciate that as this technique is so powerful, in order to be absolutely certain of parentage, each puppy in the litter would have to be tested in order to be sure of the sire in case a double mating and conception to both dogs had taken place. Using DNA fingerprinting, conceptions to two or more dogs can be sorted out.

OTHER USES FOR FINGERPRINTING

It may be possible to trace the evolution of the breeds that we recognise today, as closely related animals will have more bands in common than those that are not. Forensic work may also be helped. For example, in prosecuting dog fighters, hair and blood from a fighting dog matched with tissue from an owner's coat or from their dogs may prove useful evidence. Verification of the dog in cases where frozen semen is used, or indeed to identify the frozen semen itself, may be helpful in the odd case. In point of fact there are more safeguards on the identification of dam and sire when using frozen semen than when employing natural mating.

USE OF FINGERPRINTING IN THE TREATMENT AND ELIMINATION OF DISEASE

Whilst it is unlikely that with inherited diseases replacement of defective genes will be directly researched in the dog, it is likely that this will be the case in man. It may be possible, if the same gene occurs in dogs, to use the human gene treatment for affected dogs. It is possible that in the next 10 years or so, given the finances, it will be possible to detect defective genes. Thus it may be possible to pick up carriers of diseases which are known to be due to a single inherited defective gene, e.g., progressive retinal atrophy or epilepsy. Hip dysplasia will be more difficult as it seems to be due to the interaction of more than one 'defective' gene and also to other factors. Instead of carrying out 'test' matings and progeny testing and waiting for months or years to detect affected offspring, tissue from the puppies at birth will provide sufficient material (especially from those breeds that are docked, as the DNA can be isolated from the muscle and skin in the piece of tail) to use with specially designed DNA probes. These probes will be similar to those used for the fingerprinting, but detecting gene sequences rather than individual specific sequences. Thus it should be possible to pick up affected and carrier animals long before they develop the disease.

CONCLUSION

The technique of DNA or genetic fingerprinting provides a unique and powerful tool in the way we can discriminate between animals. We are now in a better position than ever before to prove definitively the parentage of an offspring, and in the future the use of molecular genetics in the diagnosis and treatment of disease holds particular promise.

General Management

5

DOG BEHAVIOUR – DEVELOPMENT AND TRAINING

Dog society

Wolf ancestry is everywhere to be seen in the ways dogs behave. They are committed to the social life of pack or family to the extent that an individual follows, shares and would even die for a member of the pack.

The social organisation of the wolf and dog has many parallels with that of the typical human extended family or tribe. The size is comparable, varying between five and 20 individuals. They share a similar system of leadership, which we call status in humans, but a dominance hierarchy in social animals like the wolf. The essence of dominance hierarchies is that they *reduce* physical conflict between pack members, by the application of consistent rules for the division of privileges and resources like food. 'Be humble, wait your turn and you will get a share of the carcass'! Without a stable hierarchical organisation, dogs or wolves would engage in battle at every meal and would sustain serious injury. Wolves rarely injure one another, because, if they did, they would not be able to co-operate in the hunting of big game.

Dominance hierarchies can be studied and graphically displayed in a pack of dogs as follows:

A
↓
B
↓
C
↓
D

This is a linear hierarchy, where each dog knows his or her dominance or subordinance to another. Such an arrangement is unusual, it being more common to find some pack members who are uncertain of their relative dominance, shown like this:

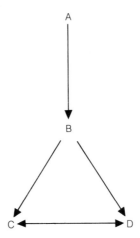

Dog 'A' above is dominant over 'B', who is dominant over the equally ranked 'C' and 'D'. The top-ranking individual may as likely be a bitch as a male in either wolf society or amongst domestic dogs. If it is a male, the bitch he mates acquires added social status to the extent that she can suppress reproductive activity amongst remaining bitches of the pack. If 'A' is female, no other bitch can be reproductively active and she can select one or several males as a sexual partner.

An additional complication about dominance hierarchies in dogs is that they are not always fixed, but can vary according to time, place or context. For instance, the dog that leads a hunt may be different from the dog which is best able to defend territory. In human social psychology this is called role-playing and dogs are very adept at it. How many times is a dog obedient and submissive away from home, but decidedly the master at home? The flexibility in the rules of canine dominance hierarchies can be exploited by owners to overcome problems posed by some dominant dogs.

Basically, owners should challenge, train and lead their dogs in contexts where it is easier to do so (perhaps outdoors), then gradually transfer to other situations, such as indoors, where it is more likely to be resisted by a dominant dog.

Sounds, signs and signals

We humans mostly feel comfortable in the company of dogs because they are easy to 'read'. The facial expressions, tail movement and position, bark and urine mark are all familiar to us in their general expression, though their detailed integration into an expressive language may not be understood. This is a big subject which has attracted internationally known scientists to its study. In practice, an owner becomes highly skilled in detecting the smallest changes in their dog's well-being and likely next move, just by trial and error. Eberhard Trumler's *Understanding Your Dog* portrays canine language for those curious about dogs in general, their own in particular. A brief description of canine vocabulary is given here:

(a) Vocalisation

Bark: On surprise, defence of territory
Yap: In play, to solicit attention
Bark-whine: In distress, to attract attention
Howl: 'Here I am', a contact call
Growl: Threat, a dominant challenge
Growl: In play, mock dominance
Whimper: In submission, to appease

Sound analysis of dog vocalisations reveals many variations of these basic calls for each dog, and further variations between individuals, breeds and possibly between sexes.

Figure 36a Body language of dogs is entirely based upon the natural model of the wolf, seen here checking out a Rottweiler/Collie cross

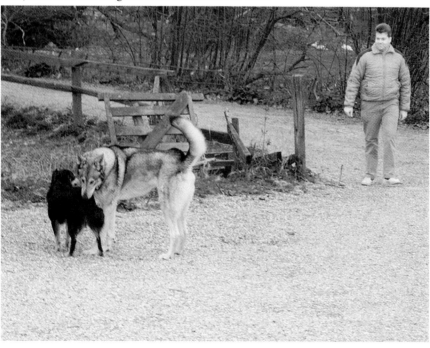

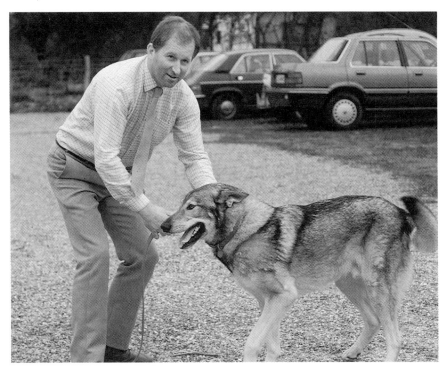

Figure 36b   Facial gestures and body language of man and dog are remarkably similar in their behavioural meaning

(b) Visual signs

Ears: Forward/back
Lips: To hide/reveal pigmentation
Eyes: Lid opening and pupillary dilation
Neck: Angle and hair erection
Back: Height and hair erection (the 'hackles')
Tail: Hair movement and height – a thousand variations.
Body: Stand, squat, roll-over (inguinal display)

The complexity of body language of dogs is both intellectually challenging to understand and beautiful in its consistency. The process of domestication and selective breeding of dogs has changed some details of body display. For instance, Boxers and Bulldogs have shortened noses and prominent lip pigmentation. The Lhasa Apso and Old English Sheepdog have a complete covering of hair over their head so that ears, lips and eyes are hidden. In some countries ears may be cropped to stand artificially erect. Other breeds 'lose' their tails and with it goes a medium for expressing emotions. Such changes to face, hair and tail do alter how a dog is received by others.

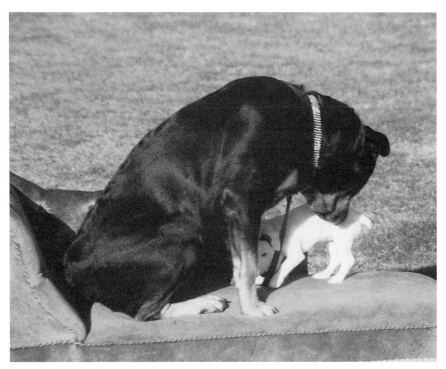

Figure 36c   Getting to know you through ano-genital sniffing

(c) Chemical signs

Urine: The daily news for all dogs, denoting individual identity, sex, diet
    and possibly the time deposited.
Faeces: A visual mark, plus a personal perfume
Saliva: Attracts investigation and licking
Skin: Numerous sebaceous glands over body
Foot-pads: Between the digits, specialised glands

The olfactory sense of dogs is remarkably developed. They are able to
follow 'trails' of a dog or a human that might be 24–48 hours old,
consisting of up to one molecule per cubic metre of a body chemical such
as lactic or propionic acid. That is why dogs linger in their sniffing and
licking of one another and of humans, checking us out for contact with
other dogs, people, food, sex, etc. There are no secrets to be kept from a
dog!

DEVELOPMENT

The changing capacity of puppies to perform certain behaviours is largely
determined by genetic influences over the central nervous system.

Nevertheless, the environment of the puppy before and after birth also affects the development of behaviour. Since good breeders and conscientious owners can influence the environment in which a puppy develops, we will here explore a good versus bad practice for raising puppies.

Prenatal influences

Compared with the human baby, the puppy has only two-ninths the time for prenatal development. It is thus born at a relatively early stage of development, unable to be as independent as, say, a calf or foal. It has been shown that unborn human babies react to sounds, taste stimuli and touch from five months after conception. By comparison, at birth the puppy is only reactive to the sweet taste, touch (proprioception) and cold stimuli. The eyes are closed at birth and neurological studies show that there is no co-ordinated response of the brain to light, sound or smells.

The most interesting event to affect a puppy's future in the womb is its sexual differentiation: to become a male or female. The cells which eventually reside in the testicles of mature dogs begin to secrete testosterone about five weeks after conception. The presence of tiny quantities of this masculinising hormone fundamentally changes the brain of dogs so that a male rather than female potential is created. This process of sexual differentiation is complete at birth, when the obvious anatomical differences in genitalia can be seen, but the more subtle differences in personality between dog and bitch are still hidden.

Birth – 2 weeks

The priorities for a new-born puppy are warmth and food, to which the thermal, proprioceptive and taste reflexes are all committed. Movements of puppies away from their mother show an interesting trial and error quality, as they sample for temperature gradients and take the warmest option. Contact with the head against the mother or another puppy stimulates a rooting reflex or burrowing movement, which should eventually create contact with the breast area. Location of the nipple is achieved by both touch and taste sensitivity to the sugar in milk.

The bitch is highly concerned to keep puppies together in a group and will nuzzle and lick them close to her belly. Puppies at this age will make a mewling vocalisation when separated from the group, when cooled or pinched. Interestingly, these distress vocalisations do not much affect the bitch: sight rather than sound is her guide to maternal care.

2–5 weeks

The world of a puppy markedly changes when its eyes open at 8–11 days and the visual system of eyes and brain function at 3–5 weeks. Functional hearing is evident from 2.5–3 weeks and the sense of smell follows at 4 weeks. Movement becomes more co-ordinated and directed as both nervous system and sensory systems mature. Thus, by 4 weeks of age, following of the mother and play between puppies occurs. The reflexes to urinate and defaecate mature at 3–4 weeks, so that the puppy can now eliminate without assistance from the bitch. By 4–5 weeks of age, the puppy moves to the edge and beyond the nest to toilet, thereby beginning the process which we owners refer to as toilet training.

The period of 2–5 weeks is the time in which there needs to be a significant interaction between puppy and people if the puppy is to become a well-adjusted member of the family. Numerous scientific studies have shown that gentle handling and stimulation of puppies should begin from 2.5 weeks of age, starting with 1–2 minutes a day, increasing to several sessions of 5 minutes or more a day. The effect of such handling is complex, but it hastens development of the neurological and endocrine mechanisms that deal with stress and imprints the puppy on people. This process of imprinting was first described in goslings; in puppies it occurs later and involves both visual and olfactory contact. Thus, the smell of humans is utilised by puppies to the extent that a Dutch scientist recommends that young puppies be anointed with the underarm odours of their prospective owners!

5–12 weeks

From 5 weeks of age we can recognise the full range of canine expressions or language and the puppies' nutritional habits are moving from pestering for mother's milk to the taking of solid food. Feeding by a litter of puppies is a competitive business, a time when the mechanisms and benefits of dominance hierarchies are learned. Play fighting can seem to be quite violent and the evidence suggests that puppies able to take the lead in play or possession of a bone become the more dominant adult dogs.

Puppies not only have to learn how to be dogs but also they must be committed, primed or socialised to man. The period between 5 and 12 weeks has been referred to as the critical period of socialisation. Contact with man prior to 5 weeks finds the puppies' central nervous system and senses unable to react to and remember incidents, whilst later contact with man does build upon earlier social skills.

The socialisation process is like a process of software programming: once in place it can be applied to any situation where dog meets man. Thus there are very major practical implications on how puppies are raised. Research and practical experience suggests that puppies should be given much sustained 'quality' contact with people up to and beyond 3 months of age. They should also be socialised with other species such as cats and poultry, even the motor car! This work also points out the optimum time for acquiring or rehoming a new puppy, which should certainly be before 12 weeks and usually about 8 weeks of age. The precise 'best' age to get a puppy will be determined by many factors; breeds differ

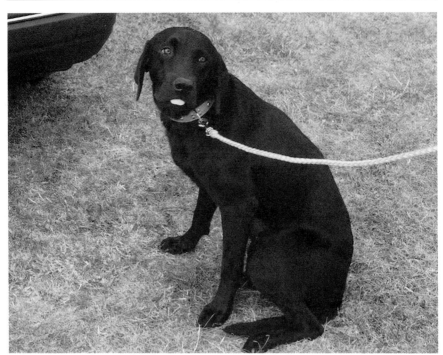

Figure 37a   Under socialised puppies can't cope with change as seen in this fearful Labrador

in their rate of development (e.g., small Terriers fast, Great Danes slow), the time, resources and attitudes of the breeder and prospective puppy owner. Some would argue that continuing contact with the bitch and litter mates would ideally continue alongside socialisation towards human beings: that one need not exclude the other. However, if in doubt, the best advice is always to take a puppy earlier rather than later.

One recent complication to the ideal socialisation of puppies has been the infectious agent parvovirus. Protection of the puppy from contact with other dogs is vital in the period between waning maternal antibodies and acquisition of active immunity from vaccination. An owner must adhere to veterinary advice on this issue, but compromise where possible to supplement the puppies' social experiences. There is much that can be done to socialise puppies before parvovirus immunity is achieved. For instance, take the puppy back to play sessions at the breeders with dam or litter mates. *Carry* the puppy to parks. Take it for car trips to remote fields or woods not frequented by dogs. Allow it to play or meet with other species such as cats, poultry or sheep (none of which carry parvovirus). Invite visitors and especially children home to play with the puppy. It is worth while discussing the necessity of socialisation with your veterinarian since it is more vital in some breeds than others.

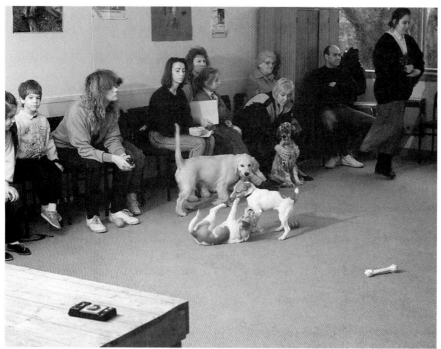

Figure 37b Socialisation of puppies through play can help prevent many behavioural problems in adult dogs

Training

It will be apparent from the earlier part of this chapter that puppies are continuously learning from at least 2 weeks of age, if not earlier. By implication, they are also being trained. Training is not some formal process that only takes place in halls or paddocks, it occurs all the time we are together with a dog. Learning is a matter of probabilities that a particular behaviour will be repeated or forgotten. Habits are acquired because earlier performances had a rewarding outcome, such as warmth, food, water, play, etc. Punishment may be tangible like pain, or more subtle like the *withdrawal* of the company of owners or other dogs.

What is a punishment for one dog may be a reward for another. For instance, some dogs hate to be sprayed with water or are afraid of high-frequency sounds; others love them! This chapter cannot be a detailed training manual for dog owners nor need it be, because training dogs is actually very easy. These are the rules:

(a) One step at a time: keep the task simple
(b) Commands: teach sounds or words, not sentences
(c) Distractions: avoid competing activities
(d) Reward success: repeatedly

(e) Punish rarely: ideally never
(f) Consistency: in all things, by all family members

There is a general approach of educational psychologists and teachers of mentally retarded pupils known as Errorless Learning. The aim here is to structure tasks so that they are broken down into small components which are easily taught. Teaching is by example, repetition and reward. The components of the tasks are so easily acquired that there is never a need to punish. The educator then links the separate lessons together and *eureka*! a complex task has been mastered. The dog should, of course, be rewarded on its successful completion. The dog has been shown by scientists and workers at the author's Animal Behaviour Centre to respond very well to this principle of Errorless Learning. I will illustrate the point by example.

TOILET TRAINING

The natural tendency of a puppy is to move away from its nest area to urinate and defaecate. Therefore, the aim should be to regulate the puppy's freedom to leave the nest at times we do not wish it to toilet. This is practically achieved by using a crate of the sort which soon becomes the puppy's safe retreat or den. When there is a possibility of the puppy soiling the surrounding area and it cannot be supervised, confine to the crate.

After feeding, the probability of toileting is greatly increased. Accordingly, remove the puppy from the crate as soon as it stops eating, lead or carry it to the intended toilet spot and wait. The toilet spot can be the location the owner wants to use as the long-term midden. Maybe it will be an area of open soil, a compost heap or man-made dog-toilet. Play with the puppy *before* and after toileting, muttering a special word or sound. This word will become the future signal or command for toileting – it must be quite different from any other word.

The owner now begins to assume control over where and when the puppy toilets, for life. After this formal visit to the garden, there should be the normal play sessions indoors with the puppy, then return it to the crate for calm rest or sleep. This whole process of removing the puppy for supervised toileting should be performed at one-hourly intervals in the 6-10-week-old animal, two-hourly intervals thereafter. Make the times accurate by using an oven timer.

Notice that newspaper has not been mentioned. The traditional method of house training encourages puppies to perform indoors on paper. By moving the paper outdoors it is hoped the habit will follow. Research at the Animal Behaviour Centre indicates that it often does not follow and the juvenile dog continues to prefer the corner where once newspaper lay.

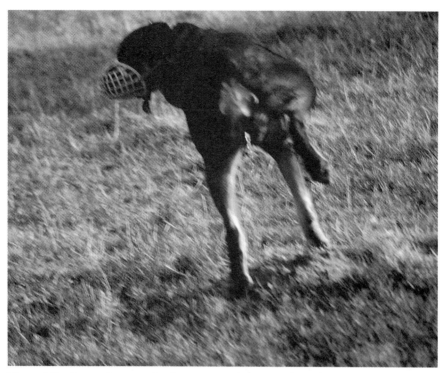

Figure 37c Dog urine contains important information for other dogs, like reading a newspaper

Finally, there is no role for the use of punishment in efficient toilet training. This would not be applied to a wolf pup nor should it to a puppy. Rather than a sharp word, a smack or, worse, to rub his nose in it, it is better to reprimand oneself for getting the timing of the training programme wrong.

OBEDIENCE TRAINING

Every dog needs to know the responses 'come', 'sit', 'down' (or 'lie'), and 'heel'. These behaviours are easily taught to puppies in the period 6–12 weeks, and a useful 'stay' immobility response by, say, 15 weeks of age. The principles of Errorless Learning described earlier can greatly simplify training to perform these responses, first as individual actions then as a chain or sequence of behaviour.

Choice of equipment is a key part of dog training. A wide, soft collar which spans approximately two cervical vertebrae of the puppy, is the first priority. Note that a choke chain or check collar is not recommended because it induces pain and disrupts learning. Link the collar to a long rope or, more conveniently, to an extending lead.

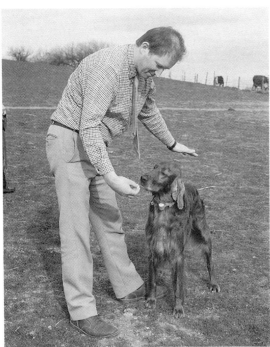

Teach SIT by pressing the rump down in prospect of a food reward.

Figure 38a

Figure 38b

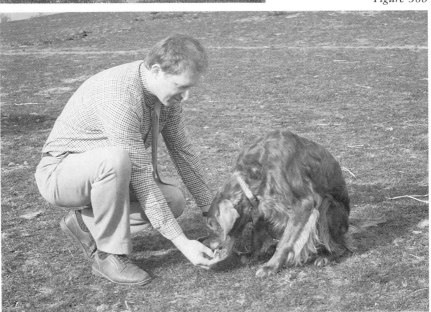

Teach DOWN by integrating the SIT with a natural lying posture, with or without pressure to the shoulder region. Alternatively, have the dog follow a titbit down his chest to ground level.

Teach the COME response as part of a young puppy's (less than 12 weeks) natural desire to follow a moving person. Call his name, then COME! Always reward, and repeat frequently on and off an extending lead.

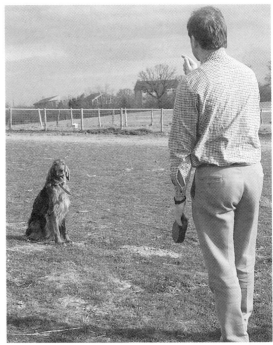

Figure 38c

Figure 38d

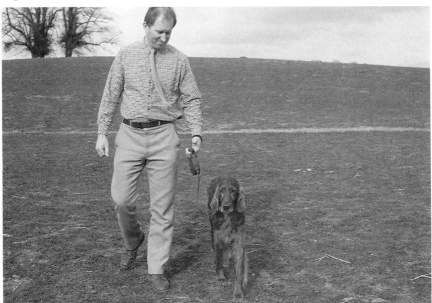

HEEL is part of a teaching process to walk the dog on a lead. The puppy should feel happy and secure to be beside the human, insecure if ahead. The simplest source of insecurity is a click of the ratchet on an extending lead, or a light, thrown chain ahead of the puppy. Synchronise this punishment with the HEEL command, then reward for being close when walking, using praise, touch or occasionally titbits.

All of these manoeuvres are easily taught to the puppy, but become much more demanding in the 6-months-old juvenile. For these older dogs, use of a canine head collar (of which the best known is the HALTI)* makes training and especially leash-training easier. Some dogs have such enthusiasm for walks that they will always try to pull on the outward trip from home. For these 'pullers' a head collar is the natural solution.

EXERCISE, STIMULATION AND PLAY

Mature dogs have an absolute requirement for physical exercise and social contact with other dogs. In practice, the once- or twice-daily walk (one hour total) provides the minimum necessary. Part of that walk should ideally be under formal control (on lead), but part off-lead for free contact with other dogs. Interruptions to regular liaisons with other dogs may reduce the social skilfulness of a dog at communicating and establishing his or her place within the dominance hierarchy. Failure to 'get on' with other dogs is sometimes a feature of adolescent male dogs or dogs that have themselves been attacked by other dogs. Specific therapy is suggested in the following chapter on behavioural problems.

Figure 39   Playgroups in the park are therapy for dogs and owners alike

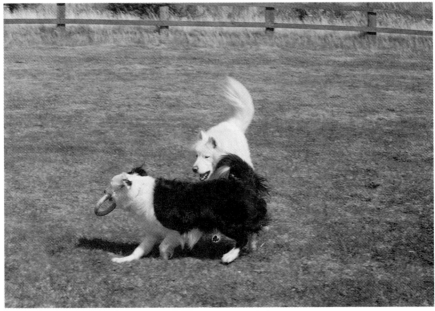

Finally, dogs of all types and ages need to play with their owners, because that is part of the social dominance-testing and attachment process. Chase-ambush, object-retrieval and scent trailing are all appropriate character-forming games, whilst tug-of-war, rough and tumble and other uncontrolled games teach inappropriate, dominant expectations of the dog towards man.

MANAGEMENT IN THE HOME

Owners are free to create any rules they wish for their dog's behaviour in the home; problems usually arise only when one attempts to change the rules. Particular dogs with a strong and dominant tendency may need specialised treatment which will be discussed in the next chapter, but most dogs seem to cope with 'humanisation' remarkably well. There are certain actions, activities and environments which are known to become points of contention between family members and they may cause behavioural problems. These are listed below:

(a) *Feeding at the table*

Dogs normally share their food with pack members, but it can be a messy salivary experience. Once programmed to expect food at the table, the begging habit will continue for years without further reinforcement. On balance, it is better never to feed a puppy or dog *at the table*. For gluttons, split the dog's daily ration of food into as many meals as are the habit of the household and feed them just before the humans, away from the table.

(b) *Sleeping on the bed*

Wolves and social animals like pigs sleep together to conserve body heat. Why should not dogs sleep with people? It is purely a matter of personal taste and consideration of what the dog has chosen to roll upon recently! About 60 per cent of British owners sleep with their dogs for some or all of the night and may continue to do so unless they have a dominant dog. Do not let an ambitious, manipulative dog into your bed, or one day he may bite you.

(c) *Diet*

Recent research has shown some interesting effects of diet upon behaviour. First, we know that dogs acquire a willingness to steal our human food if given an indulgent diet. In this context indulgent means a typical human diet and the scraps that remain. Therefore it is better to feed a complete, commercial diet which is different in character from our menu.

*Available from pet shops or the Animal Behaviour Centre, PO Box 23, Chertsey, Surrey KT16 0PU.

Secondly, the composition of diets affects canine behaviour as much as it does human behaviour. Aside from the occasional and rare dietary allergy, the fibre content and frequency of meals affects the onset of hunger. In general, frequent (2–3 times daily) small meals of high-fibre content smooth out the hunger/satiety swings. Fibre is easily added from bran, tissue paper or boiled cabbage.

Thirdly, diets high in protein or containing poor-quality protein (perhaps due to excessive processing or bad storage) can elicit changes in some dog's behaviour. Most cope well with high-protein diets; a few become disoriented, aggressive or otherwise unpredictable. The simplest test is to try a dog on several diets and stick with the one that suits. Reliable low-protein diets are available in prepared form from most veterinary surgeons. Alternatively, a home-made low-protein diet of 80 per cent boiled rice, 20 per cent boiled meat can be tried for one or two weeks.

MANIPULATIVE DOGS

Dogs are successful companion animals because they are fun to have about, are fairly predictable, usually safe and they are themselves good students of human behaviour. In other words, dogs are continuously trying to manipulate us by their expressions, touch and antics. What they want more than anything (even food) is our time. They are dependent upon us and can be over-dependent (see section on destructive dogs, page 75).

Accordingly, it is sensible to raise a puppy with sufficient independence not to panic when separated from us, using the crate-training method described earlier. Accustom it to doors being closed and separations of one-hour duration for puppies, longer for adults.

Considering the hunger of the dog for company, long periods alone may be an unreasonable deprivation. A pair of dogs or a canine-oriented cat will release the humans from the pack, albeit temporarily.

6
CANINE BEHAVIOURAL PROBLEMS

Everybody's dog occasionally lets its owner down: maybe it steals the steak, gets lost in woods or barks at a policeman. About 15 per cent of British dogs present a more serious problem to their owners, causing inconvenience, danger and sometimes financial and legal liabilities. The most serious category of behavioural problem is presented by the dog which is aggressive: perhaps towards its owner, visitors or other dogs. These three types of aggression are discussed in detail later.

We saw from the previous chapter that dogs are social animals that form strong attachments or dependencies upon their owners. Excessive attachment is at the root of the most common reason for young dogs being rejected, rehomed or, sadly, euthanased. The several symptoms of excessive attachment are also attractive features of the pet dog; loyalty and affection to excess lay the basis for destructive dogs and dogs that bark or toilet when left alone.

Toilet training can be rapidly and easily accomplished by some puppy/owner teams; in others it can take months of unpleasantness. The previous chapter gave general guidelines on how to exploit the natural response tendencies of a puppy within a programme of toilet training. Later, we will see how to tackle the persistent adult offender.

Finally, the subject of coprophagia is discussed in detail, because, surprisingly, it regularly features as the number one problem in surveys of dog owners.

The reader will see that quite simple procedures are advocated for most problems. They are based upon very good scientific theory and have been well tested at the Animal Behaviour Centre. The therapies suggested are no more than a first general approach to specific problems. A particular canine behavioural problem may require a more structured and individual solution.

The first professional to approach for help with canine behavioural problems is undoubtedly the veterinary surgeon, he or she having the training to evaluate both medical and psychological causes and treatments. Only on the advice of a veterinary surgeon should one seek additional guidance on behaviour from a qualified scientist or specialist in the field. Dog trainers do not necessarily possess any such qualifications, and dog training classes might be quite irrelevant to the problem. However, a training club environment is often quite useful to socialise with people and dogs, and events such as agility competitions can (or should) be fun for all.

DOMINANT DOGS

The dominant dog is often a larger-than-life figure, a character who makes good company for *most* of the time. Unfortunately, the dominant dog can also literally bite the hand that feeds it and choose a variety of settings in which to challenge the authority of a human as pack leader. We saw in the earlier chapter that the canine pack is run along rather despotic and undemocratic lines, and the owner must win battles with his or her dog.

Dominant dogs are often male (70 per cent of cases presented to the Animal Behaviour Centre) and usually males make their bid for leadership at about puberty. However, dominant dogs are always testing their owners, and problems may arise at any age. If a juvenile male is exceptionally dominant, it is sensible to have him castrated as early as possible, since this helps reduce the probability of problems later.

The rules whereby one can turn the tables on a dominant dog are well established, and are as much about attitude of mind as active training. The key points are as follows:

(a) Don't allow dominant dogs on your lap, chairs or beds, since height off the ground confers greater status.
(b) Dominant dogs are often exceedingly friendly, in a 'hail fellow well met' manner. Ensure that he does not initiate affection, but rather that you do. Likewise, do not leap to his service when food, water or walks are demanded.
(c) It is most important that your every command is enforced, so choose your moment for commands carefully.
(d) Do not play exciting games such as tug-of-war or rough and tumble. Games are a rehearsal for real-life confrontations.
(e) Obedience training is often useful, but cannot be delegated to others. Use of the HALTI* or other canine head collar can ensure the dog literally walks behind you, an important lesson in subordinance.
(f) Diets must not be of the indulgent and palatable type, but rather be basic, dry-food nutrition. Of course, do not allow begging at the table.

*See page 69.

If there is to be confrontation, be sure that you have the physical means and determination to carry it through, safely. Otherwise, think again. Use of a muzzle is often sensible with dominant dogs when they must be challenged, such as to have nails clipped, be groomed, etc.

Considerable assistance can be given by a veterinary surgeon with dominant dogs, especially in the use of progestagens (hormones), which give a brief reduction in dominance. For the long term, male dogs are best castrated, though spaying of a bitch is unlikely to alter her dominance much.

FIGHTING DOGS

Dogs have the right to select their company, but first encounters between strange dogs can involve bloody conflict. A succession of wins by a dog encourages more such fighting, with quite evidently disastrous implications for the welfare of other dogs. It is much more likely to be a male which engages in such fighting, and fighters should be castrated at the earliest opportunity. However, additional training or behavioural therapy is usually required:

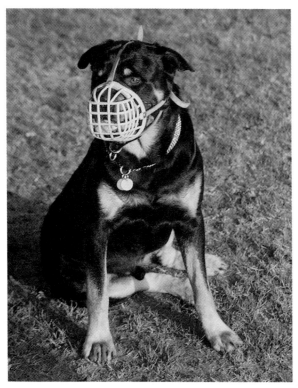

Figure 40 Dogs wearing comfortably fitted muzzles do what they would normally do but with no danger if things go wrong

(a) Keep the aggressive dog on an extending lead, thereby reducing risks of uncontrolled contact with other dogs. Do not keep your dog close to you, since they usually behave worse than when on the fully extended lead. In addition, a muzzle might be a sensible precaution. The formed plastic or nylon types are quite comfortable for wearing over one-to-two-hour periods.

(b) Use a head collar (Halti) attached to the extending lead to obtain accurate control of your dog's head, preventing him from making a dominant stare and head-on charge at an unlucky opponent. The head collar removes the need for great strength and skill in dog training.

(c) Do not shout or otherwise physically punish your dog for aggression. Rather, use humiliating procedures such as control with the head collar, a loud sound alarm (e.g., the dog stop) or thrown water. *Yanking on a choke chain always worsens aggression between dogs.*

(d) Reward your dog for tolerance of others, and develop friendly contact and play after the initial threats have subsided.

It is important that your dog be exercised amongst as many other dogs as possible both at training clubs, amongst friends and with strangers at the park. Explain your problem and seek their help. Of course, avoid contact with other dogs which are themselves aggressive. This is most definitely a type of behavioural problem where use of the correct equipment dramatically simplifies therapy. To repeat, the key equipment is an extending lead, a head collar, muzzle and anti-mugging sound alarm.

TERRITORIAL AGGRESSION

The presence of a dog in a house markedly reduces the risks of burglary, and we all feel safer in the company of our dog, be it large or small. However, most of us want a compromise where our dog tolerates or welcomes friends but deters enemies. The majority of dogs learn this difficult distinction, but some do not. Excessive territorial aggression should be avoided by active socialisation of puppies, as suggested in the previous chapter. However, if one owns an aggressive, large-breed dog, such as a German Shepherd, great caution must be exercised in applying the treatment outlined below:

(a) For the sake of safety, make sure a dog which might bite a visitor to your home wears a muzzle or at least put him on a lead whereby you can control him with certainty.

(b) Do not inadvertently reinforce your dog's antagonism towards visitors by touching or speaking gently to him. You should be off-hand and dominant towards your dog.

(c) Encourage visitors to come equipped with titbits and briefed not to stare at your dog or otherwise act hysterically. If in doubt, better to introduce your visitors to the dog inside his territory (e.g., sitting in the lounge) or outside on a public area. *Dogs are always most territorial at the point of entry to the home.*

(d) Train your dog to lie down (initially leashed near the wall) so that he cannot launch an attack upon visitors. As a visitor arrives, titbits can be thrown to him.

(e) After initial introductions, your visitor might be requested to walk your dog, on a solo basis, thereby acquiring authority through leadership on the lead. To give added control and authority to your visitor, equip your dog with a head collar so that he must follow and not pull ahead.

Punishment for territorial aggression should never be physical, but rather a surprise such as from a loud alarm or flick of water, always emanating from you, the owner. Visitors must always be associated with pleasant experiences, never punishment.

The territorial dog is easily avoided by having your house an open and welcoming home to all. Most dogs quickly recognise that their best advantage lies in contact with outsiders, rather than defence of a canine fortress.

DESTRUCTIVE DOGS

It is quite natural, even desirable, that dogs chew; they need it for their teeth and gum health. However, chewing should be directed towards food items and carefully selected safe objects such as rubber toys, hide chews etc. Puppies should obviously be discouraged from playing with slippers and objects made of textiles or wood, since toys will otherwise be confused with objects of value to owners.

Real binges of destructiveness nearly always occur when the owners are out: not because there is no fear of discovery, but rather through desperate distress at the loss of human companionship. When left alone, these dogs are destructive because chewing is a displacement activity which distracts them from the worries of the world. The focus of treatment is not upon what is chewed, but rather upon the general relationship with the owner. The following policy is usually helpful:

(a) Develop a cooler and more detached relationship in general with your puppy or dog. Crate-training is helpful in accustoming the dog to brief separations from you, and give fewer of those indulgent cuddles.

(b) Try to leave the dog on an unpredictable note, so that he cannot be certain you may not return in a few moments. It is often helpful to make several 'mock' departures prior to a genuine departure.

(c) Leave the dog as much run of the house or freedom as possible. It may be helpful to leave a radio, TV or tape recording of the owner's voice running, together with access to favourite chairs, even the bed to sleep on.

(d) *Never* punish a dog on return to discover damage done. Such a reaction is always mistimed and misunderstood by the dog, who will be more panicky on his next session alone.

The key to resolving problems of over-attachment principally lies in the relationship created by the owner. Excessive dependence is enhanced due to lots of time together. The objective should be to spend some 30 per cent of the owner's time at home separated from the dog by a door or some other physical barrier.

Particular breeds are exceptionally prone to being destructive. Of these the Labrador is perhaps the most notorious. The precise reason why some breeds are destructive and others rarely so is not understood. This is a relatively easily resolved problem. If success is not achieved by applying the rules outlined above, seek professional guidance from your veterinary surgeon. On no account should such dogs be expelled to the street and be 'latch-key' pets. The survival rate for dogs on the street is low and can result in injury not only to the dog but to others as well.

TOILET TRAINING

Most dogs are keen to deposit their urine and faeces away from feeding and living areas. This tendency makes house training straightforward, but there are exceptions. Sometimes problems arise with entire males keen to urine-mark within their own territory or when visiting another property. Such marking behaviour is under the influence of testosterone, and is reliably reduced by surgical castration.

Other dogs mislearn the owner's intention to use a particular location or substrate (e.g., lawn rather than carpet) as a toilet. It is for these dogs with inappropriate place or substrate preferences that the following advice is given:

(a) Supervise or confine the dog through much of the day by keeping him to one room or an indoor kennel/crate.

(b) At regular intervals (e.g., every 2 hours) take the dog to a garden or outdoor area where exercise can be supervised.

(c) Play with the dog, watch and wait for the usual signs of toileting behaviour (e.g., sniffing and circling). When the urinatory or defaecatory sequence begins, praise and repeat a special word reserved for this activity.

(d) Reward successful toileting with profuse praise, even a titbit and further play.

(e) The timing and composition of meals has a great influence upon the timing of defecation. If overnight toileting is the problem, feed the dog early in the morning on a low-residue diet. Equally, daytime toileting is best managed by feeding in the evening.

(f) Never punish your dog for indoor toileting episodes unless actually witnessed. The best deterrent to indoor toileting is to be fed at that location in the future.

There has recently been a marked change in public attitudes towards dogs and dog owners that deposit faeces on pavements and in public areas. The idea of scooping up behind pets is now well established and an entirely hygienic and socially acceptable habit. Rather than have a dog toilet in public areas, it is easier to train a dog to urinate and defecate to command, at a location defined by the owner and at a time convenient to the owner. Thus, the benefit of training puppies to eliminate as suggested in the previous chapter.

COPROPHAGIA

It is quite normal for dogs to supplement their energy intake by 'recycling' their own faeces, or by eating the faeces of other animals. Normal though it may be, this behaviour is usually distasteful to owners. There are no real health hazards from contact with such dogs and they need not be a source of zoonotic disease. The problem is one of aesthetics, especially of smell from faecal particles in the mouth. The problem can be considerably eased by the following strategy:

(a) The dog should be fed several meals per day of a high-fibre diet, to reduce the sensation of hunger, which initiates coprophagia.

(b) The dog should be trained to defecate on command and rewarded for doing so (see above). The faeces should then be removed immediately.

(c) The more exciting a life the dog has, the less likely it is to eat faeces. Thus, plentiful training, exercise and play with specialised toys reduces the urge to seek additional sensations in faeces-eating.

(d) The attractiveness of faeces can be somewhat reduced by the addition of chemicals to the diet. Most simply this involves iron supplements with tablets of the sort recommended for pregnant women. Alternatively, sulphur-containing amino acids may be used to supplement the diet and make it taste less pleasant. See your veterinary surgeon.

(g) Remote punishment of dogs for witnessed faeces-eating can be helpful, using a thrown light object, such as a choke chain. The punishment must seem to come from the faeces rather than from the owner. Alternatively, a specialised conditioned-aversion technique has been developed by the author which makes the dog feel ill after consuming faeces.

Dietary management is a key part of therapy for coprophagia in dogs. The tendency towards concentrated low-fibre diets, high in protein, has probably worsened this problem. The excellent complete, dry diets tend to be somewhat higher in fibre content than canned foods and can be offered on a virtually *ad libitum* basis, thereby decreasing the motivation to eat faeces.

Behavioural problems are better avoided than treated. Significant factors in the risk of owning a problem dog are selection of breed or genetics and early experiences of the puppy. Appropriate strategies for puppy-rearing are described elsewhere (Chapters 1, 2 and 3 address these problems), but selection of breed and breeder is a matter for the owner. Before making this most critical decision, a consultation with a veterinary surgeon is highly recommended, to act as a 'devil's advocate' and point out the hereditary tendencies of the various breeds being considered by the prospective owner. Genetics are as relevant to behaviour as they are to the physical ailments suffered by dogs. Do not go in for a dominant, guarding breed if you really want a lapdog!

Nutrition and Feeding

7

NUTRITION AND FEEDING

Dogs require food in order to stay alive and healthy. All the energy and raw materials they need are called *nutrients* and these are provided in a convenient but complex molecular form in their food.

At any given time in a dog's life it will have a specific requirement for each individual nutrient. The study and understanding of this subject is called *nutrition*.

Digestion

Digestion is the name given to the chemical process whereby food that has been eaten is broken down into simpler compounds which can be used by the body as sources of energy, for growth, maintenance or tissue repair.

In mammals, digestion takes place in the digestive, or alimentary, tract, which can vary from the relatively complex structure of the 'cud-chewing' ruminant, with its long intestinal tract and multiplicity of stomachs, to the relatively simple monogastric system found in the carnivore (meat eater) and the omnivore (meat and plant eater). Thus dogs, in common with other omnivores (e.g., man and the pig) and true carnivores, such as cats, have a straightforward digestive tube with only one stomach and comparatively short intestines. This basic system is capable of handling most foodstuffs, with the exception of some plant materials such as cellulose. This is one of the reasons for the longer and much more complicated digestive system found in herbivores such as the cow.

The three components of foods which require digestion are:

1 carbohydrates
2 fats
3 proteins

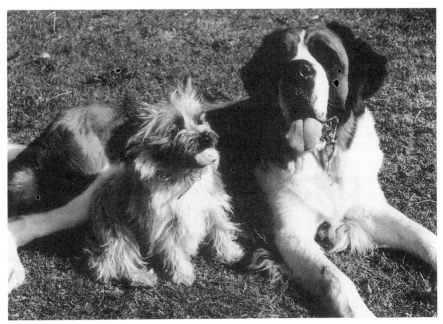

Figure 41 St Bernard and Cairn. Despite their great variation in shape and size, all dogs have a relatively straightforward alimentary tract

Table 1 shows their basic structure and the result of their digestion. The chemical process by which this is achieved is called 'hydrolysis' (splitting by water) and the rate at which it occurs is increased by organic catalysts, which are chemicals that promote the necessary reactions but are not changed themselves. These are called *enzymes* and are synthesised by the body.

The other nutrients (minerals, vitamins and water) are absorbed more or less in the form in which they are found in the food.

Table 1   Structure of nutrients

Class	Common forms in food	After digestion
Carbohydrates	polysaccharides (e.g., starch) disaccharides (e.g., sucrose) monosaccharides (e.g., glucose)	monosaccharides ('simple sugars')
Proteins	protein	peptides amino-acids
Fats	neutral fat	glycerol fatty acids some glycerides

THE DIGESTIVE TRACT

Whether you are an earthworm or an eel, a duck or a dog, your digestive tract can be considered to be a long, hollow tube, parts of which have evolved to have a specialised structure and function. The 'tube' begins at the mouth and continues via the oesophagus to the stomach, on to the small and large intestines, and finally to the rectum, where waste matter is stored before its evacuation. Each of these sections, shown assembled in Fig. 42, will be considered separately in the order in which they occur anatomically.

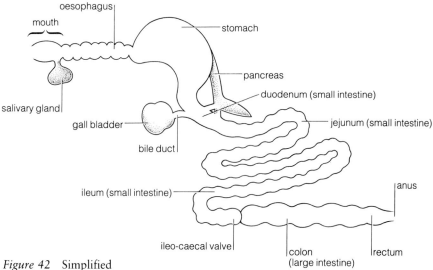

Figure 42 Simplified canine digestive system

Food enters the digestive system at the *mouth*. In many animals, chewing begins the physical breakdown of food before it is swallowed, but dogs are well known for 'bolting' their meals and in some breeds little chewing takes place. However, by virtue of their well-developed cheek, or carnassial, teeth, dogs are well equipped for chewing, cutting and crushing. For, although they are not obligatory meat-eaters, they still have the dentition associated with a carnivorous way of life.

The other important structures found in connection with the mouth are the *salivary glands* (Fig. 43). These are stimulated to secrete saliva by the smell and taste of food and are responsible for the 'dribbling' and 'lip smacking' often seen at mealtimes! Saliva contains mucus, which is a much more effective lubricant than water in aiding swallowing. In some animals, the starch-digesting enzyme amylase (ptyalin) is present in saliva, but in the dog its contribution to digestion is negligible.

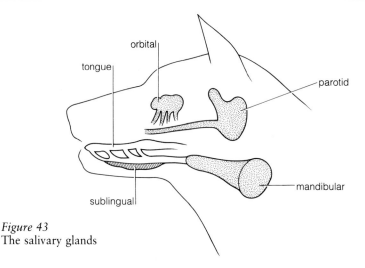

Figure 43
The salivary glands

Swallowing transfers food to the *oesophagus*, through which it passes to the stomach in a few seconds. A wave motion called 'peristalsis' pushes the food towards the stomach and prompts the relaxation of a band of muscle which usually constricts the oesophagus immediately before the stomach and, except in vomiting, prevents regurgitation of stomach contents into the oesophagus. No enzymes are added as the food passes between the mouth and the stomach, but the cells lining the oesophagus add more mucus to ease movement.

The *stomach* has several functions (Fig. 44). It is a storage organ, allowing food to be taken in as meals rather than continuously; it is a muscular mixing bag where further digestive enzymes are added and

Figure 44
Stomach of
the dog

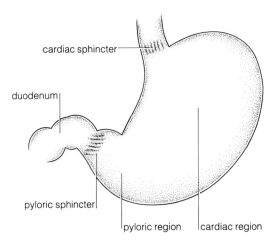

incorporated; and it is a regulator valve which controls the rate of flow into the small intestine.

Functionally, the stomach can be divided into two parts: the cardiac and the pyloric regions. The cardiac region is the largest. It has elastic walls to accommodate storage of large quantities of food and its mucosa (lining and underlying tissue) contains many glands which secrete enzymes, hydrochloric acid and mucus. Digestion of protein begins here.

Protein-digesting enzymes, called proteases, require an acid environment in which to function effectively and this is provided by the secretion of hydrochloric acid. However, the stomach consists largely of protein itself; so as protection from the activity of the enzymes it secretes a continuous stream of mucus to coat its walls. The secretion of acid, mucus and enzyme depends on the composition and quantity of food eaten and is regulated by both hormones and nerves.

Mixing peristaltic waves originate in the cardiac area of the stomach, gradually increasing in strength as they reach the pyloric sector. The pyloric region is the most muscular part of the stomach, where food is thoroughly mixed with the digestive juices that have been secreted. By this stage, the mixture is a thick milky liquid called *chyme*.

The rate at which the stomach releases chyme into the first part of the small intestine, the *duodenum*, is influenced by several factors, allowing optimum conditions for digestion. The mechanisms are basically very simple.

At the far end of the pyloric region of the stomach is a muscular ring called the *pyloric sphincter*, which, when stimulated by very strong peristaltic waves, relaxes to allow the passage of food. The presence of acids, irritants, fats and chyme in the duodenum inhibit the peristaltic waves and thereby reduce the rate of emptying. When chyme is very liquid it moves more easily through the sphincter and therefore when the contents of the stomach are well mixed and fluid, they are allowed into the small intestine, particularly if there is nothing there already.

In the duodenum, more enzymes are added to the chyme. Most of these originate from the *pancreas*, a very important organ which releases enzymes and sodium bicarbonate into the gut and also insulin into the bloodstream to control blood sugar levels.

The sodium bicarbonate neutralises the acid chyme and provides the right functional environment for the pancreatic and intestinal enzymes, which include amylase for carbohydrate digestion, lipase for fat digestion and some more proteases to continue protein digestion. Regulation of pancreatic enzyme output is largely under the control of two hormones called secretin and pancreozymin, secreted from cells in the wall of the duodenum and small intestine.

Bile from the gall bladder enters the duodenum through a duct that, in the dog, is sometimes shared with that of the pancreas. Bile salts are not enzymes but 'detergents' which emulsify fat by splitting it into tiny globules upon which the lipases can then act. They also aid the absorption of the fat-soluble vitamins A,D,E and K. Bile salts are produced continuously by the liver and stored in the gall bladder until required to digest fat.

The small intestine takes its name from its narrow bore: although it is much longer than the large intestine, in cross-section it is much smaller. It is the principal site of digestion and absorption. The surface area over which absorption can take place is increased dramatically by folds and by numerous finger-like projections called villi (Fig. 45). In the average dog, this absorptive area may be as large as the floor of a small room!

Figure 45
Diagram of a villus

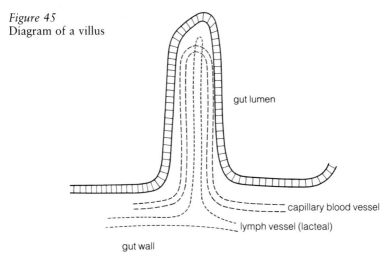

gut lumen

capillary blood vessel

lymph vessel (lacteal)

gut wall

The absorption process may be either passive, along diffusion gradients, or active, requiring the expenditure of energy to drive 'pumps' and 'carriers'. The cells of the small intestinal wall also produce enzymes which complete the process of digestion, and there are mucus cells performing a similar protective function to those in the stomach.

The products of digestion, amino acids, peptides and sugars, are absorbed directly into the bloodstream via the capillaries in the villi, whereas the end products of fat digestion are absorbed into the lacteal, a tiny lymph vessel in the core of each villus, to be transferred later to the bloodstream.

Little of the food taken in at the mouth ever reaches the large intestine. In this part of the gut, water is absorbed and in the *caecum* some fermentation of cellulose (plant fibre) occurs. It is the production of gas as a result of this process that is often responsible for flatulence!

Faeces consist of water (normally about 70 per cent), undigested food, some inorganic material and dead bacteria from the large intestine. They are stored in the *rectum* until an appropriate evacuation time.

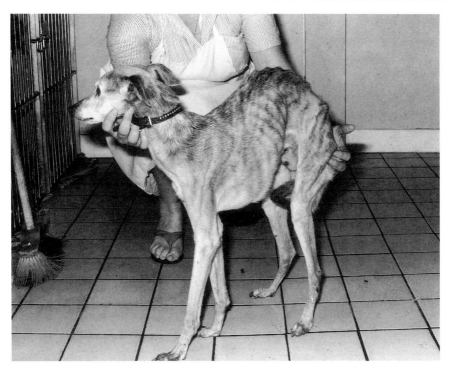

Figure 46 Persistent diarrhoea and vomiting are serious and can result in rapid dehydration

. . . AND WHEN THINGS GO WRONG

A working knowledge of the digestive system helps you to understand gastrointestinal disease. Thus diarrhoea may be the result of poor water absorption from the gut, increased water secretion into the gut or just an increase in the speed with which food is travelling through the digestive tube. In contrast, if too much water absorption takes place, faeces become hard and difficult to evacuate and constipation occurs.

Vomiting is often the result of irritation of the stomach wall, sometimes by toxins or poisons, or as a result of physical obstruction of the gut by a swallowed foreign body such as a large fragment of bone or a stone. Occasionally pyloric disease will cause vomiting too (see Disorders of the Digestive System), page 125.

Persistent diarrhoea and/or vomiting, because of their dehydrating effect and the loss of salts, are serious and can prove fatal. They indicate that veterinary attention should be urgently sought. However, occasional transient vomiting and diarrhoea, in the absence of other clinical signs, may be the result of nothing more than a sudden change of diet, a period of overeating or a scavenging raid on the compost heap!

Foods and feeding

Selection of suitable foods for a dog demands an awareness of two major factors: firstly, the raw materials available for its diet and, secondly, the type of dog and the nature of its life stage and style.

Carbohydrates can be classified into three categories: (i) the monosaccharides, such as glucose; (ii) the disaccharides, such as sucrose or cane sugar; and (iii) the polysaccharides, such as starch. They are a convenient source of energy for dogs, although starch must always be cooked to make it digestible.

Some dietary fibre, consisting of the relatively indigestible carbohydrate cellulose, is useful in the diet to prevent diarrhoea and constipation. It acts as a bulking agent and helps maintain regular gut movements.

Fat is important for several reasons: it provides more than twice as much energy per gram than either carbohydrate or protein. This is particularly valuable at times when a 'concentrated' energy source is needed, such as for growing puppies or lactating bitches. Indeed it is an important natural energy source for the dog.

Unsaturated fats contain certain 'essential fatty acids' (EFA's), a lack of which results in a dull coat, slow healing of wounds and possibly poor reproductive performance.

Fats are also carriers of the 'fat-soluble' vitamins A, D, E and K; and the inclusion of fat in dog food also improves its palatability, and hence the dog's enjoyment and willingness to eat.

Proteins are complex molecules made up of chains of simpler units called amino acids, rather like a necklace consists of a string of individual beads. There are effectively 20 different amino acids required by the dog, half of which are called 'essential amino acids' and must be taken in as part of the diet because they cannot be synthesised in the body.

Proteins are needed for growth, tissue maintenance and repair. They also form an important structural component of enzymes and hormones.

Minerals can be divided into two groups depending upon their concentration in the diet. Major, or 'macro', minerals are usually present in milligram (1/1000 g) quantities and include calcium, phosphorus, sodium, potassium and magnesium; while trace elements, or 'micro-minerals' are usually present in microgram (1/1,000,000 g) quantities and include iron, copper, zinc, manganese and iodine.

Minerals have many important functions in the body (see Table 2). **It is vital to remember that the balance of minerals in the diet is just as important as the range and absolute quantity.** For example, the correct ratio of calcium to phosphorus must be maintained. These two elements are closely linked nutritionally and metabolically, and problems can arise if this balance is seriously disturbed, as occurs when puppies are over-supplemented.

Table 2   Minerals

Mineral	Dietary sources	Main functions	Results of deficiency	Results of excess
Calcium	Bones, milk, cheese	Bone formation, nerve and muscle function	Poor growth, rickets, convulsions	Very high levels – bone deformities
Phos-phorus	Bones, milk	Bone formation, energy utilisation	Rickets (rare)	Symptoms of calcium deficiency
Potassium	Meat, milk	Water balance, nerve function	Poor growth, paralysis, kidney and heart lesions	Muscular weakness?
Sodium/chlorine	Salts, cereals	Water balance, muscle and nerve activity	Poor growth, exhaustion	Thirst, high blood pressure (if intake maintained)
Mag-nesium	Cereals, bones, green vegetables	Bone formation, protein synthesis	Anorexia, vomiting, muscular weakness	Diarrhoea
Iron	Eggs, meat (liver), green vegetables	Part of haemoglobin (oxygen transport)	Anaemia	Weight loss, anorexia
Copper	Meat, bones	Part of haemoglobin	Anaemia	Anaemia in other mammals, hepatitis in Bedlington Terriers
Zinc	Meat, cereals	In digestion, tissue maintenance	Hair loss, skin thickening, poor growth	Diarrhoea
Man-ganese	Nuts, cereals	Fat metabolism, many enzyme functions	Reproductive failure, poor growth	Poor fertility in other mammals, albinism, anaemia
Iodine	Fish, dairy produce	Part of thyroid hormone	Hair loss, apathy, drowsiness	In other animals, symptoms similar to deficiency
Selenium	Cereals, fish meals	Associated with Vitamin E metabolism	Muscle damage	Toxic

Dogs may also require molybdenum, fluorine, tin, silicon, cobalt, nickel, vanadium and chromium in very small amounts.

Table 3   Vitamins

Vitamin	Dietary source	Main functions	Results of deficiency	Results of excess
Fat Soluble Vitamin A	Fish oils, liver, vegetables	Vision in poor light, maintenance of skin	Night blindness, skin lesions	Anorexia, pain in bones and malformation
Vitamin D	Cod-liver oil, eggs, animal products	Calcium balance, bone growth	Rickets, osteomalacia	Anorexia, calcification of soft tissues
Vitamin E	Green vegetables, vegetable oils, dairy products	Reproduction	Infertility, anaemia, muscle weakness	n/k
Vitamin K	Spinach, green vegetables, liver, (in vivo) synthesis	Blood clotting	Haemorrhage	n/k
Water Soluble (B group) Thiamin (B_1)	Dairy products, cereals, meat	Release of energy from carbohydrate	Anorexia, vomiting, paralysis	n/k
Riboflavin (B_2)	Milk, animal tissues	Utilisation of energy	Weight loss, weakness, collapse, coma	n/k
Niacin	Cereals, liver, meat, legumes	Utilisation of energy	Anorexia, ulceration of mouth (black tongue)	n/k
Pyridoxine (B_6)	Meat, fish, eggs, cereals	Metabolism of amino acids	Anorexia, anaemia, weight loss, convulsions	n/k
Vitamin B_{12}	Liver, meat, dairy products	Division of cells in bone marrow	Anaemia	n/k
Folic acid	Offals, leafy vegetables	As B_{12}	Anaemia, poor growth	n/k
Pantothenic acid	Animal products, cereals, legumes	Release of energy from fat/carbohydrate	Slow growth, hair loss, convulsions, coma	n/k

Table 3 continued

Vitamin	Dietary source	Main functions	Results of deficiency	Results of excess
Biotin	Offal, egg yolk, legumes	Metabolism of fat and amino acids	Loss of coat condition (scaly skin, scurf)	n/k
Choline	Plant and animal materials	Nerve function	Fatty infiltration of liver, poor blood clotting	n/k

n/k = not known in dogs

Vitamins are basically divided into two groups (see Table 3): the fat-soluble vitamins A, D, E and K: and the water-soluble vitamins B and C. A balanced diet containing a range of meats and fresh vegetables, or a good-quality prepared pet food, will supply all the necessary vitamins for growth, development and maintenance. Only very small amounts of vitamins are required for health, and once these requirements have been met there is no value in further supplementation. Any excess of the fat-soluble vitamins is not only wasteful but may be dangerous, since they are stored in the liver.

Water intake in dogs depends on several factors of which food type is probably the most important. Fresh meat and canned foods have a high moisture content (about 75 per cent), whereas that found in dry foods is much lower (about 8 per cent). Carbohydrates, fats and proteins all produce water when they are broken down in the body tissues. This metabolic water can make a significant contribution to the overall water turnover of the body (see Table 4). For example, the oxidation, or 'burning', of 100 g of fat by the body results in the production of a greater weight of water (107 g) than the original fat.

Table 4 Metabolic water

Class of food	Water yield on oxidation of 100 g
Protein*	40 g
Fat	107 g
Carbohydrate	55 g

*Not always completely oxidized

If the environmental temperature rises, the dog, especially if it is fairly active, will need to drink more water. The physiological state of the animal will also affect water requirement: during lactation, for instance, the bitch's water intake will increase dramatically.

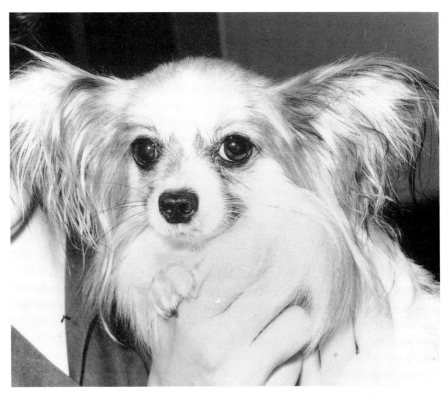

Figure 47 Energy requirements depend on a dog's size. This little Papillon requires more food per kilo bodyweight than a St Bernard

ENERGY

In nutritional terms, the major determinant for controlling food intake is the energy content of the diet, i.e., the number of calories it contains. All other nutrient components, including vitamins and minerals, must be balanced and directly related to the so-called metabolisable energy (ME) of the food. The ME is measured in kilocalories (kcals).

The dog's energy requirements depend upon the body size and age, as well as the life style, of the individual animal. Big dogs have a smaller energy requirement per unit of bodyweight than small ones (see Table 5); adults within a breed have smaller energy needs per unit of bodyweight than their puppies. In other words, a 60 kg Newfoundland doesn't need five times as much food as a 12 kg Beagle!

Remember too that all dogs within a breed are individuals and have their own precise energy requirements. This means that you may have to 'fine tune' the guidelines given on the cans and bags of prepared pet foods to allow for this. Other factors, such as age, exercise and the climate have an effect too, and hard-working dogs will clearly require more energy than the average pet dog. Indeed, working dogs should be considered as puppies during periods of training or extreme exercise and they will need two to three times the maintenance intake in several concentrated feeds.

There is a significant correlation between climatic temperature and energy requirements. Decreasing the ambient temperature from 16°C (61°F) to 10°C (50°F) results in a 20–30 per cent increase in the energy needed to keep warm and maintain bodyweight. It is worth remembering that 10°C is still quite mild, and many dogs housed in outside quarters may experience much lower temperatures. Ironically, rises in ambient temperature above 16°C also necessitate increased calorie intake to provide energy to keep cool by panting and sweating as well as maintaining bodyweight.

PREPARED PET FOODS

Prepared pet foods are available in several forms and may either be considered in relation to their intended role in the diet or they can be conveniently classified by their water content or method of preservation:

Dry food	5 to 12% water
Semi-moist food	15 to 50% water
Canned food	72 to 85% water
Frozen food	60 to 75% water

Whatever their form, such foods may be formulated and sold either as the whole, or part of, the diet for a dog.

Complete foods are capable of maintaining life and health of adults and also support growth, reproduction and work as well when fed without any other food except water.

Complementary foods are not intended for use as the only food, or to provide the total diet. They may be rich in some nutrients, but inadequate in others. Their major role in the diet is to provide a relatively cheap source of energy, and as such they complement the low energy, high protein of most canned meats.

PRACTICAL FEEDING

Adults

Healthy adults dogs can be fed on one complete food only or with a number of varieties. However, sudden changes in diet should be avoided as this may lead to diarrhoea. The total daily nutritional requirement can be given as one meal a day in adult dogs, although most owners prefer to feed more often; but at the same time, to suit their routine.

Table 5   Average energy needs of healthy adult dogs and amounts of mixed feeding regimes needed to meet them

Weight of dog (kg)	Typical breed	Energy requirement (kcal/day)	(g/day)
2	Yorkshire Terrier	115	128
8	Fox Terrier	460	512
14	Cocker Spaniel	806	895
20	Border Collie	1151	1279
26	Basset Hound	1496	1662
32	Labrador Retriever	1841	2046
40	Deerhound	2302	2558
50	Bull Mastiff	2877	3197
70	Irish Wolfhound	4028	4476

Mineral and vitamin supplements must be added to the diet in the correct proportion to ensure that nutritional balance is achieved. Energy densities of foods will vary depending on the source. For the purpose of this table typical energy densities have been assumed as follows: Tripe 0.9 kcal/g; Mixer 3.5 kcal/g; Mince 2.0 kcal/g

Table 6   Average energy needs of healthy adult dogs and amounts of different types of prepared pet food needed to meet them

Weight of dog (kg)	Typical breed	Energy requirement (kcal/day)
2	Yorkshire Terrier	115
8	Fox Terrier	460
14	Cocker Spaniel	806
20	Border Collie	1151
26	Basset Hound	1496
32	Labrador Retriever	1841
40	Deerhound	2302
50	Bull Mastiff	2877
70	Irish Wolfhound	4028

Energy densities of prepared foods will vary depending on the recipe used. For the purpose of this table energy densities have been assumed as follows:

| Canned food | 0.7 kcal/g | Semi-moist food | 3.05 kcal/g |
| Mixer | 3.5 kcal/g | Complete dry food | 3.5 kcal/g |

Food to provide this amount of energy			
Tripe+Mixer equal weights		**Mince+Mixer equal weights**	
tripe (g/day)	*mixer* (g/day)	*mince* (g/day)	*mixer* (g/day)
26	26	21	21
105	105	84	84
183	183	146	146
262	262	209	209
340	340	272	272
419	419	335	335
523	523	419	419
654	654	523	523
915	915	732	732

Food to provide this amount of energy Canned food + mixer 3:1 by weight, approx. equal volumes		*Semi-moist food* (g/day)	*Complete dry food* (g/day)
meat (g/day)	*mixer* (g/day)		
60	20	38	33
240	80	151	132
420	140	264	230
599	200	377	329
779	260	491	427
959	320	604	526
1199	400	755	658
1499	500	943	822
2098	699	1321	1151

Tables 5 and 6 provide a summary of the energy needs of adult dogs, together with the amounts of food required to meet these needs, either as prepared pet foods or on typical home-prepared diets. The tables are only intended as guidelines and the actual amounts needed by individual dogs will have to be determined by careful observation and regular weighing.

The proportions of canned meat to mixer biscuit fed should be equal amounts by volume or approximately 3:1 meat:mixer by weight.

Breeding bitches

Most growth of the foetus takes place during the last three weeks of pregnancy and although there is considerable development of mammary and uterine tissues before this, the extra need for energy and nutrients is quite small. All that is necessary is to increase the total food allowance by 10 per cent each week from the sixth week of pregnancy onwards, so that the intake at whelping is between 40 and 50 per cent more than at mating (see Fig. 48). However, if the bitch is at all overweight, it is probably better not to increase food intake until after whelping has occurred.

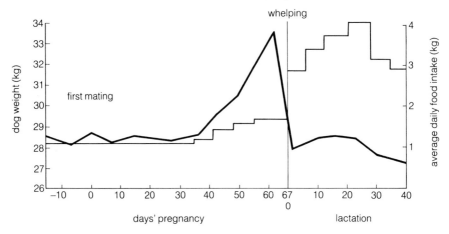

Figure 48   Typical food intake and weight change of a breeding bitch during pregnancy and lactation

Sometimes a pregnant bitch with a large litter may have such an enlarged abdomen, and her general activity may be so reduced, that her appetite falls during the last 10 days of pregnancy. In these cases it is sensible to feed several smaller meals and to introduce amounts of concentrated food of the sort which will probably be used in lactation anyway. The objective is to have a bitch at parturition which is not overfat and which has maintained her appetite.

After whelping and throughout lactation the bitch must eat, digest, absorb and utilise very large quantities of nutrients in order to produce

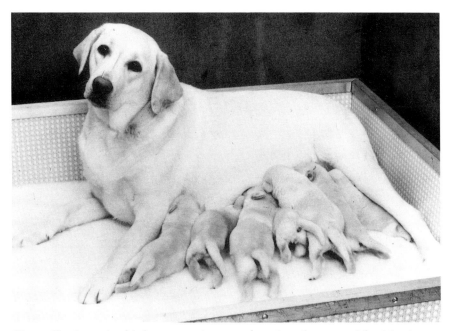

Figure 49 A nursing bitch may require up to four times her normal food intake to provide sufficient milk to satisfy energy and growth requirements of her offspring

sufficient milk of adequate composition to support the growth and development of several puppies. If canned food and mixer is the usual diet, then it is necessary to increase the proportion of biscuit used to achieve satisfactory energy intakes. Sometimes, because the sheer volume of food required to provide all the calories is too great for the bitch's gut to physically hold, it is necessary to feed concentrated prescription diets or puppy foods, relying on fat as the main energy source.

As a guide, it is usual for a bitch to be eating up to four times her normal maintenance requirements by the time she reaches peak lactation, at about 3 weeks post whelping. The breeding bitch does not need special vitamin/mineral supplementation if a correctly balanced diet, such as a good-quality complete prepared pet food, is used in the first instance.

Puppies and growing dogs

Feeding the puppy begins at weaning. This process will begin naturally when puppies are three to four weeks old and exploring their surroundings. At this age they will readily take soft, wet foods that are easy to ingest. Although many people assume that milk and milky foods should figure prominently in a weaning regimen, they are not essential.

Puppies will eat minced or chopped moist food and litters should be fed together from one or more trays, depending on litter size. Highly palatable,

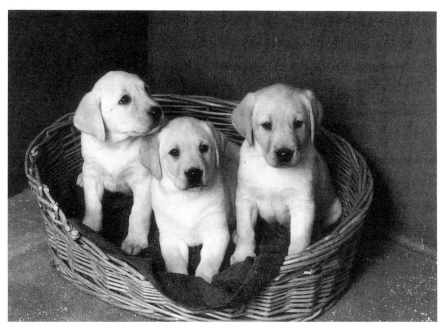

Figure 50　Labrador puppies. Weaning occurs from 3–6 weeks of age and should produce healthy inquisitive individuals independent of Mum

energy-and-nutrient-dense foods are most suitable for weaning and there are some prepared foods which have been specifically formulated for puppies.

In the early stages of weaning, it is important to remember that the bitch's milk is still the most vital source of nutrients while the puppies' digestive and immune systems are learning how to handle new sources of food. After this period, the intake of other foods quickly increase and most litters will have been weaned on to a varied diet, or a single complete food, by the time they are six weeks old.

Once weaned, puppies grow at a rapid rate and need to ingest very large amounts of energy and nutrients in relation to their size. As a guideline, young puppies require two to three times the energy intake of an adult of the same bodyweight. It is therefore essential to use more concentrated foods and to offer meals three or four times a day. This can gradually be reduced to two meals as the animal approaches its mature bodyweight.

As puppies get older, their energy requirement (and hence their overall food intake) slowly decreases. An approximate rule is as follows: when the puppy is 50 per cent of its mature bodyweight, it should be eating its adult maintenance requirement plus 60 per cent; when the puppy is 80 per cent of its mature bodyweight, it should be eating its adult maintenance requirement plus 30 per cent.

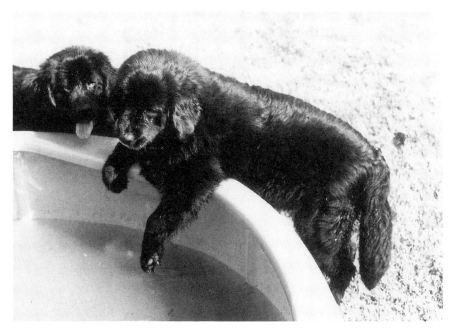

Figure 51 Newfoundland puppies. Do remember puppies of large breeds of dogs remain in puppyhood much longer than those of smaller breeds

And *do remember* that puppies of large breeds of dogs remain in puppyhood for much longer than those of the smaller breeds. Small and toy breeds reach their mature bodyweight at 6–9 months of age, whereas giant breeds are not mature until they are at least 18–24 months old (see Fig. 52).

There is no advantage in overfeeding puppies in order to try to make them reach their adult weight more quickly. 'Steaming up', as it is called in canine circles, has produced more problems than ever it solved! Controlled feeding of a balanced diet is the most likely way to produce optimum growth and good strong bone structure.

Rearing motherless puppies is a very demanding task and should not be undertaken lightly. However, it does sometimes happen that dog owners are faced with the situation in an emergency and the following points will be of interim use until full veterinary advice can be sought.

Always keep orphan puppies warm – between 21 and 26°C (70 and 80°F) depending on age.

Bitches' milk is much richer in fat and protein than cows' milk and also contains far more calories. If a commercial source of a bitch milk substitute is not readily available, a good alternative is to mix four parts of evaporated milk with one part of boiled water.

All bitch milk substitutes should be given at 'blood heat' 38°C (100·4°F)

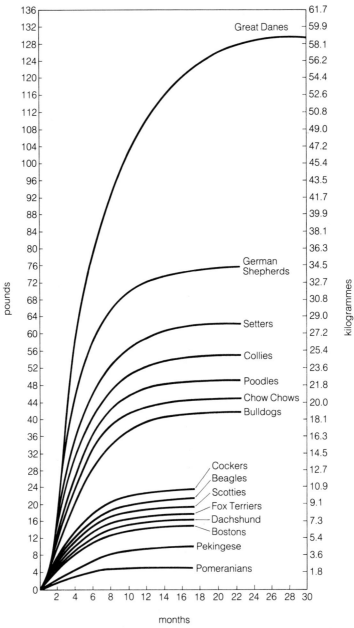

Figure 52 Growth rates of different breeds (from *Current Veterinary Therapy III* edited by R.W. Kirk)

and administered by means of a small syringe, dropper or a puppy feeding bottle. Feeds should be given slowly, in small quantities, at frequent intervals – perhaps every 1–2 hours shortly after birth.

Finally, after puppies have been fed it is important to simulate the mother's tongue action on the ano-genital area in order to elicit defecation and urination. This can be done by gently stroking with a piece of moist cottonwool or by running a dampened forefinger along the abdominal wall. After this procedure, each puppy should be carefully cleaned.

When the puppies are about three weeks old, they are able to relieve themselves without stimulation. By this time they will also be exploring their surroundings, drinking milk substitute from a shallow dish and starting to eat solid puppy foods. Playing with the orphans, at the same time as introducing the new foods, is a gentle and fulfilling way of weaning from milk.

Working dogs

Working dogs are invariably adult dogs involved in a wide range of activities, from acting as guide dogs for the blind at one end of the scale

Figure 53 Workloads of police dogs, like guide dogs, are often intermittent compared with the sustained work of sled dogs

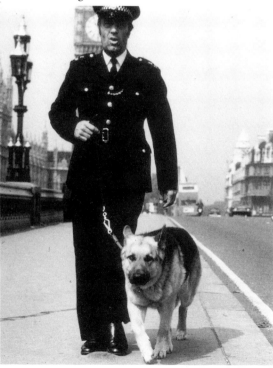

to pulling heavy sledges in the polar regions at the other. Just as the work loads of guide dogs and police dogs are often intermittent compared with the sustained efforts of sled dogs, so extra energy needs are also widely variable, often being critically affected by the factors mentioned earlier (see Energy page 92).

In general, working dogs may need up to two to three times the adult maintenance requirement, fed in a regimen that fits in with their work schedule. It is necessary to feed hard-working dogs with high-fat diets to ensure that sufficient calories are consumed and it is often useful to include puppy foods, which are more energy-dense, as part of the overall feeding programme.

Old dogs

When dogs become older, their needs are really no different from those that have existed throughout adult life. Because they may take less exercise, their total energy requirement may be less, and it is often a good idea to divide their daily food intake into several small, highly digestible meals. Most of the nutritional problems encountered in old dogs stem from the presence of some other disease or geriatric changes elsewhere in the body, e.g., kidney failure or a tendency to put on weight as a result of reduced

Figure 54　With veterinary help diet can be adjusted to minimise some of the problems of old age

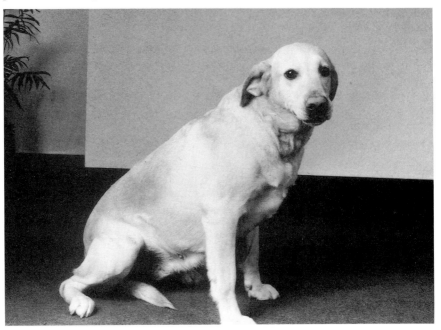

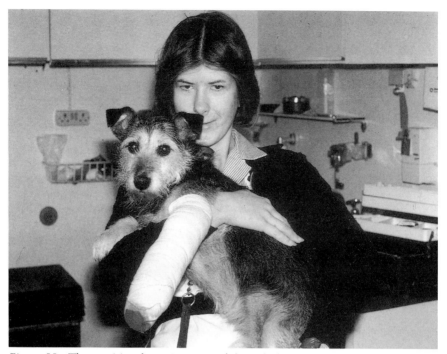

Figure 55 The nutritional requirements of the sick dog are actually higher than those of a healthy animal

physical activity. Diet can, under veterinary supervision, be adjusted to reduce these problems.

Sick dogs

One of the major problems encountered when dogs are ill is loss of appetite. Ironically, this is at a time when the requirements of the sick animal are actually higher than those of a healthy one. There are a number of measures which can be taken to encourage dogs to eat.

1. Ensure that the diet is complete and balanced, particularly with respect to its vitamin and mineral content.
2. Foods of high energy and nutrient density minimise the quantity the animal has to eat to obtain the essential nutrients.
3. High digestibility makes sure that the best use is made of the components of the diet.
4. Feed on a 'little and often' basis, dividing the daily intake into three or four meals.
5. Warm food to body temperature 38°C (i.e., approx 100°F) if necessary (but not above).
6. Include small quantities of animal fat in the diet. This is a rich energy source and helps to increase the palatability of the food.

7. Feed foods with a high moisture content because they tend to be more palatable than dry foods.
8. Remove food that is not eaten after 10–15 minutes. Fresh food offered later is often more likely to be eaten.

SPECIFIC CONDITIONS

Obesity

At least 25 per cent of the dogs seen by veterinary surgeons are *overweight* (i.e., their bodyweight is noticeably more than is usual for their type, their rib cage is not easily seen when they walk and it is difficult to feel their bone structure), and about a quarter of these are *obese* (i.e., in addition to the features of an overweight dog they have large amounts of fat which can easily be grasped in folds of skin and they show an obvious incapacity as a result of the accumulation of body fat). Overweightness/obesity represents the most commonly occurring nutritional problem seen in dogs. The reason is very simple:

Energy taken in exceeds energy needed

Result: Extra calories converted to fat and stored in body

Consequences: Excessive weight, arthritis, heart disease, breathing difficulties, diabetes mellitus, reduced liver function, impaired digestive function, reduced resistance to disease and shorter life expectancy.

Profile of an overweight dog
Eating behaviour:
   • Bolts food and asks for more
   • Begs for food at family mealtimes.

Activity:
   • Sleeps instead of playing
   • Refuses to walk more than short distances
   • Pants heavily if made to run
   • Has difficulty negotiating steps and slopes.

Weather effects:
   • Seeks shade, pants and lolls around in warm weather.

Physical shape:
   • Cannot feel ribs
   • No 'waist' when viewed or felt from above . . . pads of fat instead
   • Abdomen sags when viewed from the side.

Treatment
Controlled calorie reduction, which should be carried out after discussion

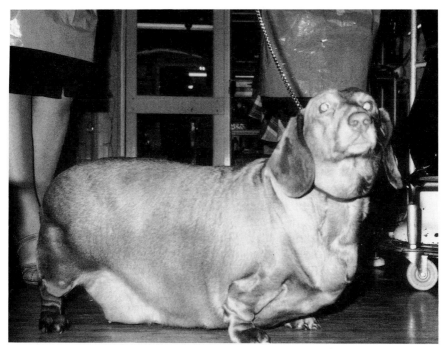

Figure 56 The most commonly occurring nutritional problem seen in dogs is obesity

with your veterinary surgeon. By using the following method the target weight should be achieved within 8–10 weeks.

Method

1. Make sure that everyone, including the children and the next-door neighbours!, understands the seriousness of the problem and agrees to co-operate.
2. Weigh the dog and set an initial target weight. This should be no more than 15 per cent less than the dog's current weight. (If necessary the programme can be repeated to ultimately achieve normal bodyweight for the breed and the size of dog.)
3. Feed a diet providing 60 per cent of the calculated maintenance requirement at the target weight. (Special prescription diets are available from your veterinary surgeon who will also help and advise you on setting appropriate target weights, etc.)
4. Weigh the dog weekly, at the same time of day and using the same scales on each occasion. Plot progress on a graph. Every time there is no loss of bodyweight reduce the food allowance by 20 per cent.
5. Give no titbits, snacks or treats.

6. Use food with a high moisture content so that 'hunger misery' is reduced to a minimum.
7. Feed frequently, not exceeding the total calculated daily intake.
8. Gradually increase exercise in line with progressive weight loss.

Other conditions

Although standard prepared foods are sufficient to enable the majority of dogs to cope with life's ups and downs, there are times when special dietary management is necessary to assist with the treatment of specific disease. Examples of this include kidney failure, bladder disease and some skin infections. In these cases it is important that a correct diagnosis is made by your veterinary surgeon so that the appropriate diet can be prescribed. It is for this reason that commercial 'special' diets can only be obtained through a veterinary surgeon in order that inappropriate foods are not fed. For example a 'fat dog' could conceivably be pregnant or have fluid retention caused by heart or kidney problems as well as being just plain 'fat', and dietary management in each case should be radically different.

The Organ Systems

8

THE DIGESTIVE SYSTEM

The digestive system consists of organs whose purpose is to grasp, digest and absorb foodstuffs (and water) and eliminate residual materials. Associated with the main organs, which make up a tube running from one end of the body to the other, are other structures and organs which make an essential contribution, principally the teeth, tongue, salivary glands, pancreas, liver and gall-bladder.

Food is required both to produce new tissues (i.e., for growth in young animals, and repair) and for the production of energy, which is constantly needed by all cells. A digestive system is necessary because most of the food is taken into the body in a form which is too complicated in its structure to be utilised directly. Proteins, fats and carbohydrates are made up of molecules which are too large to be absorbed, i.e. taken through the wall of the intestine into the rest of the body. They must first be broken down into simpler substances *which can* be absorbed, and this breaking down process constitutes digestion. The splitting of complex food molecules is carried out by enzymes present in the digestive juices which are passed, in large quantities, into the digestive tract. Other components of the diet – water, mineral salts and vitamins – do not require digestion and can be absorbed intact. (See Chapter 7 on Nutrition.)

Functional anatomy

Mouth (oral cavity)

In the dog the mouth is a large cavity with a correspondingly wide entrance surrounded and closed by the lips (Fig. 57). It contains the teeth, tongue and the openings of the salivary glands.

Food is taken into the mouth by being picked up with the front (incisor) teeth, or in the case of softer foods using the tongue. Large pieces (e.g., chunks of meat, biscuits) may be torn or crushed by the teeth into pieces small enough to be swallowed, but chewing is a very cursory affair. Saliva

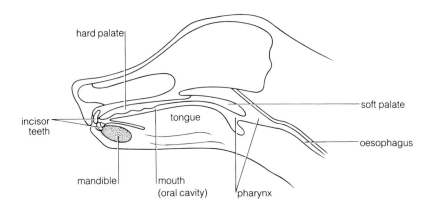

Figure 57   Section through the head of a dog to show the position of the major
structures

in copious amounts coats the food, thereby providing lubrication for
swallowing, and the tongue moves the food material around the mouth
(i.e., between the teeth for such chewing as is required) and eventually
passes it into the pharynx to be swallowed.

The roof of the mouth largely consists of the hard palate, ridges of
membrane overlying bone, but at the back there lies a membrane-covered
flap of soft tissue, the soft palate.

Teeth

Each side of the upper jaw of the adult dog bears (from front to back)
three incisor teeth, one large canine tooth, four premolar and two molar
teeth (Fig. 58). Similarly the lower jaw carries three incisor teeth, one
canine tooth, four premolar and three molar teeth. This makes a total of
forty-two permanent teeth in the mouth. (See Chapter 29 Canine
Dentistry.)

The puppy is born without teeth, which begin to erupt at three to four
weeks of age. These deciduous (or 'milk') teeth comprise, on each side of
the upper and lower jaws, three incisors, one canine and three premolar
teeth (a total of twenty-eight). The permanent teeth erupt, and displace the
deciduous teeth, between three and seven months of age.

The incisors (front teeth) are small teeth used for picking up pieces of
food and 'nibbling' the flesh off bones. The long, conical, pointed canine
teeth ('fangs') are used for tearing flesh, and the premolars and the molars
(most of which have two or more roots) are used for such chewing and
grinding as is necessary.

As well as their functions in digestion the teeth are also used to carry
objects (including puppies), for attack and defence and for grooming. The
muscles used to close the jaws are extremely strong, e.g., they allow the

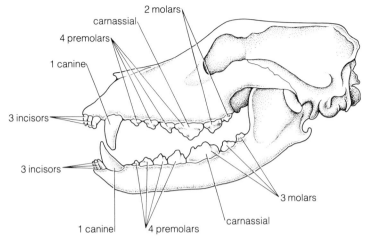

2 molars
carnassial
4 premolars
1 canine
3 incisors
3 incisors
3 molars
carnassial
1 canine
4 premolars

Figure 58   The arrangement of permanent teeth in one side of the upper and lower jaws

animal to crack bones. The largest teeth (the fourth premolar in the upper jaw and the first molar in the lower jaw) are referred to as *carnassial teeth*.

Tongue

This long, muscular structure in the floor of the mouth is attached at the sides to the lower jaw and at the back to the hyoid bone in the throat. The surface of the tongue is covered by a thick mucous membrane with numerous small projections (papillae), some of which carry the specialised nerve endings, the *taste-buds*. The free end of the tongue is broad and can be curved to form a ladle which allows it to lap liquids. The tongue scoops up liquid and throws it to the back of the throat.

Salivary glands

Four pairs of salivary glands are situated around the head and secrete saliva, which passes along ducts into the mouth. The sight, smell and taste of food, and the feel of it in the mouth, cause saliva to flow. It consists chiefly of water plus some mucin (a protein) and it lubricates the food, facilitating swallowing. It also helps to release the flavour from dry foods. Unlike in man, the dog's saliva contains an insignificant amount of the enzyme amylase used to digest starch. However, saliva in the dog is just as important as in man due to its lubricating properties and its ability to prevent drying of the tongue and lips.

Pharynx (oro-pharynx)

This muscular compartment lies behind the mouth, and food in sufficiently small pieces, coated with saliva, is passed into it by the tongue. This initiates the swallowing process, causing the muscles in the wall to

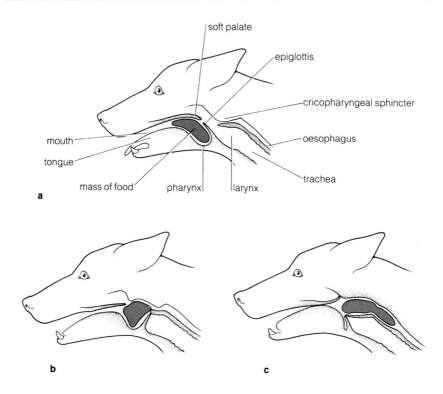

Figure 59   The act of swallowing:
(a) A mass of food is moved from the back of the mouth into the pharynx by the tongue acting like a plunger
(b) Contraction of the pharyngeal muscles propels the food into the opening of the oesophagus, simultaneously closing the other openings
(c) The food enters the first part of the oesophagus. Subsequently a peristaltic wave (wave of muscular contraction) squeezes the food along the length of the oesophagus and into the stomach

contract, thereby forcing food into the opening of the oesophagus (Fig. 59). Simultaneously the other openings into the pharynx are closed, i.e., into the nasal cavities (closed by the soft palate), the mouth (by the root of the tongue) and the larynx (by the epiglottis). This closure of other openings is important because the pharynx is a 'cross-over point' in the digestive and respiratory tracts, and without it problems would arise, in particular food could pass down the trachea, causing choking.

Oesophagus

This is a muscular tube (gullet) running down the neck and through the upper part of the chest, passing through the diaphragm and opening into the stomach. Immediately food enters the oesophagus (from the pharynx) a wave of muscular contraction (peristaltic wave) develops behind it and pushes it without interruption all the way along the oesophagus, so that it is delivered into the stomach. Once swallowing has been started, by food passing into the pharynx, the subsequent movement of food out of the pharynx and along the oesophagus follows automatically.

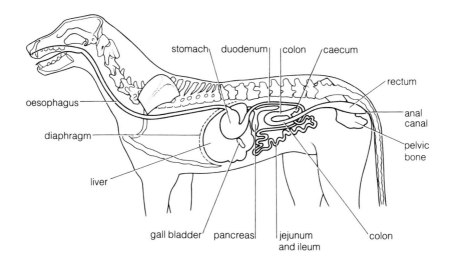

Figure 60 The position of the organs which constitute the digestive system. For the sake of clarity the jejunum and ileum are shown as shorter and less coiled than in real life (compare Fig. 62)

Stomach

The stomach of the dog is a large dilated organ at the front of the abdominal cavity which receives the food, liquefies it by thoroughly mixing it with gastric juice and then passes it out in small amounts, into the duodenum (Fig. 60). Because the food that makes up a meal enters the stomach during a relatively short period of time, but is passed out over a much longer period, it can be regarded as a temporary food reservoir.

There are rings of muscle or valves which guard the entrance and exit of the stomach. That at the entrance, the cardiac sphincter, is weak, but that at the exit, the pyloric sphincter, can close down tightly, preventing food passing out until it relaxes (Fig. 61).

The internal wall of the stomach is thrown into prominent folds and contains microscopic glands – the gastric glands – which produce gastric juice. This digestive juice consists of water and hydrochloric acid and the enzyme pepsin, which begins the breakdown of protein molecules.

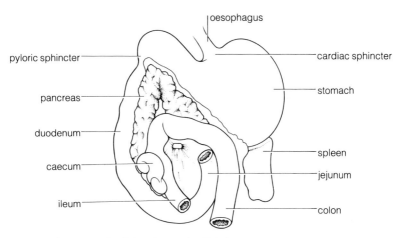

Figure 61 The stomach of the dog and adjoining organs

Small intestine

This is a long muscular tube with a lining containing numerous intestinal glands. It is subdivided into three parts, which in the order that food passes through are the *duodenum, jejunum* and *ileum* (Fig. 62). The first of these is fixed in position in the upper part of the abdomen, but the other two sections are more freely attached and lie in large loops within the abdominal cavity, occupying a good deal of its total capacity.

Within the small intestine food is slowly passed along by waves of muscular contraction known as peristaltic waves. Unlike those in the oesophagus, these waves do not pass completely from one end of the intestine to the other because the intention is not to move the food rapidly but slowly enough to give adequate time for digestion and absorption. A wave of contraction slowly builds up in a length of intestine, moves food along a short distance, and then gradually fades away. At any one time a number of such waves may be present in the bowel.

Throughout the small intestine the food is present in a very liquid form because a large volume of digestive juices has been added to it; these consist of pancreatic juice coming from the pancreas along the pancreatic ducts, bile produced in the liver and stored in the gall bladder, from where it is conveyed along the bile duct, and intestinal juice produced by the intestinal glands in the wall of the intestine. The ducts conveying pancreatic juice and bile open into the first part of the duodenum, but the intestinal glands are present throughout the small intestine.

All three digestive juices contain bicarbonate, which is required to neutralise the stomach acid and to produce an alkaline environment necessary for the correct functioning of the enzymes present in the juices. Pancreatic juice contains three enzymes – trypsin, amylase and lipase – to

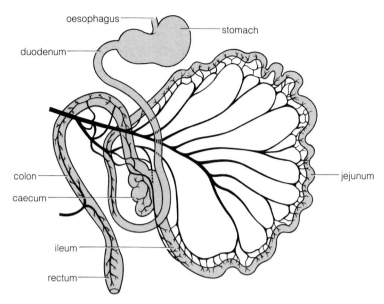

Figure 62 The components of the small intestine – duodenum, jejunum and ileum – showing their total length in comparison to the stomach and the large intestine (caecum, colon and rectum)

digest protein, starch and fats, respectively. Bile possesses no enzymes, but contained within it are bile salts, which are essential to digestion because they emulsify the fat globules (i.e., break them up into numerous smaller globules in a similar way to detergents, allowing them to be more readily acted upon by lipase) and also bile pigments (which are breakdown products of haemoglobin having no useful function but giving the green-orange colour to bile). Intestinal juice contains a number of enzymes which complete the digestive process so that proteins are ultimately broken down into their molecular components, amino acids, carbohydrates into simple sugars (such as glucose) and fats into fatty acids and glycerol.

Having been broken down into these smaller molecules the food can be absorbed in the small intestine, which necessitates the molecules passing through the wall of the intestine into the small blood and lymphatic vessels. To greatly increase the surface area available for absorption, the lining of the gut carries a large number of microscopic, finger-shaped projections called villi. The liquefied food comes into contact with thousands of villi as it is churned up and passed along by peristalsis. So-called villous atrophy, in which the villi are reduced in height, or even completely absent, greatly diminishes the area available for absorption, with the result that absorption is incomplete. This is one of the causes of the malabsorption syndrome.

Figure 63 The microscopic, finger-shaped projections, villi (*singular:* villus), which line the small intestine, considerably increasing its internal surface area. Digested foodstuffs pass through the enclosing layer of cells and into the inner blood and lymphatic vessels; a process termed *absorption*

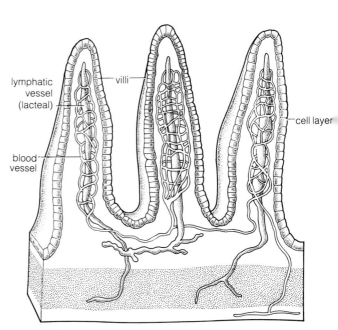

lymphatic vessel (lacteal)

villi

cell layer

blood vessel

The majority of the water which has been added in the digestive juices is also absorbed in the small intestine, although the material which is passed on into the large intestine is still relatively liquid in consistency. It leaves the small intestine by passing through a muscular valve, the ileo-caecal valve.

Large intestine

This is subdivided into the *caecum, colon* and *rectum*. The caecum, which comes directly after the ileo-caecal valve, is a relatively short, blind-ended tube which represents a cul-de-sac off the main tube. There is no appendix at the end of this organ as there is in man and therefore, not surprisingly, the dog does not suffer from appendicitis. The remainder of the large intestine (which is termed large not because it is longer than the smaller intestine but because it has a greater diameter) forms a tube which passes backwards to reach the exterior at the anus. The external opening is normally closed by the anal sphincter, another ring of muscle, which is only opened to defaecate. That part of the large intestine contained within the pelvic canal (i.e., enclosed within the bones which make up the pelvic girdle) is called the rectum.

No digestion or absorption of food takes place within the large intestine; its main function is to absorb most of the residual water, so that the material which finally enters the rectum, as the faeces, motions, or stool has a semi-solid consistency. Movement through the large intestine is much slower than through the small intestine.

Intermittently a mass of faecal material is passed into the rectum from the colon, stretching the wall of the rectum and triggering nerve endings (pressure receptors) which make the individual aware of the need to defecate (pass a motion). Given a suitable opportunity (in house-trained animals) the dog adopts a crouching posture with tail raised, tenses its abdominal muscles and relaxes the anal sphincter, causing the faeces to be expelled. Although in part a voluntary act, there is also reflex control of defecation and it cannot be delayed indefinitely.

Anal sacs

Popularly called 'anal glands', these are two small pouches situated on either side of, and a little below, the anus (i.e., at about the 4 o'clock and 8 o'clock positions). They vary in size from a pea to a walnut, depending on the breed, though in a medium-sized dog they are about ⅖ in. (1 cm) across. A small tube or duct passes from each sac to open at the anus, Fig. 64. In the wall are numerous glands producing a secretion that is stored in the sacs and used as a scent. Some of this liquid is deposited on each stool as it is passed so that other dogs can identify it; this is important in inter-canine communications.

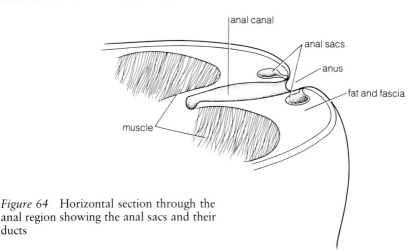

Figure 64 Horizontal section through the anal region showing the anal sacs and their ducts

Peritoneum

This is a thin, transparent membrane that lines the abdominal cavity and covers the organs that lie within it.

Pancreas

The pancreas is a V-shaped glandular organ lying close to the duodenum in the upper part of the abdomen (Fig. 61). It consists of a large number of secretory cells, producing the pancreatic juice, arranged around tiny ducts, which ultimately join together to form the two main pancreatic ducts. These convey the pancreatic juice to the first part of the duodenum.

In addition, scattered within the gland are small groups of hormone-producing cells, the islets of Langerhans, but these have an entirely separate function and are not associated with digestion. These hormones, like all others, are secreted directly into the blood (see Chapter 14, The Endocrine System).

The liver

The liver, a large, reddish brown organ (the largest gland in the body), is situated at the front of the abdomen directly behind the diaphragm (Fig. 65). It is divided by deep fissures into several lobes and has a rich blood supply, including that coming from the small intestine in the portal vein, which brings absorbed foodstuffs to the liver (Fig. 66).

The liver is the chemical factory of the body and its cells carry out a large variety of metabolic functions, including the conversion of fats, the storage of glucose as glycogen (or animal starch) and its re-conversion if required, the production of most plasma proteins (with the exception of the antibodies), the storage of iron and vitamins A, B and D, the production of clotting factors necessary for blood clotting, the breakdown of surplus amino acids and of haemoglobin and the detoxification of many substances, e.g., drugs and anaesthetics (i.e., breaking down these potentially harmful substances into compounds which can then be excreted). In addition it produces the bile pigments (from a constituent of haemoglobin) and the bile salts, which are important in digestion. These two are secreted, together with sodium bicarbonate and water, as bile, which is conveyed to the gall bladder, where it is stored.

Gall bladder

This is a pear-shaped bag situated between the lobes of the liver. It receives bile from the liver, stores it and discharges it when necessary (i.e., when food is present in the small intestine) along the bile duct into the duodenum. It acts as a reservoir for bile, and during storage removes some water from it, thereby concentrating it.

Disorders of the digestive system

Mouth

Inflammation (stomatitis) may be a result of infection (with bacteria, viruses or fungi) injury (trauma), often caused by bones, splinters, hooks or needles, burns, caused by corrosive agents or chewing at live electrical

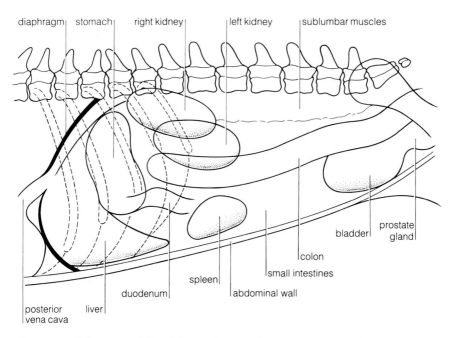

diaphragm | stomach | right kidney | left kidney | sublumbar muscles

posterior vena cava | liver | duodenum | spleen | abdominal wall | small intestines | colon | bladder | prostate gland

Figure 65 Side views of the abdominal cavity (head towards the left) to show the arrangement of organs as seen on a radiograph (i.e., an X-ray film)

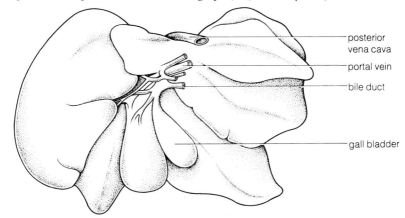

posterior vena cava
portal vein
bile duct
gall bladder

Figure 66 Liver (partially divided into several lobes) and gall bladder

cables or flexes, auto-immune disorders (in which the body produces antibodies against its own tissues) or as a result of generalised disease, especially the uraemia accompanying chronic renal diseases. As well as showing reddening, the structures of the mouth, including tongue, gums, lips, and palate, may show ulcers and/or pinpoint haemorrhages.

The two halves of the hard palate may not fuse during the animal's development, resulting in a *cleft palate*, which allows milk and food taken into the mouth to pass out through the nostrils.

Tumours (growths) may occur in the mouth, as elsewhere, but two types are specific. *Oral papillomatosis* is a condition in which multiple cauliflower-like warts (papillomas) develop, firstly on the tongue or lips, and later spread to the rest of the oral structures. The cause is a viral infection that affects young dogs, particularly around one year of age. The warts regress spontaneously and therefore the extensive excision which would be required to remove them is unnecessary.

Secondly, a *benign oral tumour* affecting the gum can arise from the lining of a tooth cavity. It is termed an *epulis* and may proliferate extensively, resulting in bleeding, ulceration and the loosening of teeth to an extent requiring surgery. It arises from middle age onwards, especially in Boxers.

Teeth

Periodontal disease is the most common dental disease in dogs, affecting *all* animals over five years old. The accumulation of oral bacteria (bacterial plaque) on the teeth, which is encouraged by a soft, sticky diet, is followed by a change in the type of bacteria and then calcification of the plaque, forming calculus (tartar). Initially there is inflammation of the gums (gingivitis) where they meet the teeth, producing on them a bright pink, or red, line. At first the tartar looks like an orange-grey upper rim on the teeth

Figure 67 Extraction of the upper carnassial tooth (fourth premolar)

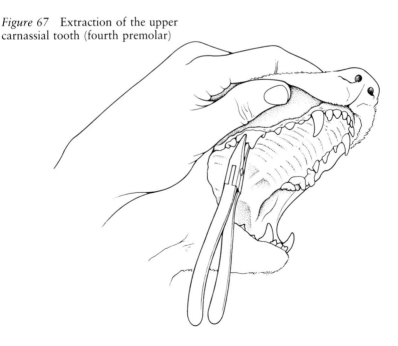

(especially the canines, premolars and molars), but in time large masses accumulate which can eventually completely cover a tooth. With further deposition the inflammation gets worse, the gum swells, the tooth loosens and bacteria may enter the tooth socket and even cause abscess formation (Fig. 67). Dogs with periodontal disease (very common in toy breeds) are depressed, have foul breath (halitosis), salivate more than usual and often experience pain on eating, especially hard foods.

Tartar should be removed at an early stage with a dental scraper or ultrasonic scaler, otherwise teeth may need removal.

A hard diet minimises plaque accumulation, but regular cleaning with a soft nylon toothbrush or even cotton wool (with or without tooth powder, or special toothpaste) is the most effective control method, especially if combined with the use of a chlorhexidine mouthwash.

Other dental disorders

Caries (demineralisation of the tooth enamel), common in man, is unusual in the dog, mostly affecting the first upper molar tooth.

Exposure or infection of the pulp cavity within the tooth may follow periodontal disease or advanced caries or result from fracture of a tooth. The result is a tooth that is painful to chew on, often requiring extraction. This condition (periapical disease) may lead to an abscess, particularly at the roots of the upper fourth premolar tooth (carnassial abscess) which often drains externally, i.e., through an opening on to the skin just below the eye.

Excessive wear may be seen in dogs that regularly chew stones or other hard objects, there may be *retention of the milk teeth* alongside the permanent teeth (requiring their removal) and there may be *defects in the enamel* attributable to damage caused before the teeth erupted (particularly brown-stained irregularities due to early distemper infection, or yellow/ brown staining due to tetracycline therapy). These conditions can all be treated successfully today without resort to extraction if the condition is treated early in its course, although the procedures are often expensive!

Tongue

The tongue can become *lacerated* (e.g., in dogs who lick out tin cans), *stung* by bees or wasps, become slowly and *progressively severed* by a rubber band placed around it (usually by malicious children), or *burned* by chewing electric wires or eating hot food.

Damage to the nerve supply to the tongue can cause it to be *paralysed* so that it hangs from one side of the mouth and is damaged when the animal attempts to eat. Lapping is impossible and the animal requires a deep bowl so that it can learn to suck up water. This ability is learned remarkably rapidly by the majority of animals.

Salivary glands

Inflammation, though painful, is unusual and most often follows trauma, e.g., bite wounds. More common is a *salivary mucocoele*, a cyst-like swelling caused by a collection of mucoid saliva that has leaked from a damaged salivary gland. The most common sites are beneath the tongue on the floor of the mouth (such a structure is termed a ranula) or in the neck below the jaw (termed a cervical mucocoele, or popularly a cervical cyst). The cause may be difficult to establish, but trauma from foreign bodies in the mouth is often suspected. Treatment involves careful dissection and removal of the cyst and the associated salivary gland.

Pharynx

Pharyngitis or inflammation of the pharynx, is less common than in man. It may occur with infectious diseases, follow the swallowing of foreign bodies or irritant chemicals, or result from the irritation of an overlong soft palate in the flat-nosed (brachycephalic) breeds of dog. It can give rise to snorting attacks ('reverse sneezing') due to severe forced inspiration.

The associated *tonsils* are often also inflamed (*tonsillitis*) in these cases, but their removal (tonsillectomy) is usually not advised unless an abscess forms or cancer is suspected. Pharyngitis and tonsillitis cause difficulty in swallowing and in extreme cases may even provoke vomiting.

Oesophagus

Inflammation and tumours of the oesophagus are unusual. Occasionally *foreign bodies* (usually bones) that have been swallowed lodge there and have to be removed, and sometimes the damage they cause results in narrowing (stricture) as healing of the oesophagus, with scar tissue formation, takes place.

Stricture, or narrowing, may also result from pressure from outside the oesophagus (e.g., caused by tumours or abscesses), or, in the region of the heart, from being encircled by a vascular ring. Essentially that problem is caused by the persistence of one or more blood vessels that normally disappear during early embryonic development.

The most common is persistence of the right aortic arch, which 'traps' the oesophagus within an encircling ring of blood vessels. Liquid (e.g., milk) is able to trickle through, but solid food cannot pass, and at the time of weaning persistent regurgitation (i.e., return of the food) begins. Gradually the oesophagus in front of the stricture dilates (i.e., stretches) to accommodate the food, which takes progressively longer to be returned (Fig. 68). Affected puppies are poorly nourished and weak. Surgery is the only effective treatment and should be carried out early to be successful, for once the oesophagus has dilated permanent problems can result.

True vomiting, or emesis, is the return of food from the stomach, but

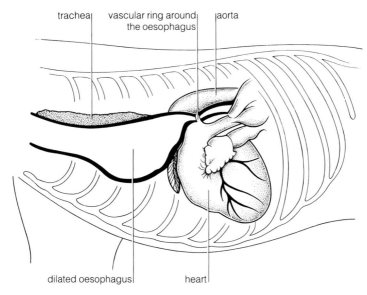

Figure 68 Persistent right aortic arch. Blood vessels encircle the oesophagus above the heart ('vascular ring'), constricting it at that point, and gradually cause a dilatation to develop further forward

the return of food in this case is strictly termed regurgitation, since it has not had a chance to reach the stomach.

Regurgitation of food is also a feature of *cricopharyngeal achalasia* and megaoesophagus. The former condition is unusual and appears to be due to a failure of the cricopharyngeal sphincter (at the entrance to the oesophagus – Fig. 59) to relax during swallowing to permit food to enter the oesophagus from the pharynx. Food is returned immediately, often with gagging and retching.

Megaoesophagus is a more common condition and appears to be inherited (in German Shepherds, Miniature Schnauzers and Great Danes – Fig. 69). It may be present from birth or it may develop in a mature dog that has had no problems as a puppy. One-third of affected puppies spontaneously recover, but mature animals do not do so. Essentially there is a defect in the nerve supply causing a lack of the peristaltic wave which pushes food along. *There is not*, as used to be thought, any difficulty in opening the cardiac sphincter into the stomach. Food comes to rest in that portion of the oesophagus which passes horizontally through the chest above the heart, and it is subsequently regurgitated. With time, the wall of the oesophagus stretches, like a 'perished' rubber hose pipe, so that food is held longer before it is returned. Surgery and drugs have little effect in the long run, and treatment involves feeding small amounts of liquefied food frequently, with the animal standing in as near vertical a position as

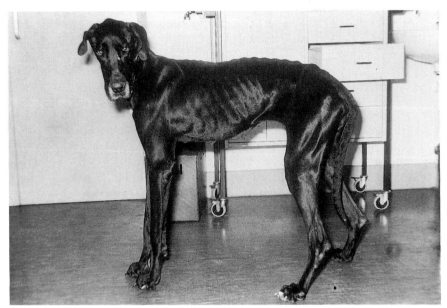

Figure 69 An emaciated young Great Dane, unable to retain solid food because of the presence of a megaoesophagus

possible. To maintain these animals, tremendous commitment is necessary. Feeding on the stairs or actual hand feeding becomes a daily routine.

In all cases of regurgitation (as with persistent vomiting generally), diagnosis is greatly assisted by the use of the X-ray techniques of *radiography* and *fluoroscopy* to observe exactly what happens to material after swallowing. Because food is not being made available for digestion, affected animals, depending on their age, fail to gain weight or will lose weight. A further hazard is that eventually some of the returned food will be inhaled, causing an inhalation pneumonia.

Stomach

Gastritis (inflammation of the stomach) is common in dogs, especially *acute* (short-lived) *gastritis* due to eating contaminated or decomposing food, trash, bones or grass, etc. Vomiting is the principal sign, which if severe may lead to dehydration. Usually withholding food for twenty-four hours, and limiting liquid to small amounts at any one time, allows the problem to resolve itself with little or no therapy, though at times drugs to control vomiting are helpful, as are the modern ionic solutions to replace the sodium, potassium and other ions lost with the vomiting.

In vomiting, which occurs relatively commonly in dogs, the stomach plays a passive role. It is the strenuous action of the abdominal muscles, combined with the negative pressure in the chest, which results in expulsion of the stomach contents. Following a period of nausea with restlessness, salivation, licking of the lips and repeated swallowing, the animal lowers its head and the forceful contraction of the muscles in the abdominal wall presses the abdominal contents against the stomach (which is now relaxed and flaccid), squeezing out its contents.

Chronic (i.e., long-term) *gastritis* is much less common and the cause is often obscure, though a number of causes are recognised. Among these are chronic renal disease, foreign bodies present in the stomach for a long time (such as stones and coins) allergic and immune disorders and cancer.

Examination of the stomach lining (mucosa) is possible today using a flexible fibre-optic endoscope with a light source. This may show the mucosa to be thickened and may reveal the presence of peptic ulcers. These are erosions extending part-way through the stomach wall and showing raised margins. Any of the causes of gastritis may be responsible for ulceration, but also severe stress and a particular type of tumour, the mast cell tumour (mastocytoma), are important causes. In the dog, ulcers are most commonly associated with tumours. Treatment is with drugs to neutralise or limit the formation of gastric acid, or surgical removal of the affected part of the stomach. Immediate surgical intervention is required if the ulcer perforates, i.e., extends completely through the wall, allowing stomach contents to pass into the peritoneal cavity, because this is followed by peritonitis, which could prove fatal.

Failure of the pyloric sphincter, at the exit of the stomach, to open adequately (*pyloric stenosis*) may be a further cause of persistent/ intermittent vomiting and consequent poor nutrition. Surgery is the preferred treatment i.e., a pyloromyotomy is performed, the circular ring of muscle being cut to allow it to open more fully.

Acute gastric dilatation (i.e., rapid enlargement of the stomach) may be due to overeating, especially in young dogs, which often provokes vomiting, but in older animals the cause is not so clear. There is an accumulation of fluid and gas; the latter may be air which animals may gulp in when eating rapidly or, it has been suggested, it may come from the fermentation of carbohydrate foods. The abdomen becomes distended and tense, and gurgling sounds may be heard. In the large, deep-chested breeds of dog the dilatation may result in rotation of the stomach within the abdomen, causing a twisting of the entrance and exit, which prevents the escape of gas into the oesophagus or the duodenum (Fig. 70). Distension interferes with the blood supply causing the onset of shock and the condition may rapidly become fatal. Urgent veterinary attention is necessary to release the trapped gas by passing a stomach tube if possible and/or to return the stomach to its normal position by a surgical operation. In addition it is imperative that the dog is treated for shock.

In an emergency a hypodermic needle or even a sewing needle can be inserted into the stomach through the skin to release the potentially fatal build-up of gas.

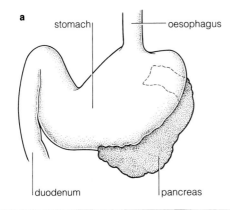
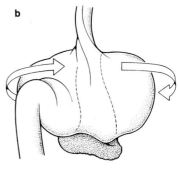

Figure 70 (above)
(a) Normal position of the stomach
(b) Rotation of a dilated stomach effectively closes the oesophagus and duodenum, preventing the escape of gas (so-called *gastric torsion*)

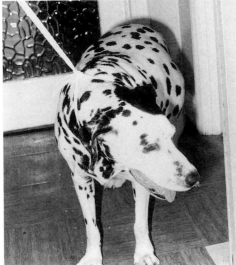

Figure 71 (left) Acute gastric dilatation quickly results in a painful distended abdomen requiring urgent veterinary attention

Small intestine

Enteritis (inflammation of the intestine) usually results in diarrhoea, and when present long-term (i.e., chronic diarrhoea) there will be a loss of weight.

Diarrhoea is a common problem with the pet dog and one for which the veterinarian is frequently consulted. The term *diarrhoea* includes both the excessively frequent passage of motions, and motions that are unusually soft or liquid. It also indicates an increase in volume. Normal dogs pass motions between one and three times a day and the stools are formed, i.e., retain their shape.

So-called *non-specific acute diarrhoea* is common in dogs. It may be due to consuming food heavily contaminated with bacteria, or food containing preformed bacterial toxins or the products of food decomposition (food poisoning). This can be common in animals which scavenge. Such diarrhoea generally last for only a few days before clearing up spontaneously.

Some bacteria are recognised as important causes of acute diarrhoea, e.g., Salmonella and Campylobacter – organisms which can also cause serious enteritis in humans. Other causes are irritant poisons, dietary allergies and viral infections such as canine distemper and parvovirus infection. In the last named condition the diarrhoea is usually preceded by vomiting and is so severe as to cause marked dehydration. The watery faeces frequently contain blood. This is true dysentery. Another condition where vomiting and haemorrhagic diarrhoea (resembling raspberry jam) appear suddenly and animals rapidly become dehydrated is commonly known as *haemorrhagic gastro-enteritis*. The cause is not definitely known, but seems likely to be an allergic response to toxins produced by bacteria in the bowel, probably *E. coli*. Young adult dogs of the small breeds seem most at risk, especially Miniature Dachshunds, Poodles and Schnauzers and also Yorkshire Terriers. Again urgent veterinary attention is required to reverse the very rapid dehydration which accompanies the condition.

A lot of water in the form of digestive juices is added to the food as it passes through the digestive tract, more than two pints for every 25 lb bodyweight (1 litre for every 11 kg), although almost all of this is later reabsorbed. However, if the gut is irritated (by viruses, bacterial toxins, irritant poisons, dietary allergies, etc.) the material may be moved through the intestines so rapidly that much of this water cannot be removed. Usually material takes between five and ten hours to pass completely through the digestive tract, but where there is increased motility this can be reduced to as little as 20 or 30 minutes. Also with increased motility there is insufficient time for bile pigments to be converted to stercobilin (which gives the brown colour to the motions) so that the motions appear yellow-orange.

Chronic diarrhoea If food cannot be properly digested or absorbed it will remain in the intestine and attract water in just the same way as a saline laxative (e.g., Epsom salts) works. The dog will pass soft motions and will remain hungry despite eating more and will gradually lose weight. The residual undigested materials can ferment in the bowel, producing large amounts of gas, which the animal passes. The disorders most often responsible for this situation are *exocrine pancreatic insufficiency* (which is dealt with under the heading of pancreatic disorders) and the various types of *malabsorption*. Sometimes 'flatus' due to fermentation will occur with one particular type of commercial diet and not with another, so it is always worthwhile endeavouring to find a diet which suits your dog and then above all sticking to it unless the dog starts to refuse it. In this way a lot of dietary problems are minimised.

Malabsorption is the failure of the bowel adequately to absorb digested foodstuffs. The causes can be complex. It can be due to long-standing inflammation, where the wall of the bowel is infiltrated by specific types of cells. This occurs, for example, in eosinophilic enteritis and granulomatous enteritis. In some cases poor immunity allows excessive multiplication of bacteria in the small intestine, which interferes with food absorption. This is called bacterial overgrowth. Some animals develop a sensitivity to certain foodstuffs, for example wheat sensitivity in Irish Setters, which then impairs the absorption of all foods. Usually in these disorders an improvement can be obtained with appropriate therapy.

Villus atrophy is a reduction in the height of the villi through which absorption takes place or sometimes their complete absence. When this occurs there is little hope of a beneficial response. Similarly, if the bowel is extensively affected with cancer, commonly lymphosarcoma, not only may absorption be interfered with but there may actually be a loss of protein from the blood through the 'leaky' intestinal wall into the bowel contents.

At times the small intestine may be *obstructed by foreign bodies* that the animal has swallowed, particularly in the region of the jejunum, which is the narrowest part. These can vary from peach stones to pebbles, plastic toys to precious mementoes, and unfortunately some dogs possess this habit more than others. Obstruction can also result from *intussusception*, in which a short (tubular) section of the bowel telescopes into an adjoining section, thereby producing a treble thickness of bowel wall over this length. This at times occurs in puppies and young dogs who have diarrhoea with straining for any reason. Both conditions require prompt surgery, because if either is allowed to persist the animal will rapidly decline. Do not delay in contacting your veterinarian if worried.

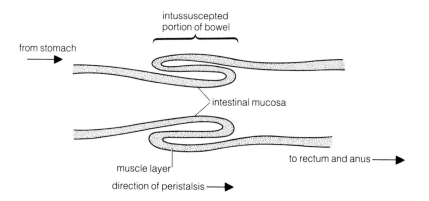

Figure 72   Intussusception of the intestine, which results when a short length of bowel telescopes into the following section, producing thickening and obstruction

Intestinal parasites (see Chapter 23) that may occur in the dog in the UK consist of worms (ascarids [roundworms], hookworms, whipworms and tapeworms) and on occasion the microscopic protozoal parasites known as coccidia. In the main these parasites do *not* produce illness in an infected animal and signs are seen only when large numbers of parasites are involved and the host is either debilitated or very young. All of them live in the small intestine with the exception of the whipworm, which is found in the large intestine, particularly the caecum. This parasite may, rarely, be a cause of colitis.

Rupture of the diaphragm The diaphragm is the muscular partition which separates the abdomen and chest cavities. Tearing or disruption of the partition is known as rupture of the diaphragm. Sometimes this rupture allows loops of bowel or other organs to pass forwards into the chest and this can cause laboured breathing. This is referred to as a *diaphragmatic hernia*. Both it and a diaphragmatic rupture require specialist surgical correction.

A hernia strictly describes the abnormal protrusion of part of an organ through an opening in the structures which normally contain it. Thus there can also be an umbilical hernia, inguinal hernia, or perineal hernia, all of which involve the contents of the abdomen.

Large intestine

Colitis is strictly inflammation of the colon, but usually involves the rectum as well. It can occur in all breeds, and at any age, but it especially affects the Golden Retriever, Rough Collie and Shetland Sheepdog. In many instances it is present from puppyhood. Since the disorder involves the large bowel, i.e., after the digestion and absorption of food has taken place, marked hunger and weight loss are not characteristic features. The loss of the normal ability to reabsorb water means that the motions are liquid, and usually they contain mucus (jelly-like material) and even fresh blood (dysentery).

Motions are passed frequently and with considerable straining. In the early stages signs appear for a time and then abate, only to reappear later, until eventually they are present continuously. The straining often causes owners to confuse this condition with constipation which is the infrequent, or difficult, passage of motions, because here, too, straining is a feature. Of course, in constipation the bowel is not being efficiently emptied, whereas in colitis emptying is complete but inflammation of the nerve endings in the rectum cause the animal to *feel* that it has a full bowel, and therefore it frequently tries to empty it.

True *constipation* is relatively uncommon in the dog, but it may arise from eating hard materials (e.g., bones) which impact in the bowel. Other causes include lack of exercise, debility or loss of the nerve supply, as can occur with 'slipped discs'. Mechanical obstruction can be due to the pressure from a tumour, an enlarged prostate gland or a fracture of the pelvic bone and can result in chronic constipation. Defecation can be painful because of inflammation or wounds around the anus, and the animal may be inhibited from trying to pass a motion. *Foreign bodies* may lodge in the rectum – having successfully passed through the rest of the digestive tract they may turn and lodge in the final segment.

Prolapse of the rectum is protrusion of the lining membrane through the anus, and it can occur in animals that habitually strain to defecate.

Anal sacs and anal abscesses In many dogs the anal sacs fail to empty properly, often because the duct becomes blocked and the secretion accumulates and distends the glands. Pressure on adjacent structures causes discomfort and the animal frequently rubs its rear end, or tries to lick or bite the anus, to relieve the irritation. If present for a long time the secretion may solidify (i.e., become *impacted*) and it may become infected, giving rise to a painful abscess alongside the anus, an *anal abscess*. Many dogs need to have their anal sacs emptied at frequent intervals, and may be subjected to repeated abscesses. If so surgical removal of the anal sacs may be recommended as a permanent solution to the problem.

Tumours of the small glands around the anus (*circumanal adenomas*) are relatively common in old male dogs. These can be successfully treated today, but to prevent recurrence castration is usually necessary.

Peritoneum

Peritonitis is inflammation of the peritoneum. It may be the result of infection, particularly if wounds penetrate the abdominal wall (e.g., deep bite wounds, gunshot wounds, puncture by sharp objects) or if there is perforation or rupture of the bowel, allowing leakage of its contents. This disorder is extremely serious, causing intense abdominal pain and shock, with diarrhoea and vomiting that leads to dehydration. Even when treated promptly it may not be possible to save the patient in every case, but prognosis is much worse if treatment has been delayed.

Pancreas

Apart from the endocrine disorders affecting the secretion of insulin, there are two major disorders of the pancreas, acute pancreatitis and exocrine pancreatic insufficiency.

Acute pancreatitis: this condition often, though not necessarily, follows the eating of a large, fatty meal. In its most severe form it may cause death very rapidly, often because of shock from the severe abdominal pain. Most animals are subject to recurrent attacks of lesser severity referred to as *chronic relapsing pancreatitis*. Several factors are believed to initiate the disorder, including obesity, infection and disturbances of immunity. During an attack dogs show a high body temperature, vomiting and diarrhoea, which is often blood-stained.

To relieve the abdominal pain many adopt a 'praying' position with the hind quarters in the normal standing position but the front legs and head lowered to lie along the ground. During such an attack nothing should be given by mouth because the stimulus of substances in the digestive tract only intensifies the signs; all drugs and fluids should be injected. Early treatment obviously gives a much better chance of survival.

Exocrine pancreatic insufficiency: this condition, common in the German Shepherd Dog, arises when 90 per cent or more of the cells which produce the pancreatic enzymes in the gland have been destroyed or have disappeared. This may be the consequence of repeated or persistent damage to the cells as occurs in chronic pancreatitis or it may, more commonly, follow an inexplicable wasting away (atrophy) of the cells. This latter condition of idiopathic or juvenile atrophy is common in young dogs, usually under one year of age. The animals show poor weight gain or may lose weight, despite a good or even voracious appetite. They often indulge in coprophagia (eating their own faeces) and produce large volumes of faeces having a 'cowpat' consistency that are greasy and foul-smelling. The coat of these poorly nourished animals is usually dry and scurfy.

The condition can be confirmed by carrying out laboratory tests (preferably on the blood), and treatment involves supplying, by mouth, the enzymes of which there is a deficiency, although a major problem is to ensure that the enzymes are not inactivated by acid as they pass through the stomach. These enzyme preparations will be required for the rest of the dog's life.

Liver

Damage to the liver, or interference with its functions, can have many different causes and effects, since the liver plays a role in most of the metabolic processes in the body. The *signs* of liver disease are numerous and include weight loss, vomiting, diarrhoea, depression and excessive thirst. Because of the liver's role in producing factors essential for effective clotting of blood there may be difficulty in controlling haemorrhage. In long-standing cases, accumulation of fluid in the abdominal cavity, ascites (or 'dropsy'), is sometimes seen. Ascites is attributable to two factors. The obstruction to the circulation caused by a damaged liver involves an increase in blood pressure to force blood through the tissue, which at the same time forces fluid out of the blood vessels. There is also a reduced level of protein in the blood plasma due to reduced protein synthesis by the liver. This reduced protein can be insufficient to retain fluid in the circulation by osmotic attraction.

Jaundice is the yellow coloration of the membranes and the skin. It is also a feature of liver disease, although only in the *terminal* stages. It is due to an excess of the yellow-orange bile pigment bilirubin in the blood.

Hepatitis: many liver diseases involve inflammation, i.e., *hepatitis*. When the inflammation is severe and of sudden onset it is described as *acute hepatitis*. This can be due either to infection or to toxic poisonous substances. Infection may be viral in origin, e.g., the virus of infectious canine hepatitis, or bacterial, e.g., leptospirosis.

More common is *chronic active hepatitis*. With this disease the damage and clinical signs are of lesser severity but of longer standing. Again there are a number of causes, including infections and toxins, but immune disorders can also play a part. In Bedlington Terriers and West Highland White Terriers abnormal storage of copper by the liver cells may be the cause.

Chronic hepatitis, which is long-term and progressive inflammation of the liver, can terminate in replacement of functioning liver cells by fibrous tissue. This is scar tissue and the condition is referred to as *cirrhosis*. The loss of more than three-quarters of the cells results in the liver failing to perform its normal functions, a situation which is described as *liver failure*. The liver appears small and shrunken and all of the signs of liver dysfunction noted previously may be present.

Portosystemic shunt is a non-inflammatory disorder which produces similar signs to liver failure due to cirrhosis. This becomes apparent in young animals and is a result of abnormal blood vessel development before birth. It results in the blood in the portal vein (bringing absorbed foodstuffs from the intestine) effectively by-passing the liver, i.e., being 'shunted' straight into the major vein (the posterior vena cava) returning blood to the heart (Fig. 73). In consequence the liver cells are deprived of the necessary nutrients required to synthesise plasma proteins and other substances and so the growth of the animal is hampered. Even more important, ammonia, which is also absorbed from the intestines, remains in high concentration in the blood since it cannot be converted to urea by the liver. This high level of ammonia can affect the brain. This effect is known as hepatic encephalopathy and results in a variety of signs, including vomiting, loss of appetite and mental disturbances, including convulsions. Whether or not surgical correction is possible depends on the precise nature and position of the shunt.

There are other non-inflammatory disorders of the liver. These involve the *abnormal storage* of certain substances, e.g., fat and amyloid, or a failure of the normal mechanisms for storing glucose as glycogen because of a hereditary deficiency of essential enzymes (*glycogen storage diseases*). Undoubtedly the most common non-inflammatory disorder is neoplasia, or *cancer*. Extensive destruction of the functional cells and their replacement by non-functional cancer cells inevitably results in the liver

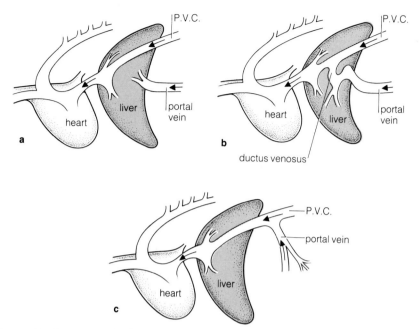

Figure 73 Portosystemic shunts:
(a) *Normally* blood carrying absorbed foodstuffs is delivered to the liver in the portal vein and percolates through the liver tissue (coming into close contact with all the cells) before entering the posterior vena cava (PVC) to be conveyed to the heart
(b) Blood from the portal vein enters an embryonic vessel in the liver (the ductus venosus) which has persisted after birth. The effect is to shunt blood directly into the PVC, which prevents the transported foodstuffs contacting the liver cells. This type of shunt cannot usually be surgically corrected
(c) The portal vein enters the PVC *outside* the liver, again preventing the liver cells having access to foodstuffs. This type of shunt stands a better chance of being successfully treated by surgery

being unable to carry out its normal functions, with the development of all the signs of liver failure mentioned previously.

Gall bladder

Although recorded, the occurrence of *gall stones* (which form in the gall bladder and may block the bile duct) is rare in the dog, as indeed is the occurrence of any gall bladder disorder.

9

HAEMATOLOGY – THE BLOOD

Every cell making up the various tissues of the body needs oxygen and energy in order to carry out its allocated task. It is the function of the blood to act as the transport system, delivering nutrients and oxygen to the tissues and removing the products of metabolism.

The blood is carried round the body through tubes which comprise the circulatory system. It is propelled through these tubes by a muscular pump, the heart, which is situated within the circulatory system and fitted with one-way valves in order to ensure that the blood travels only in one direction.

In the chapter on the Cardiovascular System, Chapter 10, problems which occur when these valves do not close properly (incompentence) or do not open properly (stenosis) will be discussed. The circulation of the blood is simple. Blood rich in oxygen is pumped from the left side of the heart, around the dog's body, and returned with depleted oxygen supplies to the right side of the heart, where it is pumped from the right atrium through the right ventricle and then via the pulmonary artery to the lungs, where it is reoxygenated as it passes through the fine capillaries. It is then returned to the left atrium and passes into the left ventricle, then, via the aorta, continues its journey once more.

In this chapter we are going to look at the main constituents of blood and the problems that occur when things go wrong with them.

WHAT IS BLOOD?

Blood is a fluid connective tissue and comprises approximately 7 per cent of body weight. It is unlike the other tissues of the body in that the matrix is fluid and called plasma, in which special cells are suspended, together with some cell fragments called blood platelets. The cells can be divided into two groups, erythrocytes, the red blood cells (RBCs), and leucocytes, the white blood cells (WBCs) (Fig. 74).

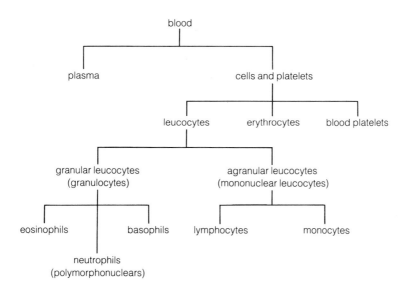

```
                              blood
                                |
        ┌───────────────────────┴───────────────────────┐
      plasma                              cells and platelets
                                                   |
                        ┌──────────────────────────┼──────────────────────────┐
                   leucocytes                  erythrocytes            blood platelets
                        |
        ┌───────────────┴───────────────┐
  granular leucocytes              agranular leucocytes
   (granulocytes)                  (mononuclear leucocytes)
        |                                   |
   ┌────┼────┐                    ┌─────────┴─────────┐
eosinophils   basophils        lymphocytes          monocytes
        |
   neutrophils
(polymorphonuclears)
```

Figure 74   Components of blood

Erythrocytes

In dogs and cats normal adult circulating erythrocytes have no nucleus. They are described as 'biconcave discs' and approximately 7 million are found in every cubic millimetre (mm^3) of blood. In size they are about 1/7,000th of a millimetre (7 nm) in diameter (Fig. 75). Canine erythrocytes have a life span in the circulation of approximately 110–120 days. Their function is to transport oxygen to the tissues and remove carbon dioxide, one of the products of metabolism. They also act as a buffer for hydrogen ions. Aged or damaged erythrocytes are continuously removed from the circulation by the action of cells (macrophages) in the spleen, liver and bone marrow. This is a continuous process and it has been estimated that about 100 million erythrocytes are removed from the circulation every minute in the average-sized dog.

Oxygen is transported by haemoglobin contained within the erythrocytes. Haemoglobin is responsible for their red colour and one of its essential constituents is iron. If the iron in the haemoglobin is depleted the animal will not be able to transport oxygen efficiently. Erythrocyte size is then usually reduced and the animal is said to be suffering from an iron-deficient anaemia (blood shortage).

When erythrocytes are broken down, iron is retrieved and recycled in the production of fresh RBCs. The remaining part of the haemoglobin is converted into bile pigment, which is ultimately excreted by the liver.

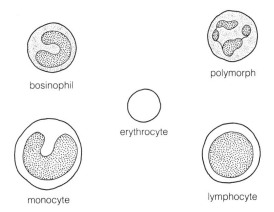

Figure 75 The blood cells

In the healthy animal circulating numbers of RBCs are kept fairly constant despite the continuous breakdown. This is due to the production of new cells at roughly the same rate as breakdown occurs.

Erythropoiesis, the production of red cells, takes place in the bone marrow, although before birth the spleen and liver are also involved. Over a period of approximately four days precursor cells in the bone marrow progress through a series of divisions to form immature erythrocytes lacking a nucleus, known as reticulocytes. These normally remain in the marrow for approximately 48 hours before release into the blood. During this time there is completion of the haemoglobin synthesis and also development of the typical biconcave shape of the mature erythrocyte. Tissue hypoxia, a lack of oxygen to the tissues, is the basic stimulus for erythropoiesis, which is also under the control of a hormone, erythropoietin. This in turn appears to be potentiated by a series of other hormones, including thyroid hormone and growth hormone. When there is a shortage of erythrocytes and concomitant tissue hypoxia the immature form, reticulocytes, can be released into the circulation and can be detected by special staining techniques, which show up the net-like arrangement of the remains of the nucleus within the cell. It is from this (reticulum – a net) that the reticulocyte derives its name.

Leucocytes

Leucocytes (WBCs) are responsible for the body's defence mechanisms. In normal healthy animals numbers can vary from about 6,000 to 18,000 cells per cubic millimetre (mm^3) of blood. They also vary according to the health of the animal.

Unlike RBCs, these cells are colourless. They consist of several cell types that can be divided into two groups, depending on whether or not there are granules visible in the cell body when viewed under the microscope following special staining techniques. Those with granules are called granular leucocytes or granulocytes and the rest are non-granular leucocytes (Fig. 74). According to the way the granulocytes react with special stains, they are further divided into neutrophils, eosinophils and basophils. The nucleus of the granulocyte is divided into lobes or segments connected by filaments, and this is termed polymorphonuclear. This is most marked in the neutrophil, which is the most common of the granulocytes, and this cell type is referred to as the polymorph or polymorphonuclear leucocyte.

Agranular leucocytes are classified into *lymphocytes* and *monocytes* (Fig. 74). The nucleus is not lobed and is very much larger than that found in granulocytes. For this reason granular leucocytes are sometimes collectively known as mononuclear leucocytes. The nuclei of lymphocytes are usually round, whereas monocytes often have kidney bean-shaped nuclei.

An important function of the leucocyte is phagocytosis, the engulfing of bacteria and other unwanted material within the body. With the exception of lymphocytes, all the leucocytes can carry out this function, but it is mainly carried out by the polymorphs outside the blood vessels, which they leave by their active movement between the cells of the blood vessel wall.

The lymphocyte is the second most common WBC in circulating blood. The main function of lymphocytes is concerned with immune response, see Chapter 20 The Canine Immune System.

PRODUCTION OF BLOOD CELLS

Bone marrow is the site of production of all blood cell types, although some lymphocytes are produced in peripheral lymphoid organs. The most primitive bone marrow stem cells have the capacity to form all six types of blood cells and also megakaryocytes, from which platelets are produced (Fig. 76). There is evidence that certain stem cells produce only lymphocytes. Other stem cells produce granulocytes and monocytes. Maturation of these various cell types is under specific hormone influence. In certain disease states the marrow will be selectively stimulated by these hormones to produce the appropriate blood cell type needed to combat the condition.

During maturation of the granulocyte the nucleus undergoes changes. It first becomes 'bandlike' and then forms the mature fully segmented nucleus. As previously mentioned, the function of the granulocyte is phagocytosis, so in the case of an acute infection supplies of granulocytes (polymorphs) will be required by the body quickly and in consequence many band forms may be passed into the circulation. These can be easily identified when examining suitably stained smears under a microscope and

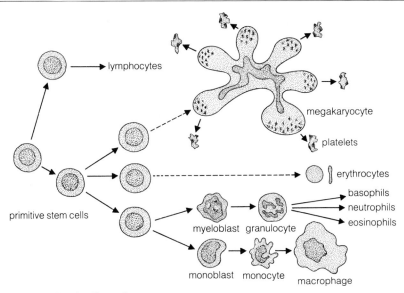

Figure 76   Blood cell production

is often the sign of an acute infection. The presence of these band or 'stab' forms of neutrophils is often referred to as 'a shift to the left'.

Granulocytes circulate in the blood for only a relatively short time (6–12 hours) before entering the tissues. About half of the neutrophils in the circulation are adherent to the walls of the blood vessels and are known as the marginating neutrophil pool, and it is these cells that are the first to pass into the surrounding tissues in order to carry out phagocytosis and so combat infection.

The functions of eosinophils and basophils are not well understood, but eosinophils appear to participate in the destruction of any parasites that migrate through the tissues. Basophils are rich in histamine and may play a part in allergic reactions.

Monocytes, after having been released from the marrow, spend a few hours in the circulation and then enter the tissues, where they mature into macrophages. These are large, mononuclear, highly phagocytic cells which often remain immobile in the tissues until they are stimulated by inflammation. They are important in phagocytosis when viruses and fungal infections are involved. Together with lymphocytes they are also involved in antibody production. They also remove old cells, devitalised tissues and endotoxins.

Lymphocytes can be broadly classified into those involving antibody production (B lymphocytes) or those involved with cell-mediated immunity (T lymphocytes) (see Chapter 20 The Canine Immune System).

Blood platelets are cytoplasmic portions of cells called megakaryocytes and they are involved in the blood clotting mechanism. The undifferentiated bone marrow stem cells form megakaryocytes, which are the giant cells of the bone marrow and have very lobulated nuclei. It is estimated that several thousand platelets are produced from the cytoplasmic fragmentation of each megakaryocyte. Platelets are also called thrombocytes and it is the number of these in the circulation that controls their further production. They usually survive for 10–12 days. At the site of damage to a blood vessel they form a platelet plug and also liberate an enzyme, thromboplastin, which ultimately results in the formation of fibrin from fibrinogen, a protein substance found in normal plasma (Fig. 77).

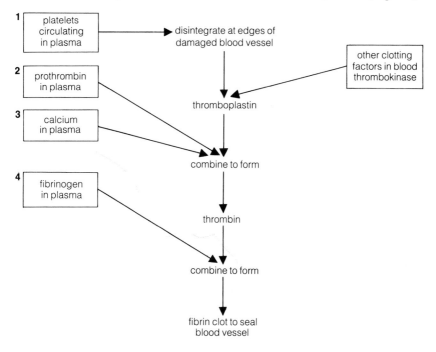

1-4 are some of the clotting factors (12 in all) found in blood

Figure 77 Diagrammatic representation of blood clotting mechanism

Fluid

Plasma is the fluid in which all these cells are suspended. It is a clear slightly yellow fluid with a very complex composition. Over 90 per cent of it is water and it also contains plasma proteins. The most important are albumen, globulin and fibrinogen. They have many functions, one of the most important of which is control of fluid balance within the body.

DISEASE CONDITIONS AFFECTING THE BLOOD

Anaemia

Anaemia is defined as a reduction in the number or volume of erythrocytes or the quantity of haemoglobin in the blood. It can be detected in the laboratory from a blood sample, and the type of anaemia can also be established.

Anaemias can be either regenerative or non-regenerative.

Regenerative anaemia

In this type the bone marrow is responding to the low erythrocyte count. This may be due to either (a) blood loss or (b) increased erythrocyte destruction (haemolytic anaemia). The regenerative response to haemolytic anaemia is usually very much more rapid than the response stimulated by blood loss. This is because there is no iron depletion, since it is being recycled from the broken-down erythrocytes.

Reticulocytes (juvenile erythrocytes) are prominent in the circulation and there may even be a few nucleated red blood cells as well.

Haemolytic anaemia is commonly caused by an auto-immune problem in the dog and is known as auto-immune haemolytic anaemia (AIHA) (see Chapter 20 The Canine Immune System.) This type of anaemia can also be due to other causes, e.g., babeiosis due to a blood parasite not normally found in Britain or haemangiosarcoma, a type of cancer involving the endothelium lining the blood vessels and heart.

Non-regenerative anaemias

Non-regenerative anaemia occurs when the red blood cells are not being replaced in sufficient numbers. This type of anaemia is usually very insidious in onset compared with the regenerative type. Non-regenerative anaemia can be divided into two types dependent upon the results of examination of the bone marrow. if the precursor cells are sparse in number it is said to be *hypoproliferative*, resulting in reduced erythrocytes (reduced erythropoiesis). If the precursors are abundant but red cells sparse the condition is associated with defective erythrocyte production (defective erythropoiesis).

Non-regenerative anaemia can be drug induced, e.g., phenylbutazone or chloramphenicol long term, and can also occur due to renal failure or the increase in circulating oestrogens, as occurs in some cases of testicular tumours or when oestrogens are administered for mismating.

Polycythaemia

Erythrocytosis (polycythaemia) occurs when too many red cells are produced. It can be relative or absolute.

A relative (transient) increase in RBCs occurs in dehydrated animals due to haemoconcentration. Contraction of the spleen just prior to blood sampling can have the same effect. This often occurs in excitable or nervous dogs.

Absolute polycythaemia, i.e., an absolute increase in the number of RBCs, occurs in certain cancers and some congenital heart abnormalities due to shunting of blood which is improperly oxygenated, thereby stimulating the bone marrow to produce more RBCs.

Platelet disorders

These can occur and result in bleeding disorders, which may be due to increased destruction or decreased production of platelets.

Increased destruction occurs with haemorrhage. There may be increased utilisation of platelets, which can occur in diseases such as disseminated intravascular coagulopathy (DIC), whereas decreased production follows the administration of drugs such as oestrogens and phenylbutazone and certain cancer chemotherapeutics, which depress the bone marrow.

Von Willebrand's disease is an hereditary defect of platelets which can lead to bleeding disorders in breeds such as Dobermanns, German Shepherd dogs and others. It results in decrease in platelet adhesion leading to coagulation problems. Other hereditary conditions which involve the clotting mechanism also exist.

Blood transfusions

Dogs, like man, have multiple blood types, but only one is strongly antigenic and can cause problems. Fortunately, naturally occurring antibodies to this blood type are rare. Blood transfusions are becoming an ever increasing part of everyday practice and undoubtedly save the lives of many dogs in an emergency. Many practices today have co-operative owners with donor dogs, usually of the large breeds. These dogs are known to not carry this particular antibody.

Conditions affecting the leucocytes

Neutrophils, as we have seen, are the most common type of leucocyte and an absolute increase is known as a neutrophilia. As explained, some of the neutrophils are marginated, in other words adherent to the walls of the vessels, and anything which causes the release of adrenalin in the body, e.g., struggling during sampling, can cause the release of these marginated neutrophils, resulting in an apparent neutrophilia of the sample. This is 'stress-induced neutrophilia' and is common in the dog. It is usually associated with non-inflammatory disorders, e.g., trauma following a road traffic accident. The administration of corticosteroids can also result in a similar picture.

The most common cause of true neutrophilia is inflammation and this represents a demand, either locally or generally, within the body for neutrophils to phagocytose invading micro-organisms.

The opposite of neutrophilia is neutropenia, a decrease in the number of circulating neutrophils. This is usually the result of a serious disorder and predisposes the animal to infection. Eosinophils are increased in the presence of certain parasites as well as in some allergic disorders. A decrease in eosinophils (eosinopenia) can be involved in the stress reaction. This includes neutrophilia, lymphopenia, monocytosis and eosinopenia and may be the result of release of naturally occurring glucocorticoids. Lymphocyte numbers can be depressed in some forms of stress and this lymphopenia often accompanies a neutrophilia associated with chronic inflammation. An increase in lymphocytes (lymphocytosis) can be associated with autoimmunity and some forms of leukaemia.

Monocytes are increased (monocytosis) with long-term glucocorticoid treatment and chronic inflammatory disorders, especially those associated with necrosis.

Leukaemia

Leukaemia is a progressive, malignant disease of the bone marrow. It is marked by distorted proliferation and development of leucocytes and their precursors in the blood. Leukaemias are divided into two main groups. Cancer involving lymphocytes is *lymphocytic leukaemia*, while that involving the non-lymphoid precursor cell line, i.e., the granulocytes, monocytes, erythrocytes and megakariocytes, is known as *myeloid leukaemia*. Thus with this type of cancer one finds abnormalities in red cells and platelets as well as a leukaemia.

FLUID BALANCE IN THE BODY

Water constitutes approximately two-thirds of the body weight. Young animals have a higher water content (75–80 per cent) than older animals (65–70 per cent).

Two-thirds of the water is contained within the cells (intracellular fluid – ICF) and this is approximately 44 per cent of body weight. The rest is extracellular fluid (ECF) and this is divided into the water within the plasma, which amounts to approximately 25 per cent of the ECF (or approximately 5 per cent of body weight) and so-called interstitial fluid, i.e., that between the cells comprising the tissues of the body. This is approximately 75 per cent of the ECF or approximately 16 per cent of body weight. Interstitial fluid is very similar to plasma except for the absence of the protein constituents. Water can readily pass into or out of the circulation through the capillary walls. The proteins in the plasma have large molecules and do not normally pass out of the circulation. They provide the blood with its so-called 'osmotic gradient', which is the process which pulls water through the capillary membranes from an area of lower concentration to one of higher concentration. This is one of the ways that the water balance of the body is controlled and is the main function of albumen, which is the most common of the plasma proteins. Globulin plays a role in the transport of hormones and in immunity. Fibrinogen, we have already seen, is involved in the clotting mechanism of blood.

Once fibrinogen has been removed from plasma, i.e., the blood has clotted, the remaining fluid is known as serum. Plasma contains many other substances, since blood transports nutrients to the cells and waste products from the cells. Many of the diagnostic aids involving blood tests measure these various biochemical products.

Although the large molecules of plasma proteins are important in maintaining the body's fluid balance, some smaller molecules also play a part. Sodium and potassium are particularly involved in this process and their levels are regulated by the kidneys, which thus play a major role in fluid balance.

The acidity of the blood is also important. This is represented by its pH, which is a measure of the hydrogen ions associated with certain organic acids. If there are too many hydrogen ions the pH drops and the blood is said to be more acidic; if too few, the pH rises and the blood becomes too alkaline. The normal pH is approximately 7.4 units, i.e., slightly alkaline or 'slightly basic'.

The pH of the blood is kept within very narrow limits due to the action of 'buffers', of which bicarbonate is the most important. Bicarbonate has the ability to give up hydrogen ions when the blood becomes alkaline and absorb them when it becomes acid. This can happen, for example, in cases of diarrhoea, when not only is fluid lost from the body but bicarbonate ions are also lost, which in turn can lead to acidosis. Both water balance and so-called acid-base balance are finely orchestrated in the body and not only the blood but also the kidneys, lungs and bowel play vital roles.

CLINICAL HAEMATOLOGY – BLOOD TESTS

In the detection of any disturbances in these finely tuned systems it is to the blood we turn for help in diagnosis, via an ever-increasing number of sophisticated diagnostic tests. This is the field of clinical haematology, 'the blood tests'. With these tests red and white blood cells and platelets can be monitored. Other tests will estimate the degree of dehydration, and following fluid replacement repeat tests will indicate when fluid and mineral deficits have been made good, so avoiding the dangers of over-infusion. These are just a few of the answers that can today be quickly established by the practice laboratory.

Using more specialised techniques many laboratories can measure hormone levels, antibody levels against various diseases and the levels of various inorganic ions, such as calcium, potassium and sodium.

Disorders of fluid and electrolyte balance

Dogs with diarrhoea and/or vomiting, anorexia (lack of appetite) and pyrexia (fever) frequently suffer from fluid depletion as well as depletion of some of the inorganic constituents of the blood. Therefore it is important that these are replaced and this is usually carried out by the administration of fluids, either orally or intravenously via a catheter inserted into a vein. This can be either the jugular vein in the neck or the radial (cephalic) vein in the forearm. In order to assess the severity of dehydration the veterinary surgeon will probably carry out certain tests, particularly those giving an indication of packed cell volume (PCV), haemoglobin concentration (HB) and total plasma protein (TPP). If an intravenous drip is administered the dog will probably be hospitalised in order that efficient monitoring can be carried out together with any further blood tests that may prove necessary. If vomiting is prolonged, large quantities of hydrogen ions are lost and therefore the animal will suffer from alkalosis, thus it is important that a fluid containing adequate chloride and potassium ions is administered. With diarrhoea, bicarbonate ions are lost in great quantity and therefore a metabolic acidosis develops, which has to be corrected with the use of the appropriate fluids containing bicarbonate or similar 'buffer ions'.

Other conditions requiring fluid therapy include gastric torsion and dilation, bowel obstruction, pancreatitis, pyometritis and renal failure. In diabetes mellitus water and electrolyte depletion, together with acidosis, often occur and until these disorders are corrected it will be impossible to stabilise the animal with insulin treatment.

Shock

In shock, cardiac output is depleted and therefore blood flow is such that tissue perfusion becomes inadequate. This results in insufficient oxygen being delivered to the tissues to meet requirements. This can ultimately lead to cell death, but initially micro emboli tend to form, which can block capillaries and cause alteration in clotting mechanism leading to dissemi-nated intravascular coagulation (DIC). It is therefore important that adequate fluid replacement is instituted as soon as possible.

Disseminated intravascular Coagulation (DIC)

This is a life-threatening condition which affects the entire vascular system. The pathological process is triggered by a variety of disease conditions, which are listed in the attached table, and is often the terminal phase of such illnesses.

These diseases cause abnormal activation of the blood-clotting system such that blood clots form spontaneously in the blood vessels. This massive, simultaneous thrombosis uses up the platelets and other clotting factors in the blood. The liver and bone marrow eventually become unable to restore these factors and spontaneous bleeding occurs from the small blood vessels into the tissues.

Clinical signs of DIC relate to the combined effects of thrombosis and haemorrhage. Small clots block the arteries within the kidneys and the lungs, resulting in acute renal failure and respiratory distress. Haemorrhages can be seen in the mucous membranes and the skin. The overall blood loss causes a drop in blood pressure, contributing to a stock syndrome which is often irreversible and results in death.

Table 7

Common initiating causes of DIC

Bacterial infections	Viral diseases
Tumours	Liver disease
Heat stroke	Severe trauma
Shock	Acute pancreatitis
Immune mediated diseases	

Therapy is aimed at treating the shock and kidney failure. Fluid therapy, including blood transfusions, should be given as well as agents to control infection, acidosis and excessive clotting. The prognosis is grave, with few animals surviving even when treated vigorously.

10

THE CARDIOVASCULAR SYSTEM

In mammals, blood is circulated to all areas of the body utilising a pumping mechanism (the heart) and a system of pipes (arteries and veins). Blood carries essential nutrients and oxygen to all tissues and removes waste products of metabolism, such as carbon dioxide. Heart failure leads to inadequate circulation and results in the poor function of all body tissues.

Figure 78   The basic anatomy of the heart showing the four chambers and the two major arteries leaving the ventricles

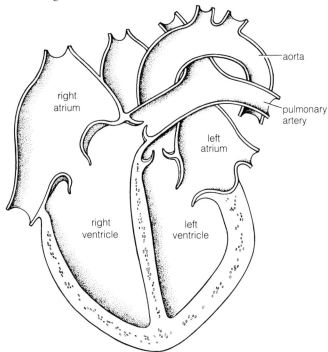

The most notable effects are fatigue due to muscle weakness and kidney failure due to a decrease in renal blood flow.

ANATOMY AND PHYSIOLOGY

The cardiovascular system

The heart is actually two pumps in series: the right side, which pumps blood to the lungs via the pulmonary circulation, and the left side, which supplies blood via the systemic circulation to the rest of the body. Most of the tissue of the heart is muscle; the myocardium. The chambers of the heart are lined by a thin membrane called the endocardium. A similar thin membrane, the epicardium, covers the outer muscle wall. The entire heart is encased in a thick membranous sac, the pericardial sac, to avoid friction and rubbing between the heart and the other thoracic organs as a result of cardiac contractions. The left and right sides of the heart each consist of a collecting chamber, the atrium, and a pumping chamber, the ventricle (see Fig. 78). The atrium has a thin muscular wall to push the blood into the ventricle. The atrial chamber is divided from the ventricular chamber by a fibrous valve called the atrio-ventricular valve. The ventricles have thick muscular walls to pump blood into the pulmonary (right side) or

Figure 79 The thoracic cavity. The head of the animal is to the left of the diagram. A view from the side shows the position of the heart within the thoracic cavity. The cavity is bounded by the spine above and the sternal bones below with the diaphragm separating the chest cavity from the abdomen. The orientation of the chambers of the heart is shown as well as the major blood vessels

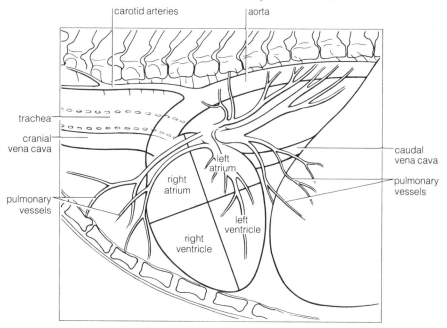

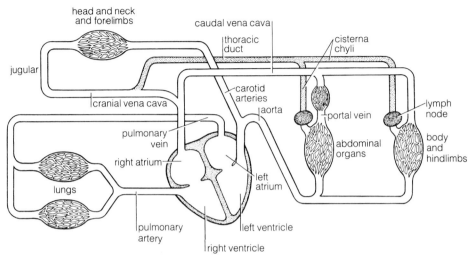

Figure 80 A diagrammatic representation of the circulation. The major blood vessels are shown leaving the heart and branching into capillary beds in various regions of the body. Veins leave these capillary beds to return blood to the heart. The portal vein is shown taking blood from the abdominal capillary bed into another one within the liver, before the blood flows back to the heart via the caudal vena cava. The lymphatic system is demonstrated by lymph nodes draining fluid from the abdominal organs, body and hindlimb areas before the lymph flows into the main blood stream via the cisterna chyli and the thoracic duct to the cranial vena cava

systemic (left side) circulations and maintain adequate blood pressure (see Fig. 79). The main pulmonary artery leaves the right ventricle and then divides to carry blood to the right and left lung lobes. The pulmonic valve prevents backflow of blood from the lungs to the right ventricle. The aorta is the artery which carries blood from the left ventricle to the rest of the body. The fibrous aortic valve prevents reverse flow into the ventricle.

Veins are thin-walled vessels which carry blood to the heart (see Fig. 80). They contain valves to avoid backflow of blood. Arteries carry oxygenated blood away from the heart. These vessels have thick elastic walls to maintain the blood pressure created by the pumping of the ventricles. Arteries terminate in small vessels called capillaries, which infiltrate all tissues and organs of the body. These small vessels then join together again to drain into veins returning the blood to the heart. Capillaries are very thin walled so that nutrients, gases and waste products can be exchanged between the blood and the body cells.

De-oxygenated venous blood flows back to the heart via veins which join to form the anterior vena cava, draining the head, neck and forelegs, and the posterior vena cava, which drains the abdomen and the hindlegs. Venous blood from the systemic circulation flows into the right atrium. It is transferred to the right ventricle, which pumps it around the lungs. Gas exchange takes place in the lungs between the inspired air and blood in the thin-walled capillaries. Carbon dioxide is given off and oxygen is taken up by the red blood cells. The oxygenated blood returns via the pulmonary veins to the left atrium, and thence to the left ventricle which pumps it into the systemic circulation to feed all the tissues (see Fig. 79).

The lymphatic system

The lymphatic system forms an additional mechanism for the return of tissue fluid to the main circulation (see Fig. 80). There is a deficit between absorption and excretion of fluid by the capillaries due to higher pressures (hydrostatic and oncotic) within the vessels than in the tissues. The excess fluid along with protein and lipids from cellular metabolism is channelled via thin-walled lymphatic vessels back into the venous system. Flow through these vessels is effected by the movement of adjacent organs and muscles and a series of one-way valves. The lymph is filtered through lymph nodes (lymph glands) before joining larger vessels, the cisterna chyli in the abdomen and the thoracic duct in the chest, which drain via the jugular veins or vena cavae into the right atrium (see Fig. 79).

Lymph nodes filter out foreign proteins for recognition by the immune system (see Fig. 81). Other lymphoid tissue in the spleen, thymus and bone

Figure 81 The position of the major lymph nodes of the dog are shown. The submandibular, parotid, prescapular, axillary, superficial inguinal and popliteal can be felt through the skin. The others may be palpated or seen on X-rays only when they are enlarged

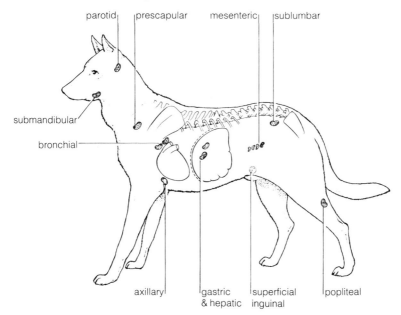

parotid   prescapular   mesenteric   sublumbar

submandibular

bronchial

axillary   gastric & hepatic   superficial inguinal   popliteal

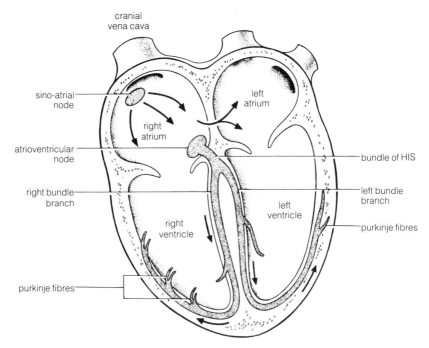

Figure 82 The conduction system of the heart. The specialized tissues of the heart are shown, which conduct electrical impulses through the heart to ensure co-ordinated muscular contraction

marrow is also involved in the initiation of immune responses. The spleen is a reddish, tongue-shaped organ which lies alongside the stomach in the abdomen. Red blood cells may be produced and stored in the spleen. The white blood cells (lymphocytes and monocytes) are also produced here. In addition the spleen is responsible for the breakdown of aged red blood cells and the recycling of their components. Bone marrow produces and stores both red and all of the white blood cell series. The thymus is a grey-white solid organ which lies in the left side of the chest in front of the heart. The thymus increases in size up to adulthood, but regresses thereafter and becomes less active. A significant proportion of the body's lymphocytes are produced in the thymus.

Lymphatic vessels are particularly well developed in the lining of the intestine. At this site they are often referred to as lacteals, and absorb most of the lipids from the gut. This fat content of lymph gives it a milky white appearance to the naked eye. There are no lymphatic vessels in the brain, spinal cord, bone marrow or muscle bellies.

Function of the cardiovascular system

The volume of blood pumped by the heart in any one minute (cardiac output) can be altered to meet the body's demands.

Cardiac Output = Heart Rate × Stroke Volume

Thus an increase in heart rate will lead to an increase in cardiac output. There are sensory receptors in the kidneys and the major arteries which alert the brain to changes in blood flow and oxygen levels. If these fall below normal, compensatory mechanisms are activated to make up the deficit. The heart rate can be increased or decreased according to the body's requirements. Thus heart rate goes up during exercise, but will drop markedly during rest or sleep. The regular contraction or rhythm of the heart is maintained by specialised cells within the heart muscle (see Fig. 82). These cells form a framework along which electrical impulses are conducted to activate the muscle fibres to contract. The electrical impulse starts in pacemaker cells (the sino-atrial node) in the right atrium, which spontaneously maintain a regular heart rate. The impulse then travels over the whole of the right and left atrial muscle to cause contractions which force blood into the ventricles. The impulse is slightly delayed at the junction between the atria and the ventricles, in the atrio-ventricular node, to allow time for atrial contraction before passing to the ventricles. Then special fibres, called Purkinje fibres, carry the impulse to all parts of the ventricular muscle to produce a co-ordinated contraction, which empties the chamber. The pattern of these electrical changes within the heart can be recorded by placing sensitive electrodes at points on the surface of the body. The recorded pattern is called an electrocardiogram (ECG) (Fig. 83). Abnormal changes in the ECG may be seen in some diseases of the heart. Large breed dogs which frequently suffer from cardiomyopathy often have

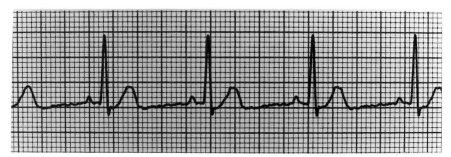

Figure 83 An example of a normal electrocardiogram trace

concurrent atrial fibrillation, which can be recognised as a characteristic irregularity of the ECG (see Fig. 84).

The stroke volume is the volume of blood leaving the ventricle with each heart beat. It can be altered in two ways. Either the volume of blood entering the ventricle during the relaxation phase of the cardiac cycle can be increased by greater relaxation of the ventricular muscle, i.e., increased

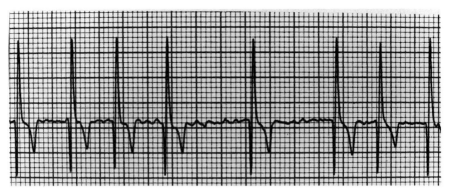

Figure 84   An ECG from a dog with atrial fibrillation. The small (P) waves at the start of the cycle are absent and replaced by many irregular small fibrillation waves

ventricular filling, or the amount of blood expelled by the ventricle can also be increased by an increased force of muscular contraction.

Heart failure results from pathological conditions that affect the normal compensatory mechanisms controlling heart rate and stroke volume.

PATHOPHYSIOLOGY OF HEART FAILURE

When the heart fails to pump sufficient blood around the body, compensatory mechanisms try to correct this imbalance. The most notable feature of heart failure is conservation of fluid by the kidneys. This increases the volume of circulating blood in an effort to maintain blood pressure and tissue perfusion. However, this increase in blood volume creates more strain on the myocardium, which becomes progressively weaker and inefficient. As a result of the sluggish blood flow, fluid tends to seep out of the thin-walled capillaries into the tissues. The lymphatics initially drain this excess fluid, but soon become overloaded so that fluid accumulates in the tissues. This produces the cardinal signs of congestive heart failure. Generally one ventricle fails sooner than the other, and in the dog, left-sided failure is most common.

As the left ventricle fails to move blood into the systemic circulation, the blood dams back into the left atrium and hence into the lungs. This increases blood pressure in the lungs and causes fluid to seep out of the capillaries into the lung tissues and air spaces. This fluid in the lungs causes coughing and breathing difficulties. When the right ventricle fails it is unable to clear the blood from the systemic circulation, which consequently becomes congested, and accumulations of fluid occur in the abdomen or the chest cavity, interfering with the function of the organs in these areas. The abdomen may become quite enlarged due to this free fluid, called ascites. The blood vessels, especially the thin-walled veins, become distended and seepage of fluid may even cause swellings of the limbs in severe cases.

HEART SOUNDS

Combinations of muscle contractions and movement of blood associated with the opening and closing of the valves within the heart result in sound waves which are audible with a stethoscope, at the external surface of the chest wall (see Fig. 85). During each cycle of cardiac contraction in the dog two sounds are normally heard: lubb-dup. The first sound, lubb, is heard when the ventricles have been filled by contraction of the atria and the atrio-ventricular valves between the chambers close. The ventricles then contract and the blood is emptied out into the aorta (left side) or pulmonary artery (right side). At the end of ventricular contraction the aortic and pulmonary valves close and this, together with the slowing up of the blood flow, results in the second heart sound, dup.

Figure 85 Auscultation of a dog's heart using a stethoscope

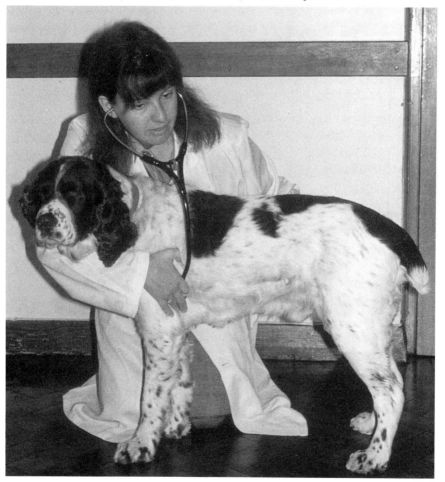

Murmurs are abnormal heart sounds caused when the usual pattern of blood flow is disturbed, resulting in turbulence. Back flow of blood through diseased valves which do not close properly leads to most murmurs heard in dogs. In addition, congenital heart defects can result in abnormal communications between heart chambers or major blood vessels. The consequential turbulent blood flow causes murmurs.

THE INVESTIGATION OF PATIENTS WITH HEART DISEASE

An accurate history detailing the type of difficulties which the dog has experienced is very useful to indicate how the investigation should progress. A dog which has become suddenly ill with severe exercise and breathing difficulties may require urgent supportive treatment before detailed diagnostic tests can be undertaken. In contrast, a dog in which a murmur has been detected without any related clinical problems should be very carefully evaluated to assess whether in fact any treatment is necessary at all.

The age and breed of the dog can be helpful indications of the type of heart disease from which it might be suffering. Animals less than three years of age are more likely to have congenital deformities, and certain

Figure 86 A lateral (or side view) radiograph of the thoracic cavity of a normal dog. See figure 79 to clarify the anatomy

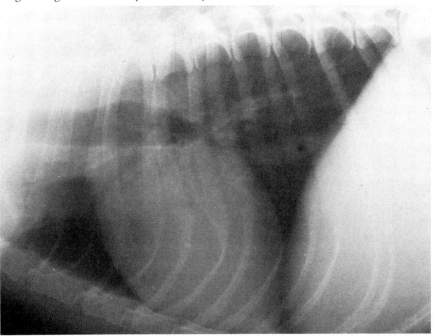

defects are known to have a genetic inheritance in some breeds. Some acquired heart diseases are more common in certain breeds. The lifestyle of the dog may also influence a clinician's decision with regard to the investigations and treatment required. The considerations may be quite different for an athletic dog from which peak performance is expected compared with a companion dog.

A careful clinical examination is undertaken to evaluate all body systems and then special note is made of signs relating to heart function. The nature and rate of the pulse is noted in conjunction with careful assessment of the heart sounds by listening at all points over the chest wall. In addition the colour of the mucous membranes of the mouth are noted and the character of the breathing is recorded. Possible signs of heart failure are assessed, i.e., distension of body surface veins, congestion of the lungs and swelling of the abdomen due to fluid accumulation.

Radiographs of the chest can be very helpful in the assessment of patients in heart failure (see Fig. 86). The heart size can be evaluated to give an indication of the severity of the problem, and the shape of the heart can imply which of the chambers or blood vessels are predominantly involved (see Fig. 87). Finally the lung fields may show varying degrees of congestion, indicating the severity of any left-sided failure.

Figure 87 A lateral thoracic radiograph of a dog with enlargement of both the right and left ventricles. See figures 79 and 86

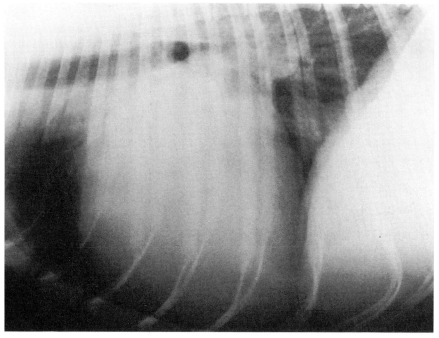

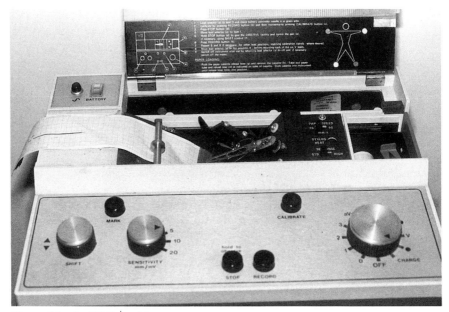

Figure 88   An ECG machine

When any irregularity of the rhythm of the heart beat is detected on clinical examination, an ECG recording is required to define the abnormal rhythm. An ECG machine records electrical impulses generated by the contraction of the heart muscle (see Fig. 88–90). For this examination the dog is usually restrained in a standing or lying position and electrodes are attached to all four limbs, and sometimes to the side of the chest (Fig. 89). A jelly is applied to facilitate electrical conduction between the dog and the electrodes. The equipment merely records electrical impulses from the dog. The animal does not experience any unpleasant sensations.

In some cases it is possible to apply the electrodes and place the recording equipment in a carrying pack for the dog, so that long-term recordings over 24 hours or more can be made. These recordings can be useful in those dogs which collapse only intermittently with an abnormal heart rhythm.

Ultrasound examinations are becoming increasingly available for evaluation of canine patients. Very high frequency sound waves are emitted by a transducer placed on the body wall. Echoes reflected back from structures within the body are picked up by the same transducer and converted to various visual patterns by a computer. These pictures are usually displayed on a television monitor during the examination and may be recorded on graph paper, photographic film or video tapes. The pictures can show either a linear patern of heart motion recorded with time (M-mode ultrasound) or a two-dimensional picture of cardiac anatomy with

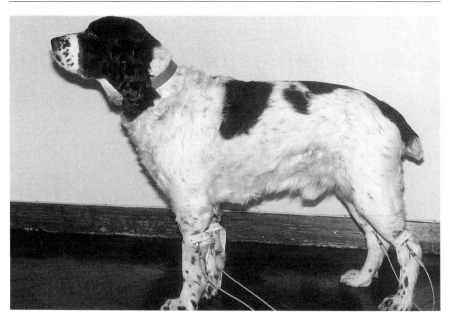

Figure 89 The ECG leads attached to a dog in the standing position

movements (real time or two-dimensional ultrasound). The actual anatomy of the heart may be evaluated to demonstrate any muscular or valvular defects and accurate measurements of heart size can be made. Doppler ultrasound is a further refinement, which enables determinations of blood flow, blood pressure and cardiac output to be made.

There is no discomfort for the animal during these examinations, although areas of hair may have to be clipped off and coupling jelly applied between the transducer and the chest wall. Ultrasound recording equipment is very expensive, so these studies are usually only undertaken at specialist veterinary centres.

All the methods of examination discussed so far are called non-invasive methods because they cause no discomfort or potential danger to the patient. More invasive methods are sometimes justified: blood samples can be used to examine the cells and other substances; blood gas levels of oxygen and carbon dioxide can be helpful in determining heart and lung function. Tests can also be made to evaluate the function of other organs, such as the liver and kidneys. In addition, some tests can indicate the severity of damage to the cells of body organs, including the heart.

Under general anaesthesia catheters can be passed into the heart chambers to record blood pressures and dyes can be injected to highlight cardiac structures on radiographs (angiography) (see Fig. 91). The catheters can be passed via the jugular veins in the neck into the anterior vena cava and thence into the right side of the heart. To catheterise the

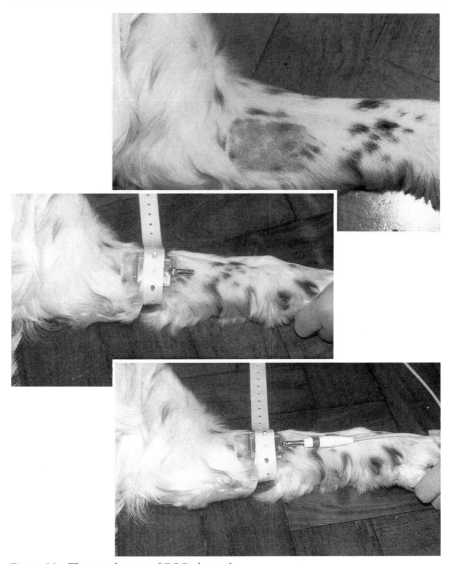

Figure 90   The attachment of ECG electrodes
(a) Hair clipped from the leg for good electrical contact
(b) The electrode coated with jelly strapped to the leg
(c) The lead to the ECG machine connected to the electrode

left side of the heart, catheters are passed into the aorta either via the carotid artery in the neck or the femoral artery on the inside of the hind leg. Angiography carries some risk and is only justified if the results are likely to indicate a better form of treatment than could be determined without this information.

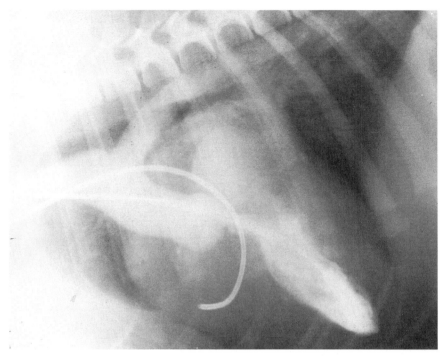

Figure 91 A lateral thoracic radiograph of a dog showing an angiogram achieved by injecting dye through a catheter via the femoral artery and aorta to the left ventricle. The dye outlines in white the aorta leaving the left ventricle and shows abnormal narrowing at the level of the arrow (aortic stenosis)

PRINCIPLES OF TREATMENT OF HEART DISEASE IN THE DOG

The major effect of heart failure is the congestive accumulation of fluid in the body tissues. Diuretic drugs which increase water loss via the kidneys form the mainstay of therapy in removing excess tissue fluid. In addition to diuretics, other drugs are available to relieve the respiratory signs of heart failure. These include bronchodilators and cough suppressants. More recently, vasodilator drugs, which cause relaxation of the arterial and venous walls, have been used to increase the volume of the circulatory system and relieve congestion. This dilation of the circulatory system helps to reduce the effort required by the heart to pump blood around. Exercise should also be reduced to decrease the workload placed on the heart. In addition, it is useful to decrease the amount of salt (sodium chloride) in the diet as the level of salt in the tissues influences the amount of water which can be held in the body.

In cases where the muscular contraction of the heart is weak, drugs can be given to increase the force of contraction. The most commonly used drugs in this group are the digitalis compounds. Abnormalities of heart rhythm can be controlled by drugs chosen from a large group of compounds known as anti-dysrhythmics. Such drugs can increase or decrease the heart rate, or regulate abnormal impulses arising from the conduction system or the heart muscle itself. Severe cases of rhythm disturbance that do not respond to drug therapy are best treated by the implantation of an artificial pacemaker to regulate the heartbeat. Some congenital heart conditions can be alleviated by surgery.

Common congenital heart defects in the dog

Patent ductus arteriosus

In the foetus the ductus arteriosus is a direct connection between the main pulmonary artery and the aorta so that the majority of the circulating blood bypasses the non-functional lungs. This vessel normally closes after birth, but if it fails to do so, some blood is pumped directly from the aorta back into the lungs. This results in pressure overload leading to left-sided failure. This condition is known to have a genetic inheritance in the Miniature Poodle. It is possible to close the vessel off surgically and so correct the flow of blood.

Septal defects

A defect may remain in the wall separating either the left from the right ventricle or the left from the right atrium – the so-called 'hole in the heart'. Blood then flows from the high-pressure left side to the lower-pressure right chamber and results in right-sided heart failure. Ventricular defects more commonly result in failure signs than atrial defects.

Pulmonic stenosis

In this condition there is an abnormal narrowing of the main pulmonary artery as it leaves the right ventricle. This means that the right ventricle has to work harder to pump blood into the lungs and eventually it fails. The signs are of right-sided congestive failure. This condition is genetically inherited in the Beagle. Several different methods of surgically enlarging the defect are now available for dogs, with encouraging rates of success.

Aortic stenosis

The abnormality in this condition is a narrowing of the aorta as it leaves the left ventricle; thus the ventricle has to increase its work to pump blood around the body (see Fig. 91). The consequent inability of the heart to maintain systemic blood pressure may lead to fainting, which is sometimes fatal. Signs of left-sided heart failure may also be noted. No surgical treatments are available for the dog and drug therapy provides only temporary respite. This is a genetic defect in the Newfoundland breed.

Dysplasia of atrio-ventricular valves

Deformities of either the right- or left-sided valves between the atrium and the ventricle can occur. These valves are incompetent, allowing blood to flow back into the atria when the heart contracts. Right- or left-sided failure respectively will result. The only available treatment is supportive drug therapy.

Tetralogy of Fallot

This is a complex deformity of the heart which so severely compromises function that it is usually fatal by six months of age. There is a ventricular septal defect as well as pulmonic stenosis. The aorta is displaced so that both the right and left ventricles pump blood into it and the right ventricular muscle becomes overdeveloped. This condition has been shown to be genetically inherited in the Keeshond.

Acquired heart disease in the dog

Cardiomyopathy

This condition affects the myocardium itself. Two types of cardiomyopathy are recognised in the dog, both of which may arise spontaneously without specific cause. In the hypertrophic form, the ventricular muscle becomes excessively thickened. The space within the ventricle for the blood to fill is thus reduced. This decreases the stroke volume, and hence the cardiac output. Signs related to low blood pressure such as weakness and fainting may be noted and ultimately left-sided congestive heart failure results. This condition has been particularly noted in Cocker Spaniels.

The second type is dilated cardiomyopathy. The heart chambers become enlarged, but the muscle walls become thin and too weak to pump the extra blood volume. These changes lead to left-sided failure, often with right-sided failure too. In large breed dogs such as Great Danes and Irish Wolfhounds, the dilation of the left atrium frequently leads to the rhythm abnormality of atrial fibrillation (see Fig. 84). Apart from the spontaneous or idiopathic form, dilated cardiomyopathy may have other causes, such as bacterial infections, secondary tumours, toxins, metabolic diseases or viral infections, e.g., parvovirus.

Both types of cardiomyopathy are progressive diseases which may be alleviated by drug therapy, principally digitalis compounds, anti-dysrhythmics and diuretics. The disease is invariably fatal, often within six months of the diagnosis being made.

Endocardiosis

This is a degenerative condition affecting the valves of the heart. The deterioration tends to be progressive with increasing age. The atrioventricular valves are most frequently involved and become deformed, with resultant incompetence. Both right and left sides of the heart become involved (see Fig. 87). Blood then flows back through the valves into the atria when the heart contracts and congestive failure results. Small breed dogs such as Miniature Poodles and Cavalier King Charles Spaniels are most commonly affected. Drug therapy using diuretics, vasodilators and bronchodilators enables most dogs to live for some years after the initial onset of the disease.

Pericardial disease

Fluid may accumulate in the pericardial sac around the heart. Pressure builds up and presses on the chambers, decreasing the amount of blood which can enter and hence decreasing the stroke volume. The fluid may be drained off to relieve the condition. This also permits analysis of the fluid to establish the cause of the problem. There are two major types of pericardial fluid accumulation in the dog. In young, large breed dogs such as St. Bernards and Labradors there is no known cause of the blood-stained fluid: the so-called idiopathic pericardial haemorrhage. Some cases are fatal, whilst others may recover completely after one or two drainage procedures. In older dogs the cause is often due to a tumour of the right atrium. Since such tumours cannot be treated, these cases are ultimately fatal.

Cor pulmonale

This is a condition of right-sided enlargement and resultant right-sided congestive failure. It occurs when diseases of the lungs create increased resistance to the pumping of blood by the right ventricle via the pulmonary arteries. Chronic airway diseases are usually associated with cor pulmonale. This condition is often seen in small breed dogs such as Yorkshire Terriers, West Highland White Terriers and Chihuahuas. Treatment is aimed at relieving the primary lung disease with drugs such as antibiotics, bronchodilators and cough suppressants.

Disorders affecting blood vessels

Porto-systemic shunts

The portal vein takes venous blood from the intestines to the capillary bed of the liver (see Fig. 80). Here the blood percolates so that the newly absorbed nutrients can be utilised by the hepatic cells. In addition, any toxic substances which have been absorbed can be detoxified and excreted either via the bile or in urine after the blood has been filtered by the kidneys.

Congenital abnormalities of the portal vein may occur such that it joins the posterior vena cava directly without dispersing the blood through the liver capillary bed. The consequent inadequate utilisation of nutrients causes poor body condition. In addition the products which have not been detoxified, principally ammonia, can affect the brain and result in over excitability or comatose-like depression. The symptoms become evident in young animals, usually less than one year of age.

Surgical correction can be achieved where there is a single anomalous vessel. Radiography following injections of dye during surgery are required to outline the abnormality. Where surgical correction is not possible the diet may be controlled to avoid excessive build-up of ammonia. A low-protein diet is advocated.

Miscellaneous

These conditions are rare in the dog:

Arterial thrombosis, often affecting one hind leg and causing lameness, has been noted in bowel disorders which result in very low blood protein levels, e.g., lymphangiectasia of the gut wall. Arterial thrombosis associated with atherosclerotic disease of the blood vessel wall is the most common form of thrombosis in man and is the major cause of heart attacks due to myocardial ischaemia. A few cases of atherosclerosis have recently been reported in dogs, often associated with inadequate thyroid gland function.

Arterio-venous fistulas are direct connections from arteries to veins without an intervening capillary bed. A patent ductus arteriosus is one such example. Others may be congenital or acquired. Cases have been reported affecting the arteries and veins running down the edge of a rib, or in limb vessels following trauma. A 'thrill' or vibration can be felt over the affected vessel and a hum or murmur can be heard. The direct connection causes high blood pressure in the venous circulation and can lead to right-sided heart failure. Surgical correction is often possible.

Hypertension (high blood pressure) has recently been recognised in the dog. The symptoms relate to renal failure and detachment of the retina, such as may be seen in severe, untreated cases in man. In common with the majority of cases in man the cause of the hypertension is unknown. Anti-hypertensive drugs can decrease the severity of the symptoms.

Disorders affecting the lymphatic system

Hypoplasia of lymph nodes

There are several situations where the lymph nodes may become hypoplastic or small. This decrease in size is associated with poor function, in particular with respect to their main role of priming the immune system to protect the body from foreign invasion. Thus animals with hypoplastic lymphoid tissue are more prone to infections.

Congenital hypoplasia has been described in some species, but is not documented in the dog. The condition is most commonly acquired secondarily to other diseases which deplete the immune response, such as prolonged illnesses, severe protein deficiency or tumours (e.g., lymphoma, multiple myeloma). Immunosuppression by anti-cancer drugs, radiation therapy or adreno-cortical steroids may also result in lymphoid hypoplasia.

Hyperplasia of lymph nodes

Enlarged, overactive lymph nodes are found secondarily to other diseases. Other lymphoid tissue in the spleen, liver and bone marrow is frequently affected at the same time. Bacterial and viral infections as well as protozoal infections such as toxoplasmosis result in hyperplastic lymph nodes. In addition, solid tumours of lymphoid tissue or leukaemias may have a similar effect.

Lymphangiectasia

This term describes the dilation of lymphatic vessels due to obstruction to the flow of lymph. This may arise due to a congenital lack of sufficient vessels to drain an area effectively. This can be seen as swelling of one or more limbs in puppies. Alternatively there may be insufficient lacteals in the intestine, resulting in oedema in the gut wall and poor absorption of nutrients, especially proteins and fats. Affected animals are in poor bodily condition and frequently have diarrhoea due to abnormally high levels of protein and fat reaching the colon.

Lymphangiectasia may also cause similar syndromes due to acquired vessel damage. Traumatic injuries and resultant scar tissue may lead to physical obstruction of lymphatics. Inflammatory disorders of the bowel wall can result in overloading of the lacteals and may result in permanent scar tissue and obstruction.

Chylothorax

Conditions which cause obstruction to the anterior vena cava or thoracic duct result in lymphangiectasia within the thorax and suppuration of lymphatic fluid (chyle) in the pleural cavity. This accumulation of chyle in the space between the lungs and the thoracic wall is known as chylothorax. The condition may be caused by tumours in the chest which press on the vascular structures or by vein thrombosis. Chest trauma as in road traffic accidents may cause rupture of the thoracic duct or scar tissue, which later obstructs lymphatic flow. It is speculated that right-sided heart failure could result in chylothorax due to effective obstruction of anterior vena cava flow. This has been seen in cats, but remains unproven in the dog.

Afghan Hounds have been shown to develop chylothorax more frequently than other breeds, suggesting a hereditary predisposition to the condition in this breed.

Dogs with chylothorax experience difficulty in breathing and lose weight. The accumulation of fluid in the chest cavity compresses the lungs and thus decreases their capacity for oxygen absorption. Obstruction to chyle entering the main circulation affects the availability of protein and lipids for cellular metabolism. Weight loss is a consequence of this.

Radiographs readily show the accumulation of free fluid in the thoracic cavity. A sample of the fluid should be collected for laboratory diagnosis to confirm that it is chyle. An ultrasound examination could be useful to demonstrate any tumours.

At present, surgical treatments for this condition in the dog carry approximately a 40 per cent success rate. Medical management consists of efforts to maintain adequate nutrition and to treat any known underlying causes. Drainage of the chest is necessary for animals in severe respiratory distress, and this may need to be repeated periodically during medical managment. Overall the prognosis for this condition is guarded.

CONCLUSION

This chapter has described the basic anatomy and function of the heart and the related vasculature, as well as the lymphatic system. The commonly available methods of investigation of heart disease in the dog have been outlined together with brief mention of the types of treatment which may be employed. The more frequently encountered congenital and acquired conditions were discussed with reference to the foregoing sections to enable the reader to understand the cause of the disease and its likely management.

11

THE REPRODUCTIVE SYSTEM

In general, dogs appear to be relatively fertile, with about 80 per cent of bitches that are mated producing puppies. However, fertility problems do occur in both individual animals and in kennels, and these can be very frustrating when they affect dogs or bitches which have excelled in the show-ring or elsewhere.

Contrary to popular belief, infections do not play a large role in infertility in dogs in the UK although in many cases it is not clear why some bitches fail to conceive.

Pet owners also have to cope with their pets' sexual problems, and these are usually different from those which affect breeding dogs. It would perhaps be more accurate to say that pet owners are sometimes inconvenienced by their pets' instinctive sexual behaviour, i.e., this is not a problem for the dog. The matters that concern the pet owner and professional breeder stem from the same basic physiological processes, and cannot easily be separated for the convenience of the reader. I can only hope that those looking for information on a specific topic can pick it out without too much difficulty.

Before launching into the complexities of the subject, it is worth mentioning the basic anatomical difference between male and female puppies. Occasionally people new to pet ownership find, to their embarrassment, that they either have to change their pet's name, or face the prospect of forever having to explain to friends why they call their male dog 'Felicity'. The common mistake is to think a bitch puppy is a dog. This is because the bitch's vulva is some distance from the anus, and may be just between the back of the thighs. In male dogs, however, the opening of the prepuce is at the front of the thighs. The dog has a bone in his penis and should have two testicles, which help to clinch the diagnosis.

A rare condition is intersexuality or hermaphroditism. In this case dogs have elements of both sexes, but as puppies they look like either normal females (commonly) or males and their problems do not become apparent until they reach puberty.

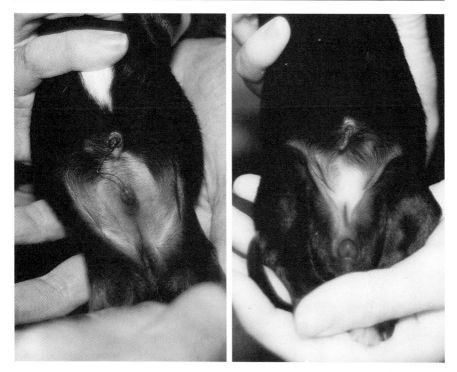

Figure 92 Sexing puppies is no problem when they are seen together (male – left; female – right)

The male genital organs

In order for a male dog to be fertile he has to be able to produce normal sperms (spermatozoa) and be capable of depositing these in the vagina of a bitch. The factors which govern these processes are complex and not completely understood, although our basic knowledge does in many cases help us to explain why faults sometimes occur.

SPERM PRODUCTION (spermatogenesis)

Sperms are produced in the dog's testes (testicles) and this process is continuous, usually proceeding uninterrupted from puberty to old age or death. During sperm production the number of chromosomes in each cell is halved so that when fertilisation (the fusion of a sperm and an egg) occurs the normal number of chromosomes (78) is restored. Many millions of sperms are produced each day and there is some controversy over the fate of those that are not ejaculated; however, they do not accumulate in the testes or its emptying ducts to produce an 'infertile' ejaculate. Sperms are roughly tadpole shaped and are propelled in a rotating manner by their

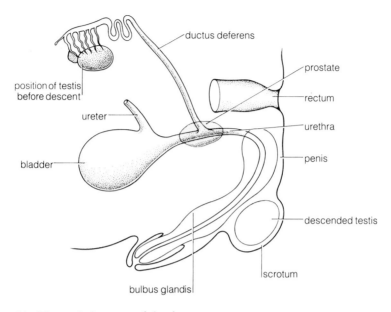

Figure 93   The genital system of the dog

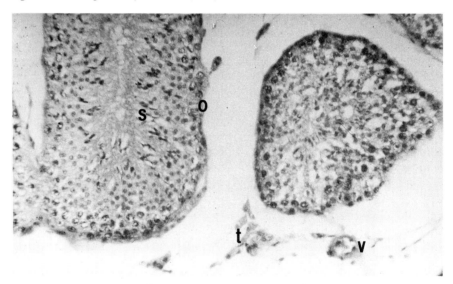

Figure 94   Cross-section of dog's testis. This shows two of the tubules in which sperm are produced. Cells on the outside (o) of the tubule divide and move to the centre, where they change into sperms (s). The heads of the sperms are the dense black structures. Between the tubules are cells (t) that produce the male hormone testosterone. There is also a small blood vessel (v). The empty spaces between the tubules are artefacts which occur during preparation of the tissues

tails. Some of the factors which affect sperm production are known, particularly the influence of temperature. Sperm production cannot proceed at body temperature. The testes are therefore housed in the scrotum, which is a little cooler than the rest of the body. The temperature of the testes is governed by two delicate mechanisms. Firstly, the artery which supplies blood to the testis from the body is surrounded by a complex of veins which are returning blood from the testes to the larger veins of the abdomen and thence to the heart; the warm arterial blood is in this way cooled by the venous blood which is returning after having percolated through the testes. Secondly, a thin layer of muscle in the scrotal skin can regulate the size of the scrotum and therefore how close the testes lie to the warmer body wall; this action is helped by a muscle, the cremaster muscle, which attaches the testicle indirectly to the body wall. On cold days the scrotum is small and the testes are kept close to the body. When the dog has an abnormally high temperature (e.g., due to a generalised infection) this control mechanism can't cope and sperm production is adversely affected.

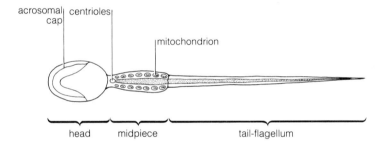

Figure 95 Structure of a sperm

After sperm have been produced they travel along collecting ducts in the testes until these ducts merge into a final 'exit' tube, the epididymis. In this tube the sperms mature, and their progression along it takes about twenty days. The epididymis is in fact very long, but it is tightly coiled upon itself and is enclosed in a membrane which fixes it to the top of the testis. The coiled epididymis is said to have a head (at the front of the testes), a body and a tail. In normal dogs the tail of the epididymis can be felt as a roughly 'pea'-sized structure on top of, and at the back of, the testis. At this point the epididymal tube becomes straight and is called the *vas deferens* or *ductus deferens*; it runs into the abdomen, along with the blood vessels and cremaster muscle, through a small opening, the inguinal canal. The two tubes, or *vasa deferentia*, cross the abdominal cavity and empty together into the urethra; this is the tube which conducts urine from the neck of the bladder to the tip of the penis. Normally the *vasa deferentia* are full of mature sperms and in dogs which do not ejaculate, sperms are constantly over-flowing into the urethra and are voided during urination. Their place is taken by new sperms being produced by the testes. Most of these processes, and the dog's sexual activity, are influenced by hormones.

MALE HORMONES

A hormone is a messenger substance which is released from one part of the body and travels to others in the blood. The main male hormone is called testosterone. It is produced in the testis after puberty by cells which lie between the sperm-producing tubes and is responsible for stimulating the development of male characteristics and for 'triggering off' male behaviour responses (Fig. 93). It also ensures that the prostate gland remains active.

Both the production of testosterone and the formation of sperms are controlled by other hormones released from the pituitary gland at the base of the brain.

NORMAL MATING

The time interval between a dog being introduced to a bitch in heat and him achieving intromission of the penis into the vagina varies greatly and depends on many factors. However, during this time the dog will mount the bitch and make thrusting movements. This causes partial exposure of the penis from the sheath and he ejaculates varying amounts of clear fluid. This is the first fraction of the ejaculate and it contains few, if any, sperms. The origin of the fluid is probably the prostate gland, which is attached to the urethra close to where the *vasa deferentia* open into it. Eventually during coitus the dog's penis enters the vulva and this stimulates him to thrust more vigorously so that the whole of the glans penis enters the vagina, and the prepuce is pushed back by the vulval lips. Up until now the dog's penis does not need to become erect because the bone which it contains provides the rigidity necessary for intromission. However, once this has been achieved, a number of things happen at the same time. Firstly, the dog's penis begins to swell. The tissue of the penis is full of potential cavities which now fill up with blood to cause a dramatic increase in size, particularly at the base of the glans penis – the *bulbus glandis* or bulb. This almost spherical swelling of the penis, aided by contractions of the vulval and vaginal walls, helps to ensure that the penis is locked firmly into the bitch's tract. Also at this time the dog ejaculates the second fraction, which is rich in sperms. These sperms come from the *vasa deferentia* and are conveyed along the penis by sequential contractions of the urethral muscle (as indeed are all the fractions of the ejaculate). The volume of this fraction is small, about ½–1 ml, and is deposited at the front part of the bitch's vagina, near to, but not at, the cervix. The other major event at this time is the dog's instinctive desire to dismount and turn so that he is back to back with the bitch; as long as the dog has achieved a sufficient erection, the penis remains in the vagina and the dogs are 'tied'. The reason why this peculiar process has evolved is unclear. It certainly seems unlikely that the dog can maintain his physically demanding perch on top of the bitch for any length of time, and the fact that the penis must bend through 180 degrees (between the bone and the attachment of the penis to the body) would restrict the blood vessels that drain the penis and help to maintain the erection.

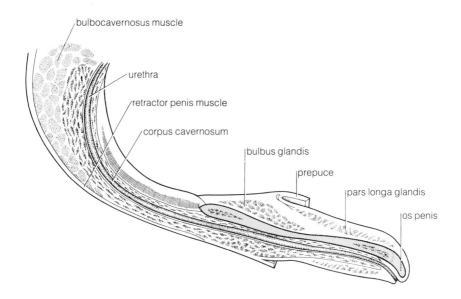

Figure 96   Structure of the penis

The 'tie' can last for any time up to half an hour or so. During this time the dog ejaculates the third fraction, which is clear fluid from the prostate gland; this is thought to wash the sperms forward into the womb. The likely success of a mating is often judged by the length of the tie, but some matings are fertile without any tie at all.

It is very dangerous to try to separate mating dogs. They should never be pulled apart as this will damage both the dog's penis and the bitch's vulva. Advice from your veterinarian should be sought after unplanned matings to avoid unwanted pups.

ANTISOCIAL SEXUAL BEHAVIOUR

Dogs do not know if they have been born or selected to be stud dogs or not, and their natural instincts are therefore not governed by these considerations. There is also a large variation in temperament in male dogs – some never show any interest in bitches, whereas others seem unable to think of anything else.

Sexual behaviour can begin at a very early age. Three-month-old puppies will sometimes practise copulatory movements on feet or inanimate objects. This behaviour should be discouraged in pets in the same way as other undesirable traits. However, take care not to be too severe with dogs which may be used at stud. Dogs of all ages will get erections, often for no obvious reason, and the swollen penis is evident in the prepuce. There is no cause for alarm!

Other antisocial behaviour which is sexually motivated includes roaming (looking for bitches) and urinating on walls and furnishings in the house (urine marking). These activities may only occur, or become more severe, when a 'local' bitch is in heat; it is amazing how far the smell of some of these bitches will travel. A dog that is worried by these smells may also stop eating. Aggression towards other male dogs is often also sexual, and this and other male problems may be treated or avoided by castration, i.e., removal of the testicles. However, the operation will not stop all undesirable behaviour in all dogs; a course of hormone treatment before surgery may give a better clue to the likely benefit of surgery.

Aggression towards people is different. Whatever the cause, castration is not the solution, although it may be tried as an adjunct to behaviour modification therapy.

DISCHARGE FROM THE PREPUCE

Some dogs develop a copious discharge from the prepuce; this soils carpets, etc., and can have an offensive smell. It is normal for all dogs to have some discharge and the definition of abnormality is difficult. Some of these discharges are very refractory to treatment, but if you are worried it is worth a visit to your veterinarian.

The female genital organs

The bitch will allow the male dog to mate her only when she is in heat, which in the majority of bitches occurs every 6 to 10 months. Just as in the male dog, the hormonal events which control the reproductive process are very complex and involve a number of body organs. Our knowledge of the hormones involved, the sequence of their release and the concentrations usually found in the blood is steadily increasing. However, to date we know little of the consequences of possible malfunction of these procedures, so that a detailed description of hormonal events will not be given in this section on the normal bitch.

PUBERTY

Sexual maturity in the bitch is usually achieved after six months of life and is marked by the bitch's first heat. At this time a small gland at the base of the brain, the pituitary gland, becomes active and releases hormones which stimulate changes in the ovaries. However, the factors which initially 'turn on' the pituitary are unknown, and some normal bitches do not have their first heat until 18 months or later; in general, bitches of the small breeds mature earliest. After the first heat there is also a great deal of variation in the frequency with which successive heats occur, and this is normal. Despite claims to the contrary, there is no evidence that irregular heats predispose to false pregnancies or pyometra ('pus in the womb').

OESTRUS OR HEAT

External signs

In simple terms heat begins with the first signs of discharge (colour) at the vulva and ends when the bitch will no longer allow mating by the dog. However, it is convenient to split this period into two parts; the first, called pro-oestrus, lasts about nine days and ends when the bitch will first allow mating. The second period, oestrus proper, is also about nine days long and is the period during which the bitch is sexually receptive. There is a great deal of variation in the lengths and intensity of these periods, and choosing the correct time for mating can be difficult in some bitches.

During pro-oestrus the discharge can vary from almost nothing to very heavy bleeding. To some extent the amount of discharge seen is dependent on how meticulously the bitch licks herself clean. At this time also the vulva is swollen and the bitch may pass small amounts of urine more frequently than usual. This has the function of washing a scent, or pheromone, from the bitch's vestibule and in that way advertising to local dogs that she will soon be receptive.

Unless the bitch is actually running with an interested dog, the change from pro-oestrus to oestrus is difficult to observe. In pro-oestrus the bitch shows some signs of interest in the male, and may flirt and 'egg him on', but will not allow mating. A reduction in the volume of discharge will sometimes be seen around the beginning of oestrus, but it is not a constant feature and relying on this sign alone can be very misleading.

During oestrus the swollen vulva also becomes softer and less turgid than before. Some bitches exhibit male-like mounting and thrusting behaviour.

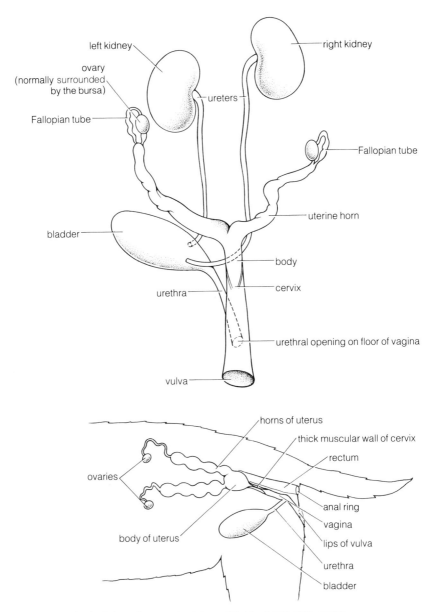

body of uterus is approximately one third the length of the vagina

Figure 97   The genital system of the bitch

It may occur only during oestrus, or at any stage of the cycle and even after spaying. It is purely a behavioural phenomenon and doesn't indicate any hormonal upset.

Internal changes

The external signs of heat are manifestations of internal changes, mainly in the ovaries. Each bitch has two ovaries and at birth they contain all the eggs (ova) that she will shed during her life, plus a lot of others that are wasted. Before the beginning of pro-oestrus some of these ova become surrounded by an organised wall of specialised cells which produce fluid into a central cavity. These fluid-filled sacs, which contain the ova, grow throughout pro-oestrus and are called follicles; they produce one of the female hormones, oestrogen. On average 6 to 8 of these follicles grow to maturity, although the number varies greatly with breed. Once the follicles have become mature or ripe, they rupture to release the egg. This process is known as ovulation. In some animals ovulation is an explosive event, with all the fluid and the ovum being expelled from the follicle, which then collapses. In the bitch the follicle doesn't collapse and very little fluid is lost – the ovum seems to be selectively extruded from the rupture point. Ovulations in an individual bitch occur over two or three days, usually at the beginning of the period of oestrus. However, the relationship between the beginning of oestrus and the time of ovulation can be quite variable.

The ovary of the bitch is surrounded by a thin-walled bag or bursa. This ensures that the ova do not get lost in the abdomen but are attracted to the opening of the uterine tube (or Fallopian tube), which is incorporated in the bursa. Fertilisation of the ovum by a sperm occurs in the uterine tube.

Meanwhile, the fluid-filled sacs which contained the ova can no longer be called follicles, but they continue to function, albeit in a different role. They produce another female hormone, called progesterone, and the gland that evolves in the old follicle is called a *corpus luteum* (Fig. 98). In fact the bitch is unusual in that the follicle starts to change into a *corpus luteum*, and to produce progesterone, some time before the ova are shed from the ovary. The *corpora lutea* continue to produce progesterone for the duration of pregnancy, or for about 60 days if the bitch does not conceive.

During pro-oestrus the follicle-produced hormone oestrogen causes changes in the uterus (womb) and vagina. The blood vessels in the womb become enlarged and red blood cells seep out of some of them. This contributes to the characteristic bloody discharge which escapes from the vulva at this time. The vaginal wall is also affected by oestrogen; it becomes much thickened, presumably so that it can withstand the trauma of mating.

Also at this time the cervix (neck of the womb) relaxes so that sperm can enter after mating. Sperms are deposited at the front of the vagina and

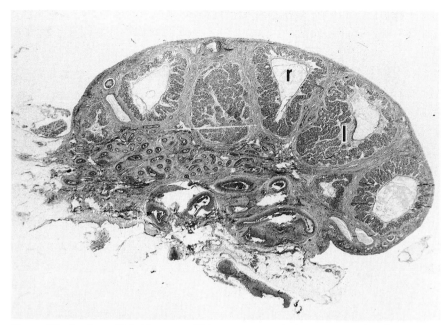

Figure 98 Section of bitch's ovary. This was removed about two weeks after ovulation. It contains the remnants (r) of the old follicles, with luteal tissues (l) developing in the old follicle wall; this latter tissue produces the hormone progesterone

are washed forward partially by the third fraction of the ejaculate but also by virtue of their own swimming movements, and contractions of the muscles of the vagina and uterus. The sperms travel along the short body of the uterus and then up either of the long, coiled uterine horns. At the tip of the horns they enter the uterine tubes and it is here that one sperm fuses with one ovum to produce the beginnings of a new individual, known at this stage as the zygote.

Chromosomes

Using specialised techniques, each cell in the dog's body can be seen to contain 39 pairs of ribbon-like protein complexes called chromosomes. At conception, one set of chromosomes was contained in the egg, the other in the sperm. Thereafter, as the new individual is formed, each cell will contain an exact replica of the initial set of chromosomes obtained from the egg and the sperm. This is important because the chromosomes contain the genetic information which controls how an individual will develop. However, sperm and eggs can only be produced after what is called a reduction division. In this process two important things happen; firstly a swapping of genetic material occurs between pairs of chromosomes so that they are then not the same as those inherited by the individual from its mother and father. Then the altered pairs of chromosomes are separated, so that each set goes into one sperm or egg. The number of chromosomes is thus halved in these cells, and neither contains an exact copy of what was inherited from the individual's parents. This is why mating two dogs of different breeds can result in a litter containing very different-looking puppies. It is also worth noting here that if a bitch mates with two dogs at the same heat she can have a mixed litter containing puppies sired by both fathers. However, the father of one litter of puppies has no influence on subsequent litters.

Pregnancy

Initially the fused cell of the zygote divides and subdivides repeatedly without there being any overall increase in size. However, after about four days it leaves the uterine tube and thereafter not only continues to divide, so that soon there are many millions of cells, but also increases in size. At this stage it is convenient to call each developing pregnancy a conceptus.

Figure 99   The developing whelp

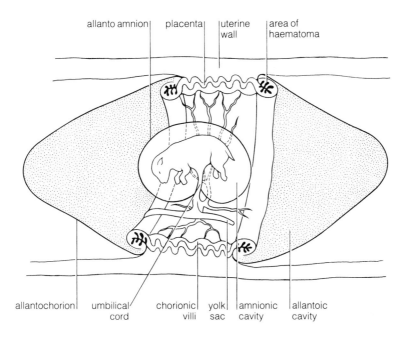

The word refers to all the products of conception, i.e., the new individual, or embryo, and its membranes which will contribute to the placenta.

Initially the conceptuses are free to move around in the uterus and it is not until 18 days or so after fertilisation that an attachment to the uterine wall begins to develop; this is relatively late compared with other animals. In general it is supposed that the conceptuses find themselves evenly spaced throughout the uterine horns, but occasionally one develops in the body of the uterus. From the 21st day or so each conceptus produces a visible bulge, or swelling, in the uterus and each swelling increases in size gradually as the pregnancy proceeds. In each swelling a conceptus has developed to the stage where there is a recognisable embryo (the new individual) surrounded by a small amount of fluid, which is contained in the inner foetal membrane or bag, the amnion. Outside the amnion is a large fluid-filled sac, the allantois, which is in turn bounded by the outer foetal membrane, or sac, the chorioallantoic membrane or allantochorion. The foetus is attached to the allantochorion by the umbilical cord, which travels through the amnion.

The outer surface of the allantochorion is held tight against the lining of the uterus, initially by the pressure of the fluid within it; later the surface of the allantochorion develops microscopic finger-like processes which fit snugly into similar-sized depressions in the uterine wall. This interdigitation between the villi (fingers) of the allantochorion and crypts (depressions) of the uterus is called the placenta, i.e., it is the intimate association between foetal membranes and uterus. Often the word placenta is used to describe just the foetal contribution to this association, i.e., the allantrochorion or 'afterbirth'. The placenta of the bitch forms a band around the equator of the allantochorion and at both edges of this band some of the blood vessels which supply the area rupture to produce what is known as the marginal haematoma; this is just a continuous blood clot along the edges of the placenta. As this blood decomposes during pregnancy a green pigment is formed, and this is often seen during and after normal births. If it is seen before any puppies have been born, veterinary advice should be sought without delay.

The placenta has two functions. The first is to physically stabilise the conceptus in the uterus. The second, and more important role is that of providing an indirect contact between the foetus and its mother. The rudimentary foetal heart is already beating by the 21st day. It sends blood down the developing umbilical cord in the umbilical arteries. When these arteries get to the allantochorion they divide and subdivide until eventually blood is flowing through extremely tiny channels called capillaries. These thin-walled vessels are massed into the villi of the allantochorion and are side by side with capillaries in the crypts of the uterus. The walls of these capillaries are porous, and allow the exchange of small molecules such as gases, salts and nutrients, although the process by which this occurs is highly complex. The result, however, is that the capillaries collect substances which are essential for the growth of the embryo, and lose the waste products which have been produced. The capillaries of the allantochorion fuse to form bigger and yet bigger vessels until they all unite to form the umbilical veins, through which the blood is returned to the embryo.

During the first 35 days or so the embryo doesn't increase in size very much because the cells in its body are still rearranging themselves and forming the precursors of the body's organs. Until this time, in the bitch each conceptus produces a firm spherical bulge in the uterus, and is separated by a tight constriction of uterus from its neighbour. However, after the 35th day growth of the new individual is more rapid, and it is now called a foetus rather than an embryo. Also the allantochorion expands so that the constrictions in the uterus are lost, and the membranes come to lie next to each other, the uterus becoming uniformly swollen. It also becomes less tense because the volume of the foetal fluids does not increase at the same rate as the expansion of the membranes. Thus as the foetus grows the amount of fluid surrounding it decreases; in early pregnancy the fluid acts as a cushion against the movement of other organs in the bitch's abdomen, or trauma from outside. As the foetus matures it becomes less sensitive to these influences because it is acquiring a skeleton and skin, and this coincides with the fluid cushion becoming less effective.

Formation of the foetal bones is continuous and they are usually dense enough to show up on X-rays by 40 to 45 days.

As pregnancy advances, the mammary glands gradually become enlarged. This is initially due to an increase in the tissue which produces milk from the blood circulating through it, and an increase in the system of little ducts that carries the milk to the teats. Eventually, just before labour (parturition) commences, the glands become grossly swollen due to the accumulation of milk.

Food intake by the bitch need not increase until after the sixth week, because before then the developing conceptuses have minimal nutritional requirements. Thereafter the bitch may find it more comfortable to eat many small meals. Supplementation should not be necessary if the bitch is fed a balanced diet, and excessive use of calcium may depress the bitch's own ability to mobilise calcium later on. Despite good feeding most bitches become anaemic in later pregnancy.

PREGNANCY DIAGNOSIS

As yet there are no hormonal methods of pregnancy diagnosis. Palpation of the abdomen, to identify the firm spherical swellings, is easiest at about 25 days. However, they can still be missed, particularly if the bitch is fat or unco-operative. After 35 days palpation becomes very difficult because the uterus becomes softer.

Ultrasound scanning is very useful, but the machines are expensive and require skilled interpretation. It can be used at 3 weeks, but is more accurate at 4–5 weeks. Even then there is often an underestimation of puppy numbers in large litters.

In the later stages X-rays (after 45 days) and listening for puppies' hearts with a stethoscope can be used. The puppies' heart rates are nearly twice that of the mother, but panting by the bitch can make confusing listening.

Recently a test for special proteins in the blood around the 30th day has shown promise as a method of pregnancy diagnosis. However, inflammatory conditions, e.g., pyometra, will cause a false positive result.

Whelping

Whelping or parturition is said to occur classically in three stages, but this definition is not easy to apply to the bitch. The patterns of normal whelpings also vary so greatly that only an overall description can be given. However, all bitches show some signs of first-stage labour. The major events occurring at this time are that mild contractions of the uterus and dilation of the cervix. These contractions appear to become more severe with time and they cause the bitch to become restless. In particular, nesting behaviour becomes intense, the bitch may lose her appetite and she commonly pants and may vomit. If the bitch's temperature is monitored several times a day it will be found to fall from normal 37.7–38°C (100–100.5°F) to about 36.6°C (98°F), but this drop may only be transient. Most bitches whelp within 24 to 48 hours after the temperature drop.

The onset of first-stage labour is impossible to define, and its length varies greatly – up to 48 hours is not uncommon.

The second stage of labour begins once the bitch starts to strain. This is stimulated by part of a puppy being pushed through the relaxed cervix by the uterine contractions. Once in the front of the vagina, it triggers a reflex mechanism which makes the bitch actively push the pup out; sometimes this seems to occur with very little effort. In most cases the allantochorion ruptures inside the uterus, but the puppy is born in the inner membrane, the amnion; the bitch usually clears this membrane from the pup, and breaks the umbilical cord.

Third-stage labour is defined as the period of time when continued uterine contractions cause the allantochorion (often loosely called the placenta at this time) to become detached and expelled. In the bitch there is an intermingling of puppy births and the passing of the placentas. After the birth of one puppy, abdominal contractions cease until another has been pushed into the vagina. The time lapse between the birth of successive puppies varies greatly and a judgement as to when things are going wrong is often subjective.

Puppies can be born head first or back legs first. The position of the limbs is rarely a complicating factor, but when a puppy is being born backwards (posterior presentation) it can become stuck if the legs are flexed at the hips, i.e., the feet are pointing forwards. This is a true 'breech presentation'.

Other things which impede the progress of second-stage labour are large puppies, or those being born head first (anterior presentation) but with the head deviated sideways or downwards.

Accounting for afterbirths can be difficult. They often do not follow individual puppies in an orderly manner and the bitch can devour them quite quickly; this often causes diarrhoea.

PSEUDOPREGNANCY

If a bitch is either not mated or doesn't conceive, she still ovulates in the normal way, and the *corpora lutea* develop in the ovary and produce progesterone in exactly the same way as they do when pregnancy occurs. Some of these bitches go on to show signs of pseudopregnancy, and once again this can occur whether mating has taken place or not. Other words used for pseudopregnancy are false pregnancy, phantom pregnancy and pseudocyesis; they all mean the same thing. The intensity of signs of pseudopregnancy varies greatly and may involve some or all of the following: loss of appetite, milk production, reluctance to go out (fear of leaving the imaginary puppies), shivering, mothering inanimate objects and territorial aggression. There are various treatments for the condition if signs become severe, but usually they disappear naturally with time. However, milk production can make the bitch uncomfortable, and aggression can be difficult to cope with in a household. It is amazing that bitches which don't eat for many days appear not to lose weight. Once a false pregnancy has been resolved it usually recurs only after the next heat. However, a small number of bitches have recurrent bouts after the same heat, and in these the timing of spaying (neutering) can be tricky if a recurrence of the condition after the operation is to be avoided.

Historically, it would appear that wild dogs came into heat only once a year, and that they all did so at the same time. The dominant bitches in the pack were the only ones to breed, but the puppies were subsequently cared for by all the bitches, i.e., they had false pregnancies; this allowed the dominant bitches to hunt for the pack. Over thousands of years of domestication, little attention seems to have been paid to selecting for or against false pregnancy, so that we have inherited the current situation.

UNWANTED PREGNANCY AND CONTRACEPTION

Misalliance (or mesalliance) refers to an unplanned mating. Pregnancy can usually be prevented by an injection of the hormone oestrogen within the next one to three days. However, repeated injections are not advisable due to possible side effects.

Hormonal preparations, both injectable and in tablet form, are available to prevent oestrus in bitches. They are very useful when used for short periods of time, but the possibility of side effects increases when their use is prolonged. A common alternative is to have the uterus and ovaries removed surgically, i.e., have the bitch spayed or neutered.

There is no universal agreement as to the most appropriate age for this operation, and the matter is best discussed with your veterinarian. However, the common side effect of having a bitch spayed is her tendency to put on weight. Some bitches require regular weighing and strict dietary control to prevent it.

Breeding problems in the dog

Infertility is difficult to define in the dog because of the sporadic manner in which many are allowed to breed. Some owners are concerned when their dog 'misses' two bitches, others when five or six have failed to conceive. However, there are some recognisable reasons why some dogs do not produce puppies.

Inability to mate

Most dogs know instinctively how to mate a bitch because the behavioural pattern which is imprinted in the brain is stimulated by the hormone testosterone. Even before puberty many dogs practise copulatory movements. However, some dogs are more sexually overt than others and there is no evidence that lack of sex drive in an entire dog is caused by a deficiency in testosterone. More likely, unwillingness to mate is psychological due to previous or current adverse stimuli. For instance, one common example of the different approach of individual dogs to mating is that some successful sires will only mate when the bitch is absolutely ready, whereas others are always keen. Treatment of the reluctant male is difficult and requires time and patience. Varying the amount of supervision, the personnel involved, the venue and the bitch are all worth a try. Collecting semen artificially from the dog in the presence of a bitch in heat may also help in some cases. Hormone treatment is not usually indicated or worth while.

Physical pain, particularly in the spine and hips, may make some dogs unwilling to mount, but the cause may not be immediately apparent.

Occasionally young dogs are unable to expose the penis due to a continued attachment (frenulum) of the penis to the sheath or because the preputial orifice is too small (phimosis). Surgical correction is usually necessary.

Poor semen quality

Persistent high temperatures and specific diseases such as distemper can interfere with sperm production, but these are seldom seen these days. A condition called canine brucellosis occurs in North America and causes inflammation of the testis (orchitis); to date it has not been recorded in the UK. Other causes of inflammation are usually trauma through injury to the testes or scrotum. (See Chapter 22 Viral and Bacterial Diseases.)

Some drugs specifically inhibit sperm production, such as the hormones which are used to depress sexual behaviour and to control enlargement of the prostate gland. It is possible that other drugs interfere with spermatogenesis, but this has not been investigated in detail.

Collecting a semen sample from a dog is relatively simple, particularly in the presence of a bitch in heat. Evaluation of an ejaculate usually reveals one of three things. Firstly the semen may be of good quality, which suggests that the dog should be fertile. Secondly, some dogs produce no sperms at all, and we call the condition spermatogenic arrest because most of these dogs have a history of having been fertile at an earlier date. The problem can occur at any age, but often as early as 18 months. Typically, affected dogs have no history of illness and are bright and healthy, ejaculate readily but produce large volumes of prostatic fluid which contain no sperms. Their testicles are soft and the tails of the epididymides are small. The condition has been shown to be inherited in some breeds, and affected dogs show signs of being immune to their own testicular tissue. As yet there is no known treatment and the condition does not improve spontaneously.

The third category of dog in this context is one that produces some sperms, but the motility is poor and/or the number of abnormalities is high. The ability to decide what is normal is rather arbitrary, but it is felt that an ejaculate should contain more than 100 million sperms and that 90 per cent of them should be normal. However, dogs which have seminal quality below this standard are not sterile, but are statistically less able to achieve optimal fertility rates.

The cause of most of these problems is unknown and no treatments have been shown to improve the semen. However, allowing the dog to mate the bitch repeatedly, at least once a day during oestrus, has given promising results.

Overuse is often given as a cause of infertility. Experiments on normal laboratory dogs, with good semen quality, have shown that ejaculation once a day, and sometimes more frequently, does not seriously reduce sperm output. However, what effect frequent ejaculation may have on the semen of an infertile dog is not known.

Cryptorchidism

This term describes a dog with one or both testicles in the abdomen – the dog is then described as a unilateral or bilateral cryptorchid, depending on whether or not both testes are affected. In most puppies the testes have descended through the inguinal canal soon after birth. They are often difficult to palpate at this time, but in most normal dogs both can be detected by twelve weeks of age. Thereafter some testes do seem to disappear and return, but as time advances their chances of achieving a proper scrotal position becomes ever reduced. Occasionally non-scrotal testes have descended through the canal but have then wandered off in the wrong direction under the skin.

Testes which are not in the scrotum cannot produce sperms, but they continue to produce testosterone. Thus bilateral cryptorchids can mate, and unilateral cryptorchids are fertile. However, due to the inherited nature of the condition these dogs should not be bred from, and it is advisable for the undescended testes to be removed, because they have a tendency to become cancerous in later life. There is no treatment for the condition, so hormone injections are an unnecessary expense.

Breeding problems in the bitch

In general, compared with other female animals, bitches appear to be very fertile. However, for various reasons, individual bitches may fail to conceive at two or more successive heats, or a kennel may experience a fall in the numbers of puppies born. There is no evidence, however, to support the assumption that parvovirus, or vaccination against it, causes infertility in the bitch.

Investigation of infertility in the bitch is difficult. Using conventional methods it is not possible to see the ovaries or uterus by X-rays, and information gleaned by the newer technique of ultrasonography is sparse. It is difficult to visualise the whole of the vagina even using sophisticated endoscopes and speculae and it is impossible to look through the cervix and into the uterus. In fact it is difficult to pass any sort of instrument into a bitch's uterus without using surgery. This leaves only examination of the cells from the vaginal wall, which can be rewarding, and measuring hormone concentrations, which is of limited application.

Delayed heats

Late puberty and long intervals between successive heats are sometimes an obstacle to breeding bitches. They do not signify an underlying disease process, but the reason for the delay is unknown. Hormone treatments give poor results and are only of use as a last resort. Keeping the bitch in close contact with others in heat may help.

Failure to mate

Bitches may resent attention by the male dog because they are nervous, because they are not properly in heat or because they are so imprinted on people that mating with a dog seems 'unnatural'. Checking for the right time with vaginal smears (see later) can be helpful, but otherwise measures taken for the unco-operative male dog can be tried. Occasionally mild tranquillization will remove apprehension.

Sometimes strictures at the vulva and further into the vagina prevent intromission and may require surgical treatment.

In some bitches in late pro-oestrus a polyp-like object may be seen protruding through the vulva. This is really the grossly swollen vaginal wall which has 'prolapsed'. It then becomes dry and damaged if it is not protected, but regresses normally once the season has finished. It may be removed surgically to allow breeding. True polyps also occur. These may be seen at the vulva at any time of the cycle, or may cause a purulent or bloody discharge.

Wrong mating time

As mentioned previously, the timing of ovulation in the bitch is not always coincident with her first acceptance of the dog. However, most people arrange to have their bitch mated 10 to 12 days after the start of pro-oestrus, and most bitches get pregnant. The reason for this high success rate with a relatively unsophisticated system is threefold. Firstly, most bitches are ovulating at around this time; secondly, if the bitch has already ovulated all is not lost because the ovum is not at that time ready to be fertilised; it takes about 36 hours to undergo a final division in the uterine tube, which brings the chromosomal number down to half those in a normal dog cell. And thirdly, if the bitch ovulates some days after mating she is still likely to get pregnant because dog semen of good quality is known to live for four to five days in the bitch's reproductive tract.

It therefore seems difficult to mistime even a single mating. However, some bitches ovulate as early as five days after the first signs of pro-oestrus, whereas others ovulate as late as the 21st day. In neither of these cases is mating on days 10 to 12 going to be fertile.

Vaginal smears

The most satisfactory method of indirectly following the hormone changes (which *are* well correlated with the ovulation time) is to study the cells which are shed from the wall of the vagina. This vaginal cytology must be carried out by someone familiar with the techniques involved, but can be very accurate in determining the best time to mate in problem bitches. Several smears may have to be taken as the cellular changes reflect the hormone changes that have occurred, but do not predict those that are likely to occur. Using glucose test papers to measure the amount of sugar in vaginal secretions is also said to be helpful.

The measurement of hormones is still in its infancy. Most of the changes are so transitory that several blood samples would have to be taken each day to detect them, and the delay in having the samples analysed in the laboratory would also be a disadvantage. In the future, rapid tests, particularly if they can be carried out on urine, may become practical. Already we can measure one hormone in blood very quickly. This is progesterone, and since concentrations of the hormone rise slowly before ovulation, it may soon be possible to look at a blood sample every two days or so and accurately ascertain the right time to mate.

Infections

Apart from canine brucellosis, which doesn't occur in the UK as yet, there is no specific bacterial venereal disease of dogs. Two viruses occur occasionally; one causes tumours of the penis and vagina, the other a mild inflammation. Neither of them is associated with infertility in the UK.

Vaginal swabs

It is common for breeders to ask for vaginal swabs to be taken before mating. However, by necessity, these swabs are taken from a site (the terminal vagina) which is a long way from the uterus, where the pregnancies develop, and even further from the uterine tubes, where fertilisation occurs. This site is known in normal healthy bitches to have a resident population of bacteria, which includes the beta haemolytic streptococci (BHS) and many others which some people worry about. Although beta haemolytic streptococci have been isolated from dead puppies, there is no concrete evidence to link them with infertility in the dog or bitch, or to support the theory that they are spread by mating.

Vaginal discharge

Occasionally vaginal bacteria travel forward into the uterus, and if the lining of the uterus has reduced resistance, as it often has in older bitches, then the life-threatening condition of pyometra develops. This starts insidiously during oestrus when the cervix is open and the bacteria can enter. After ovulation the cervix closes and the pus that is being produced builds up and slowly makes the bitch more and more ill, eventually causing loss of appetite, increased thirst and vomiting. If, at this stage, the cervix opens, some of the pus is seen to escape and the cause of illness is easier to diagnose.

Discharge from the vulva of the bitch may occur for a variety of reasons. These include pyometra, bladder infection, etc., or may be normal, e.g., during oestrus. Also, some bitches have an obvious discharge, especially after they have been in oestrus, which is not caused by pyometra. This is assumed to be due to inflammation of the vagina, i.e., vaginitis. However, the bacterial growth in the vaginas of these bitches is the same as in normal bitches, and the discharge may be refractory to treatment. Some young bitches can have a quite copious vaginal discharge which causes no ill health and clears up when they have their first heat. The cause for this is unknown and it is usually unaffected by antibiotic treatment. Nevertheless, it is prudent to take vaginal discharge in adult bitches seriously due to their association with pyometra.

Unknown causes of failure to conceive

Even in species of animals where the reproductive process can be studied much more closely than in dogs, fertilisation may fail to occur even when everything seems to have gone correctly. For example, we are still in the dark over most of the factors which govern the delicate movement of sperms and ova in the uterine tube, and the mechanisms which stop them entering the uterus too early. We also have to assume that the female reproductive tract is a very hostile environment for sperms, if 100 million are necessary to ensure six fertilisations. There may even be problems that we haven't even begun to suspect yet.

Pregnancy failure

Resorption certainly occurs in some bitches. For some unknown reason the embryos die, and the fluid of the conceptus is resorbed back into the bitch's circulation. The remnants of the embryo and its membranes are expelled later and usually eaten unobserved by the bitch. It is difficult to believe that resorption occurs in later pregnancy, i.e., after the puppies have been seen moving. The bitch has then either aborted and eaten the puppies or she was not pregnant.

Abortion occurs infrequently and may be due to bacteria. Presumably these gain entrance to the uterus via the cervix, but why it happens isn't known. Brucella canis infection, the main infectious cause of canine abortion in North America and other countries, is not a problem in the UK. Another Brucella spp. B. abortus has been reported to cause abortion in bitches in the UK. (See also Chapter 22 Viral and Bacterial Diseases.)

Whelping problems

Pregnancy length appears to be very variable in the bitch because it is measured from the first mating. In reality pregnancy is very uniform in length if we use hormone changes as a starting point. However, until it becomes practical to measure these substances, we are stuck with the problem of when is a bitch 'overdue'.

Primary uterine inertia is a condition sometimes seen in bitches with only one or two pups, or in very big litters. In these bitches the temperature falls as expected, but none of the other signs of first- or second-stage labour are seen, except that the cervix opens. This allows in bacteria, and if the condition is not recognised, infected dead pups can result, requiring surgical removal. Secondary uterine inertia occurs after one or more pups have been born, due to exhaustion of the uterine muscle. This may respond to an injection of the hormone oxytocin.

Once a bitch is in labour, two major signs that she needs help are, firstly, unproductive straining and, secondly, restlessness. Continuous straining for half an hour without result suggests that a puppy is stuck in the vagina and requires repositioning, or maybe removal by Caesarean operation. Therefore if in doubt consult your veterinarian – *do not wait to see* – it may be too late!

Restlessness and panting, especially when a full-sized litter seems to have been produced, may mean that a pup is left in the uterus. This may not be very easy to diagnose except by using X-rays or ultrasound.

The decision whether or not to use the Caesarean operation to relieve whelping problems can only be made in the light of the circumstances of the case in hand. It is often a difficult decision to make at the time, and all too easy to decide, in retrospect, what should have been done.

Post whelping problems

Acute metritis (inflammation of the uterus) is luckily rare; it is a severe infection which creates a foul-smelling discharge and a very depressed bitch with no milk and a high temperature. The first signs are often continuously crying pups. Sometimes this is associated with retained foetal membranes.

Nervous bitches may also fail to produce milk, and may continually move their puppies from place to place.

Lactation tetany can occur at any time, usually towards the end of lactation. The bitch salivates and shakes uncontrollably, and seems to 'grin'; this may progress to convulsions. Calcium treatment must be given as soon as possible by your veterinarian.

Subinvolution of the placenta is not common, but indicates that the womb hasn't contracted totally after expulsion of the pups. The bitch will have a continuous but slight bloody discharge which may last for months and is refractory to treatment. It will disappear at the next heat.

Artificial insemination

This is possible in the dog using 'raw' semen, which is inseminated into the bitch immediately after collection. If the semen has to travel some distance it can be diluted in a suitable substance and chilled; in this way it will keep for 48 hours or so. Alternatively, the semen can be frozen for use at any time in the future.

At present, AI is little used in the UK as the Kennel Club will only register puppies from such a mating if they have given prior permission. Also, due to the regulations governing the importation of biological substances into the UK, we can receive only frozen dog semen from abroad.

Before exporting dog semen it is worth contacting the Ministry of Agriculture, Fisheries and Food to ascertain any import regulations in the receiving country.

12

THE URINARY SYSTEM

Structure and function

Dogs, like all mammals, have two kidneys situated in the upper (dorsal) abdomen, just behind the liver, one either side of midline, the left being half a kidney length behind the right (Fig. 100). Although not rigidly fixed, the kidneys are fairly constant in position due to their close relationship

Figure 100 Part of a lateral X-ray film of a dog's abdomen to show the position of the left kidney ————— in relation to the right ——————. The anterior half of the right kidney is not discernible.

The length of the left kidney is equal to the distance between the first two and a half lumbar vertebral bodies

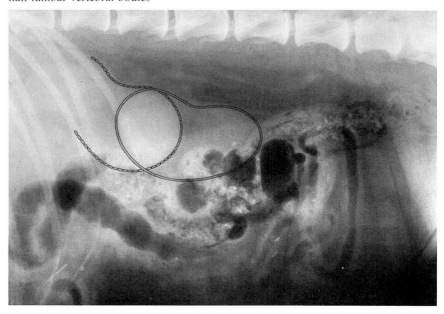

to adjacent fixed structures, especially the liver in front (anteriorly) and the backbone (lumbar spine) and its supporting (sub-lumbar) muscles above (dorsally). Palpation of the kidneys is possible in most dogs, but normal position limits this to the left kidney and the rear (posterior) portion of the right. Palpation is much more difficult in dogs which are obese and those with tense abdominal wall muscles.

Each kidney is bean-shaped and dimensions vary according to breed size, but for a 10kg (22lb) dog, each kidney weighs about 15gm (0.5oz) and is 5.5cm (2in) long, 3.5cm (1.4in) wide and 2.5cm (1in) thick. An estimate of kidney size, irrespective of breed, can be made from a lateral abdominal X-ray by comparing kidney length with the length of the first three lumbar vertebral bodies. Normal kidney length is equivalent to 2.5 to 3 vertebral bodies (Fig. 101).

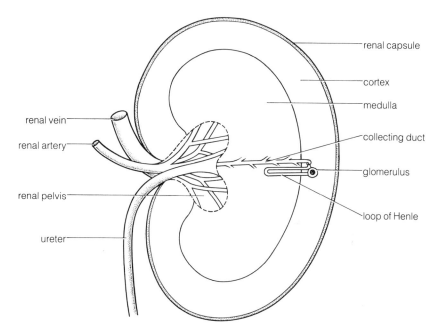

microscopic glomerulus, loop of Henle and collecting duct have been magnified out of proportion for clarity

Figure 101   Diagram of a longitudinal section through the centre of a kidney.

The kidney has a very rich blood supply, with blood entering at the hilus via the renal artery and then passing through a complex network of arteries, capillaries and veins, finally leaving at the hilus via the renal vein (Fig. 102). Intimately connected with the blood vessels is a complicated arrangement of tubules and ducts which carry fluid filtered from the

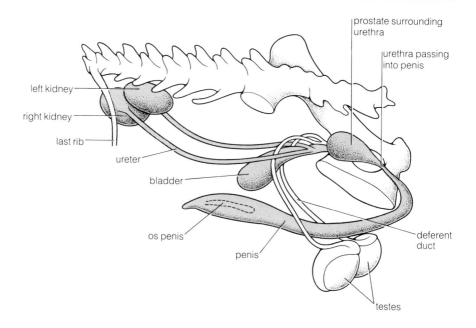

Figure 102a   Diagram to show the position of the male urinary tract in relation to the vertebral column and pelvis and the genital organs.

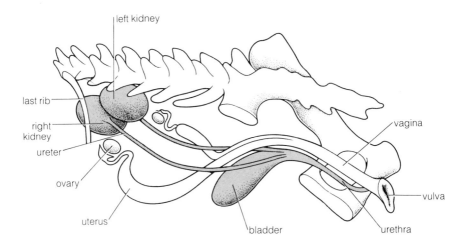

Figure 102b   Diagram to show the position of the female urinary tract in relation to the skeleton and genital organs.

vascular system. This fluid eventually becomes urine and leaves the kidney via the ureter, a thin muscular pipe which runs back through the abdomen to the urinary bladder (Fig. 100), a highly distensible bulb-shaped organ situated at the extreme posterior end of the abdomen, where urine is stored prior to being voided. Urination is the process whereby urine is expelled from the bladder following relaxation of the bladder sphincter (outflow valve) and contraction of the bladder wall muscles, forcing urine into the urethra, which in the female opens into the floor of the vagina and in the male becomes the passage through the penis.

Filtration of the blood takes place in microscopic tufts of blood vessels surrounded by the bulbous beginning of the urinary tubule system. Each tuft is called a glomerulus and this, together with its associated tubules and blood vessels, is called a nephron. The glomeruli are found in the outer part of the kidney, the cortex, while the majority of the tubules and closely associated blood vessels are deeper, in the medulla. The tubules unite to form collecting ducts which empty into the renal pelvis and thence into the ureter. The glomeruli act as blood filter units and permit the passage of water and small molecules into the duct system and, under normal circumstances, prevent the passage of blood cells, proteins and other larger molecules.

The kidneys perform several life-maintaining functions and some others which are not so vital but still very important. Urine is the final outcome of the kidney's role in maintaining the body water at the correct volume, concentration and acidity (pH). In addition to ions such as sodium and chloride, the urine contains large amounts of the soluble products of nitrogen metabolism such as urea and creatinine. The kidneys play an important part in the control of blood pressure as their finely tuned vasculature close to the glomeruli quickly recognise and respond to any variations, especially lowering of pressure. This is in part due to the fact that filtration of blood in the glomeruli can take place only if the blood pressure is sufficiently high. On the other hand, if it is too high over a period of time, damage is done to the sensitive tissues of the kidneys as well as in other parts of the body, for example blood vessels. The kidneys have a more minor function in converting vitamin D_3 to its final, useful form, thus providing a key factor in calcium metabolism, and a further function in the production of a substance called erythropoietin releasing factor, produced in the kidneys, which promotes the production of red blood cells in the bone marrow.

The ureters, bladder and urethra have no function apart from the passage, storage and expulsion of urine, although in the male, the urethra is also used for the passage of seminal fluids formed in the prostate gland and testes.

Mechanisms of kidney failure

To say that a dog is suffering from kidney disease conveys very little and may in fact be misleading. Examination of the kidneys of dogs after death has shown that a large number have suffered some form of kidney damage at some time during life, but it has been of a minor nature, probably never causing the dog to be ill. One reason for this is that the kidneys have a very large reserve capacity, so damage has to be severe and widespread before the dog shows any clinical signs. Kidney disease is therefore not the same as kidney failure. Moreover, some of the tests for kidney function, for example the measurement of the level of urea in the blood, will indicate changes that are the result of disease elsewhere in the body leading to a secondary effect on the kidneys. Thus, extreme dehydration may cause a rise in blood urea levels due to the concentration of the plasma and also because glomerular filtration is reduced as a result of the fluid depletion. If the latter is corrected by means of replacement fluid therapy, then renal function continues as normal. This form of raised blood urea (termed uraemia) is called pre-renal. In other circumstances, uraemia may develop because urea is unable to leave the body, for example in the case of a dog suffering from rupture of the bladder in a road accident. Urine is still formed by the kidneys but escapes from the bladder into the abdominal cavity from which urea is re-absorbed into the blood circulation. This is called post-renal uraemia or, more accurately, azotaemia. In both pre- and post-renal uraemia, the situation is life-threatening and requires immediate treatment, but is not primarily the fault of the kidneys. Primary renal failure occurs whenever there is a decrease in the rate of glomerular filtration due to disease, from whatever cause, actually within the kidneys. In some cases, as with the examples of dehydration and bladder rupture given above, the kidney failure is potentially reversible provided rapid and appropriate treatment is given and the animal is still capable of responding. In other cases, the uraemia is irreversible and the animal will die. The same applies to cases of primary kidney disease, where recovery depends on the severity of the condition, the nature of the damage done to kidney tissues and the speed at which appropriate treatment is applied.

If primary kidney disease is sudden and severe, the dog is said to be suffering from acute renal failure, which may be fatal, despite treatment. In some cases there is complete recovery, while in others there is ongoing insidious damage and eventual loss of sufficient nephrons for the development of chronic renal failure. Clinical signs of chronic renal failure are not usually apparent until three-quarters of the total number of nephrons have been destroyed, so the process may continue over many months or years, and by the time signs do appear, the condition is well advanced. The loss of further nephrons will lead to increasingly severe illness, but in some dogs this process occurs extremely slowly, and during

Table 8: Clinical signs usually present in dogs with renal failure

Acute renal failure	Chronic renal failure
Sudden onset illness	*Usually gradual onset illness*
dullness	reduced appetite
weakness	intermittent vomiting
loss of appetite	weight loss
dehydration	increased thirst/polyuria
congested eye mucosae	increasing dullness
swollen painful kidneys	small, firm kidneys
oliguria/anuria	anaemia
repeated vomiting	'rubber jaw'

Uraemic signs

(seen in the late stages of both acute and chronic renal failure)

uraemic halitosis (foul meaty smell, with overtones of ammonia)
brown discolouration of tongue
ulcers on tongue tip, gums and cheeks
vomiting and diarrhoea containing altered blood
muscle twitching
uraemic convulsions
coma and death

this time appropriate treatment often allows the animal to lead a reasonably normal life. Clinical signs of acute renal failure can be associated with infection with *Leptospira canicola* and they are described and compared with the signs of chronic renal failure in Table 8.

Blood and urine samples taken from dogs in acute and chronic renal failure will help to confirm the diagnosis and the important laboratory results to be expected are shown in Table 9. Other helpful diagnostic procedures, such as radiography and ultrasonography, can be used to give an indication of kidney size, shape and position, and radiography can also help in demonstrating the demineralisation of bone ('rubber jaw') that may occur in chronic renal failure due to the failure of the kidneys to excrete phosphate.

It is clearly important to distinguish between acute and chronic renal failure both in terms of the choice of appropriate treatment and in prognosis (outlook). The broad outlines of treatment are given in Table 10.

We have already said that the glomerular filter acts as a barrier to large molecules in the blood, especially protein. If the glomerulus is damaged, either on its own (glomerulonephropathy) or in conjunction with generalised kidney disease, in both acute and chronic failure states, then substantial amounts of protein may be lost into the urine. In many cases the protein leak may not cause any trouble; in some, it will contribute to

Table 9: Laboratory results commonly reported from dogs with renal failure

	Acute renal failure	*Chronic renal failure*
Blood samples		
packed cell volume	high (dehydration)	low (anaemia)
total white blood cells	raised (only if infection)	usually normal
plasma urea	high	normal* to high
plasma creatinine	high	normal* to high
plasma phosphate	high	normal to high
plasma phosphate	high	normal to high
plasma calcium	normal to high	normal to high
plasma sodium	high (dehydration)	normal to high
plasma potassium	high	normal to high
plasma chloride	high (dehydration)	normal to high
Urine samples		
volume	less	increased
protein content	variable	low to moderate
specific gravity	high	low

*the kidney can be failing in its ability to concentrate urine without rises in urea and creatinine; more than 70 per cent of the kidney mass has to fail before rises in these parameters occur.

loss in body weight, but in others, if proteinuria is severe and prolonged, blood protein becomes so depleted that the circulation loses the osmotic support that protein provides and fluid flows out of the blood vessels into the extracellular compartment of the body (i.e., the spaces between cells and the cavities of the abdomen and chest) to accumulate as oedema. When this happens, the dog is said to be suffering from the nephrotic syndrome and it may or may not accompany chronic renal failure. Prior to the development of the nephrotic syndrome the dog may have noticeably lost weight and may have been thirstier, but need not have been dull or inappetent. In dogs, the oedema fluid nearly always gravitates first to the lower parts of the hind limbs and then affects the skin of the lower body wall. In more severe cases the abdomen is swollen due to accumulation of ascites fluid and possibly breathing difficulties due to fluid in the chest (hydrothorax), together with swelling of the head, neck and forelimbs. At this point the dog looks bloated and may appear to have gained weight rather than lost it. Many nephrotic dogs behave quite normally within the limitations of the fluid accumulations, but if suffering from coexisting chronic renal failure they will show the associated signs.

Laboratory examination of blood and urine samples is particularly helpful, and typical results are given in Table 11.

Table 10: Treatment of renal failure in dogs

Acute renal failure	Chronic renal failure
Rehydration (intravenous fluids)	Drinking water freely available
Re-establishment of urine production with fluids, diuretic drugs or osmotic agents, e.g., mannitol	Low-protein diet, either proprietary or home prepared
	Vitamin supplementation
Alleviation of vomiting	Phosphate binders, to prevent absorption from intestine, e.g., aluminium hydroxide gel
Peritoneal dialysis (rarely)	
Specific treatment, e.g., antibiotic if indicated	Anabolic steroids to help promote red blood cell production
	Gastric ulcer therapy, e.g., cimetidine

So far we have described kidney disease in general terms. This is possible because the kidney can only react in a few fixed pathways to a number of different insults, whether they are congenital (a disease present at birth or resulting from an inborn error), metabolic, viral, bacterial, chemical, immune-mediated, traumatic or neoplastic in origin. While this makes diagnosis of kidney disease in general relatively easy, it seldom permits a specific diagnosis and in most cases, the latter is difficult unless kidney tissue is examined, either by biopsy in the living animal, or at post mortem. Even then, it is sometimes impossible to be precise, because the severity of the changes, e.g., in chronic renal failure, may make them indistinguishable.

Table 11: Laboratory results commonly reported from dogs with protein-losing nephropathy and the nephrotic syndrome

	Without renal failure	With renal failure
Blood samples		
plasma urea	normal	raised
plasma creatinine	normal	raised
plasma phosphate	normal	normal–raised
plasma cholesterol	raised	raised
plasma total protein	normal–low	normal–low
plasma albumin	low–very low	low
plasma globulin	normal–high	normal–high
Urine samples		
volume	normal–increased	increased
protein content	very high	high
specific gravity	normal–high	low

Other clinical signs of urinary tract disease include straining to pass urine, irrespective of the amount of urine passed, and blood in urine (haematuria). Both of these signs will be dealt with in more detail with diseases of the urinary bladder.

Congenital renal disease

Occasionally dogs are found to have only one kidney (unilateral renal agenesis), but provided the existing kidney is healthy the dog will live normally, as one kidney is more than adequate to cope with demands. More seriously, malformation of both kidneys during embryonic development can result in the presence of multiple fluid-filled cysts and these may impair renal function sufficiently for puppies and young dogs to die from chronic renal failure. A familial form of polycystic kidneys has been reported in Cairn terriers.

Familial diseases are defined as those which occur in more members of a family than would be expected by chance. They are usually genetic in origin, but the term familial is favoured to hereditary unless the exact mode of inheritance is known. Another point which must be made is that not all diseases of genetic origin are evident at birth or even in the young dog. Certainly a Cairn terrier with severe polycystic kidneys will be suffering from renal impairment at birth and will probably go into clinical chronic renal failure soon after weaning, when meat protein is introduced into the diet. However, many of the dogs known to suffer from familial nephropathies as young adults and older dogs have normal renal function at birth and often during the first few months of life. The mechanisms which trigger renal failure in these breeds are uncertain, but in breeds where inheritance patterns are known it is certain that the genetic abnormality is present from conception.

For over 40 years and in many countries, a familial nephropathy has been consistently recognised in parti-coloured Cocker Spaniels, especially blue roans, but it is only recently that it has been shown to be an autosomal recessive trait. In the last 20 years there has been a growing list of over 30 breeds in which juvenile kidney diseases have been diagnosed, but of these only a third have been shown to be familial and in only four has an attempt been made to determine the mode of inheritance. The breeds so affected are shown in Tables 12 and 13.

Clinical signs

Affected puppies and dogs will, at some time, show signs of chronic renal failure (Table 8), but the age at which they do so is variable. Some are thirsty and poorly grown from just a few weeks of age and do not survive to adulthood. Others, even though the disease is present at birth, appear

Table 12: Breeds reported to be affected by familial nephropathies

Breed	Mode of inheritance
Cocker Spaniel	autosomal recessive
Norwegian Elkhound	
Samoyed	sex linked
Dobermann	
Lhasa Apso	
Shih Tzu	
Standard Poodle	
Soft-coated Wheaten terrier	probably autosomal recessive
Bull terrier	probably autosomal dominant

Table 13: Breeds reported to have had juvenile nephropathies not confirmed as familial

Bedlington terrier	Irish terrier
Keeshond	Old English Sheepdog
Malamute	Dalmatian
Swedish Foxhound	Shetland Sheepdog
Vizsla	Boxer
Yorkshire terrier	Flat-coated retriever
German Shepherd Dog	Cairn terrier
Cavalier King Charles Spaniel	Dachshund
Miniature Schnauzer	Japanese Spitz
Scottish terrier	

to adapt to life with mild to moderate chronic renal failure and live relatively normal lives, sometimes into middle age. In these cases, the owner may remain unaware of the problem until clinical signs appear, after which the dog may deteriorate rapidly. In some breeds, e.g., Cocker Spaniels, kidney function is apparently normal from a few months up to two years before the disease process begins. When it does, clinical signs often appear soon afterwards, and affected dogs usually suffer a more severe illness than animals which have had the problem from birth.

The variable nature of the timing of the appearance of the disease means that most puppies have been dispersed before they become ill. Lack of information about breed susceptibility and the condition of litter-mates makes diganosis difficult. Moreover, owners and veterinary surgeons alike may find it hard to accept that a dog developing chronic renal failure in middle age could be suffering from a congenital, possibly inherited, illness. Nevertheless, any dog up to middle age, with chronic renal failure, should be suspected of having a possible congenital problem, and owners are encouraged to request a post mortem examination of the kidneys by an experienced renal pathologist. Suspected and confirmed cases should always be reported to breeders and/or breed clubs in order that steps may be taken to publicise the problem, investigate it and attempt to institute a control programme.

Treatment

There is no curative treatment. Management is that for any dog with chronic renal failure (Table 10). If diagnosed very early, affected young puppies will benefit for a longer period if they can be weaned on to non-meat protein. Vitamin B supplementation and prolonged courses of anabolic steroids are also helpful. Water should always be available. It is always difficult to estimate how long an affected dog will survive with chronic renal failure, as the rate of progression varies enormously. Some guide as to progress will be possible if regular (monthly or bi-monthly) checks on blood urea, creatinine and phosphate levels are made.

Urinary tract infections

Infection of the urinary tract is common, but does not necessarily lead to illness with clinical signs. The commonest infectious agents are bacteria, but viral and fungal infections are occasionally encountered. The most common bacterial agent involved is *Eschericia coli*, followed by *Proteus* sp. and *Staphylococcus aureus*. These three organisms account for about 80 per cent of bacterial isolates from the urinary tract. Other bacteria found occasionally include *Enterococcus, Klebsiella, Enterobacteria* and *Pseudomonas* sp. *Mycoplasma* sp. (organisms not classed as bacteria) have also been encountered. Bacterial infections may be of a single agent or mixtures. Tuberculosis can affect dogs and if infection localises in the kidneys, urine may contain the causal agent, *Mycobacterium tuberculosis*. *Leptospira* sp., especially *L. canicola*, can infect the kidney and may cause serious disease (see Chapter 22, page 386), but regular, routine vaccination against leptospiral infection over the last 30 years of a large proportion of the dog population has effectively reduced the number of cases seen, and in the main these only occur in unvaccinated dogs. Leptospirosis and tuberculosis are zoonoses (i.e., they can be passed from dog to susceptible human). Great care should always be taken when dog urine has to be handled, whether or not infection is suspected.

Infection reaches the urinary tract mainly by the ascending route (i.e. via the external orifices up the urethra), but can occasionally arise in the kidneys via the blood (haematogenous spread) or from infection in adjacent organs and tissues, e.g., a deep bite wound leading to a perirenal abscess. Infection may involve the whole urinary system or remain localised in the lower (bladder and urethra) or upper (kidneys and ureters) part of the tract. The establishment of infection and its disease-producing capability depends on a large number of factors, but risks are increased if there is damage to the urinary tract epithelium (lining), which can result from catheterisation of the urethra and bladder; anatomical and physiological abnormalities of the urinary tract preventing or interrupting normal urine flow and bladder emptying; dilution and alkalinity of the urine; poor general health; and specific illnesses, such as Cushing's syndrome (see Chapter 14, page 247) and diabetes mellitus (see Chapter 14, page 251).

Clinical features

(i) *Lower urinary tract:* Inflammation of the urinary system is often generalised but can be local. Thus inflammation of the prepuce and penis in males is called balanoposthitis, and of the vagina of bitches, vaginitis. Inflammation of the urethra is called urethritis, of the bladder, cystitis, and of the kidneys, nephritis. In the male, inflammation of the testes is called orchitis and of the prostate gland prostatitis. Infection leading to inflammation of the lower urinary tract usually produces a sudden onset of illness, which is relatively mild. It is often afebrile (the animal has a normal temperature) and animals usually remain well and eating. It is, however, quite distressing for both the animal and the owner, as it is accompanied by stinging irritation and pain, with frequent attempts being made to pass small quantities of urine, often containing blood. Very severe infections with pus-forming (pyogenic) bacteria, e.g., staphylococci, may lead to formation of cloudy, purulent urine, but this is uncommon in dogs.

(ii) *Upper urinary tract:* Infection in the kidneys can be localised (abscess) or generalised (pyelonephritis) and can affect one (unilateral) or both (bilateral) kidneys. The resulting disease can be sub-clinical, i.e., show no obvious illness. Nevertheless the disease may be insidious and chronic, eventually leading to chronic renal failure if untreated. In other cases, more severe bilateral kidney infection can lead to potentially fatal illness, with fever, dullness, reduced appetite, vomiting, kidney swelling and pain, and acute renal failure. In less severe cases, there may be a moderation of these signs and no renal failure. However, if treatment is not given or is ineffective (usually because it is not given for long enough), the condition may become chronic and lead to occasional acute relapses and eventually chronic renal failure.

Diagnosis

The presence of urinary tract infection is indicated by the demonstration of significant urinary tract pathogens in sufficient numbers in fresh, clean urine (i.e., uncontaminated samples in sterile containers). Infected urine may contain protein, blood, damaged epithelial cells and white blood cells (polymorphs) associated with pus formation; it is often alkaline, although canine urine is normally acidic. Blood samples may show increased numbers of white blood cells (indicating that infection is present) and evidence of renal failure if it is present. Lateral abdominal X-rays can be used to demonstrate kidney shadows, one or both of which may be enlarged in acute infections or reduced, often irregular in outline, in chronic infections. The bladder can also be easily visualised and thickened bladder walls in cases of chronic cystitis can be highlighted by the use of a pneumocystogram, which involves the infusion of air into the bladder, showing the inside of the bladder black in contrast to the white wall.

Treatment

Many simple cases of cystitis will respond to conservative management by enforced diuresis, normally achieved by promoting polyuria and polydipsia by adding salt to the food, and urinary acidification, by means of drugs such as ammonium chloride, d,l-methionine and sodium acid phosphate. In more severe cases, and in all cases of upper urinary tract infection, broad spectrum antibiotics must be used. Your veterinary surgeon will probably do an antibiotic sensitivity test on the bacteria, which may be cultured, preferably before antibiotic therapy is started. Antibiotics commonly used are ampicillin and amoxycillin, and potentiated sulphonamides. In recent years gentamicin has been used more frequently and is very effective in most cases, but is toxic to the kidneys and must be used under very careful veterinary supervision. Antibiotic therapy must be continued for long enough to be really effective and the minimum course should last 10 days, even if symptoms of illness have disappeared. Sometimes treatment has to be continued for four weeks. Recurrent episodes of cystitis require investigation for the possibility that a bladder stone (urolith) may be present.

Glomerular disease

For many years it was thought that the only disease regularly affecting the renal glomeruli was amyloidosis, in which non-inflammatory proteinaceous material becomes deposited in the glomeruli. This may be confined to the kidney, where it is associated with the breakdown of certain immunoglobulin proteins, or more widely distributed in a number of vital organs as a reaction to certain chronic, infectious, inflammatory or neoplastic diseases.

However, during the last 20 years it has been recognised that dogs can also develop glomerulonephritis, resulting from damage initiated by the formation or deposition of immune (antigen-antibody) complexes in the capillary walls of the glomeruli (membranous nephropathy) or in the mesangium – the structure holding the tuft of capillaries together – (proliferative glomerulonephritis). The underlying cause has been discovered in some cases, for example heartworm infection, in countries like the USA, where infection is endemic, some malignant tumours and generalised immune-mediated diseases like systemic lupus erythematosus. In the majority of cases the disease is of uncertain cause, for which the term idiopathic is used.

In both amyloidosis and glomerulonephritis, the damage to the glomerulus results in a leak of protein into the urine, which in many cases leads to the development of the nephrotic syndrome (see pages 195–6). At the same time, damaged glomeruli are being closed down, with the consequent death of nephrons, and resultant scarring and fibrosis. This progressive loss of nephrons and renal fibrosis leads inexorably to chronic renal failure. Thus dogs with glomerular disease develop a protein-losing nephropathy, may become nephrotic, and often eventually succumb to renal failure.

Clinical features

Clinical signs of a protein-losing nephropathy do not appear until large amounts of protein have been lost in the urine for a considerable time. When urine protein loss plus normal daily requirements exceeds daily dietary protein intake (a negative nitrogen balance) the dog begins to draw on its own protein, largely from muscle, and so begins to lose weight. Protein in the urine tends to attract water, which means the animal will urinate larger volumes more frequently (polyuria) and consequently will become thirsty (polydipsia). Unless chronic renal failure occurs early on, the only signs of a protein-losing nephropathy are therefore weight loss, polydipsia and polyuria. When blood protein falls below a critical level, variable from one animal to another, the nephrotic syndrome develops and the dog becomes oedematous.

Oedema can spontaneously regress and later recur, but more often requires to be dispersed with diuretic drugs (often called 'water tablets'). The intestine wall can also become oedematous and this may prevent absorption of digested food and water, leading to diarrhoea. In some cases of protein-losing nephropathy, large thrombi (aggregates of blood clotting factors) form in blood vessels, especially the pulmonary arteries, which carry blood from the heart to the lungs. If a pulmonary artery is occluded, then the animal develops severe respiratory distress and may die within a few hours. There is no treatment for this particular problem. Temperament changes leading to aggressive behaviour have also been noted in a few dogs with protein-losing nephropathies. At some time most dogs with a protein-losing nephropathy will show signs of chronic renal failure (Table 8) and this is progressive.

Diagnosis

The hallmarks of a protein-losing nephropathy are: (a) massive persistent proteinuria; and (b) reduced plasma albumin; and the nephrotic syndrome (a) and (b) plus (c) oedema, with or without evidence of chronic renal failure.

A definite diagnosis of the underlying disease can only be made by means of a renal biopsy, which involves either removing a small piece of kidney cortex using a special needle or cutting out a tiny wedge of kidney. The former can usually be done through a very small incision in the body wall, whereas the latter requires a laparotomy, a full surgical opening of the abdomen. Amyloid material can be readily recognised on stained sections by routine microscopy, while the immune-mediated diseases usually require examination using special stains, plus immunofluorescence and electron microscopy.

Treatment

There is no specific treatment for amyloidosis; however, dietary management may help to temporarily alleviate chronic renal failure and diuretic drugs should be used if the animal becomes nephrotic. Corticosteroid drugs are unhelpful in this condition, while for the immune-mediated diseases it is thought that immunosuppressive drugs like prednisolone (a corticosteroid) may help to reduce the number of immune complexes. Such drugs have been used in the treatment of similar diseases in man but with only limited success, and there is no real evidence that they are beneficial for glomerulonephritis in the dog.

Dogs losing protein but not in renal failure should be given increased dietary protein, either by means of extra food or improved quality, e.g., top-range cat food which normally contains more protein than dog food. However, either of these measures may precipitate diarrhoea. Egg is an ideal source of high-quality protein if the dog will eat it.

Oedema is usually responsive to diuretic drugs, frusemide being the most useful, and treatment should be stopped once the fluid has been cleared. Dogs on diuretic drugs are naturally thirstier, but excessive water intake should be discouraged in order to allow the drug to act as fully as possible on the oedema fluid. When a dog has a combined protein-losing nephropathy and chronic renal failure, treatment is more difficult because an increase in dietary protein will exacerbate chronic renal failure. However, in most cases it has been observed that as renal failure progresses, proteinuria diminishes. This is presumably because as more glomeruli are lost the surface area for protein loss is steadily reduced. In these dogs, therefore, renal failure is more of a threat than recurrence of the nephrotic syndrome, and so a reduced-protein diet is usually prescribed.

Prognosis

Most dogs with glomerulonephropathies live for only a few months following diagnosis. Those in renal failure have a poorer outlook than those with an uncomplicated protein-losing nephropathy or nephrotic syndrome, and dogs with membranous nephropathy have survived for more than a year. However, frequently recurring nephrotic episodes, intractable diarrhoea and aggressive behaviour are bad signs and often necessitate early euthanasia.

Chemical and drug toxicity (nephrosis) and renal ischaemia

Nephrotoxins can be classified in three broad groups:

(a) natural body constituents or products of metabolism which become toxic if normal levels are exceeded;
(b) drugs (including some anaesthetics) which may be prescribed, or to which the dog may gain access, or (rarely) be given deliberately; and
(c) chemical or inorganic poisons which may be inadvertently ingested (see Table 14 and also Chapter 27 Poisoning).

Nephrotoxins in sufficient amounts cause acute renal failure, which is normally severe and often fatal. In addition, acute renal failure of a similar

Table 14: Canine nephrotoxins

(a) *Toxic metabolites*
    myoglobin
    haemoglobin

(b) *Drugs*
    (i) anaesthetic – methoxyflurane
    (ii) antibiotics – aminoglycosides
                   amphotericin B
                   cephalosporins
                   sulphonamides
                   polymixin B
                   bacitracin
                   tetracyclines

(c) *Chemicals*
    ethylene glycol (antifreeze)
    heavy metals – lead, arsenic, mercury

(d) *Miscellaneous*
    injectable X-ray contrast media
    snake venom

kind can result from the effects of reduced renal blood flow (renal ischaemia) in such conditions as kidney injury, prolonged anaesthesia, severe shock, extensive burns and extremes of temperature (hypothermia and heatstroke).

In most of these conditions the kidney tubules are the prime target and lining epithelial cells are destroyed in large numbers. Epithelial cell debris blocks the tubule lumen, preventing urine flow, resulting in reduction in or absence of urine in the bladder (oliguria or anuria) and back pressure on the glomeruli reduces glomerular filtration. If the dog survives and urine begins to flow again, it is very dilute and remains so until the tubular epithelium has been re-established. However, this pre-regenerative polyuria is a good sign that recovery is taking place.

Clinical features

Toxic nephrosis leads to classical acute renal failure and the dog becomes suddenly and severely ill, with swollen painful kidneys. There is dullness, inappetence and repeated vomiting. Uraemic signs of foul breath, brown tongue and ulceration of the cheeks and tongue tip are likely if the condition lasts for more than 48 hours. Urine output is reduced or ceases completely until the recovery phase.

Diagnosis

Unless the condition has arisen because of known circumstances, e.g., a course of drug therapy, anaesthesia and surgery, severe shock, etc., or the dog has been seen to ingest toxic material, the specific underlying cause may never be discovered. Blood biochemistry will support the clinical findings of severe renal failure, but tests for specific poisons, e.g. heavy metals, are not readily available, and even if they are done, results are unlikely to be available until the dog is either dead or better. Certain poisons, e.g., ethylene glycol, one of the main constituents of anti-freeze used in car radiators, can be recognised on microscopic examination of the kidney, but again, this is usually a retrospective diagnosis. If the dog dies or is euthanased during the course of the illness, then microscopic examination of the kidneys will reveal the disruption of the tubules and necrosis of epithelial cells.

Treatment

Toxic nephrosis requires urgent and rigorous treatment. Intravenous fluid therapy for rehydration and encouragement of urine flow is vital, but must only be continued if urine flow is established. Diuresis can be encouraged by using diuretic drugs or infusions with osmotic substances like mannitol. In some cases the use of peritoneal dialysis may be considered by the veterinary surgeon, whereby a large volume of concentrated electrolyte solution is infused into the peritoneal cavity and then removed an hour later. The idea is to attract water and solutes, including urea, through the peritoneum into the dialysed fluid and these are then removed with the fluid, resulting in a reduction in blood urea levels. If the procedure is successful it needs to be repeated several times if it is to be of lasting benefit. Peritoneal dialysis requires intensive handling of the dog and may have detrimental effects on an already very ill animal; it is also very time consuming and expensive, so a careful prior assessment of its potential value in each individual case must be made.

Any drugs already in use must be stopped immediately and the dog should be given intensive nursing care. Specific treatments may be given if the underlying cause is definitely known. Repeated blood testing to measure kidney function will give a good indication as to the success or otherwise of the treatment.

Prognosis

Toxic nephrosis is always serious, but if the dog recovers from the acute illness, complete restitution of renal function is possible. In other cases there is residual damage, which, if severe enough, may lead to chronic renal failure.

Kidney trauma

Injuries to the kidneys may follow road accidents and other crushing incidents. The renal capsule may be ruptured and the kidney lacerated, or if the capsule remains intact, there may be intra-renal haemorrhage, severely increased renal pressure and necrosis. In either case the situation is serious, especially if both kidneys are affected. Badly lacerated kidneys may contribute to severe internal haemorrhage and possibly death, in addition to whatever effects there may be from reduced renal function. When only one kidney is affected, the other should function more than adequately, provided it is normal. It may be necessary to remove the damaged kidney as soon as is practicable after initial shock has been overcome.

Clinical features

These will vary according to the nature and extent of the damage and which other organs are involved. There should be a history of an accident and the dog is likely to be in a state of shock, probably collapsed, with very pale mucous membranes. The veterinary surgeon may find on palpation of the abdomen either one or both kidneys to be enlarged, bulbous, and painful or a mass in the kidney region of irregular shape. There may be mild distension of the abdomen if a large volume of blood is present. This will gradually be absorbed if the animal survives.

Diagnosis

This will be based on the history, clinical signs and evidence of free blood in the abdomen (confirmed by needle aspiration of the contents), or of misshapen kidney shadows on an abdominal X-ray. Final diagnosis may require an exploratory laparotomy operation.

Treatment

Initially treatment will be directed at counteracting shock and giving intensive care. Fluid or blood transfusions may be required and antibiotic and corticosteroid drugs administered. Surgery will be performed as soon as the animal can stand anaesthesia. Sometimes lacerated kidneys can be repaired, and subcapsular or intra-renal haemorrhages drained to reduce intra-renal pressure. In cases of severe unilateral damage, inspection of the other kidney for normality and prior renal function tests will help to determine whether or not the damaged kidney can be removed. If both kidneys are hopelessly damaged, euthanasia will be necessary. Whenever a post-traumatic laparotomy is performed, the integrity of the bladder will always be checked, as this organ is more vulnerable than the kidneys.

Prognosis

Traumatic renal damage is unlikely to heal without considerable scarring. However, this would have to be extensive and involve both kidneys for renal failure to occur and many dogs recover well. Dogs which require unilateral nephrectomy also do well provided the remaining kidney is in good condition. The outlook is poorer when both kidneys are severely lacerated or contused, or if infection is involved, e.g., following deep wounds caused by fighting.

Kidney tumours

The kidney can be affected by primary or secondary tumours. Primary tumours arise from cells or tissues within the kidney, while secondary tumours, arise elsewhere in the body and spread to the kidney, usually via the bloodstream.

Primary renal tumours are relatively uncommon and usually only affect one kidney. They tend to grow in one part of the kidney (focal) and it is unlikely that renal function will be disrupted. However, most primary kidney tumours are malignant and therefore will spread – often growing out of the kidney along blood vessels, usually the renal vein. The commonest type of primary tumour is the renal carcinoma.

Secondary renal tumours are more common and their appearance in the kidney depends on the nature of the primary tumour and both kidneys are likely to be affected. Since they have spread to the kidney from a primary site, they are by definition malignant tumours. In cases of carcinomas, i.e. tumours arising in epithelial cells, for example in the liver or ovary, secondary renal deposits tend to be focal and may only cause problems if they are many in number in both kidneys. In the case of sarcomas, i.e. tumours arising in connective tissue, spread into both kidneys is usual, and the infiltration is diffuse, i.e., the whole kidney is involved. Common secondary tumours include lymphosarcoma and haemangiosarcoma.

Clinical features

Primary tumours of the kidney may never be discovered as they may never lead to signs of renal failure. Aggressively destructive tumours like renal carcinomas may cause haemorrhage in the kidney and blood may be seen in the urine (haematuria). Occasionally an irregular-shaped kidney can be palpated and there may be local pain. Often the clinical signs may be related more to the effects of the tumour spreading out of the kidney than to the kidney itself.

Secondary tumours, because of their tendency to be bilateral and diffuse, are more likely to cause a reduction in renal capacity and lead to renal failure. The kidneys may feel grossly enlarged and misshapen but are seldom painful. However, it is unlikely that the degree of kidney failure will be more serious than effects of the tumour elsewhere in the body, e.g., in the liver or spleen, especially haemangiosarcomas, which are very vascular and fragile tumours and tend to rupture and bleed easily. Likewise lymphosarcoma can cause gross kidney enlargement and moderate renal failure, but is more likely to present as an illness unrelated to primary kidney disease. (See Chapter 28, page 481.)

Diagnosis

Primary kidney tumours may be suspected on clinical signs of weight loss, possibly mild renal failure and sometimes recurrent haematuria. Confirmation is aided by contrast radiography, ultrasound examination and exploratory surgery. Biopsy of affected kidney material should be diagnostic.

Secondary kidney tumours may be diagnosed as for primaries, or via other organs or tissues which may be involved.

Treatment

It is theoretically possible for a malignant tumour of the kidney to be successfully removed, as usually they are unilateral. However, it is unfortunate that in most cases the tumour has begun to spread by the time a diagnosis is made. If there is any evidence of metastasis, the situation is hopeless. Of the secondary tumours, lymphosarcoma is probably the only one which may respond well to chemotherapy, treatment being directed at the whole animal rather than just the kidneys. Some dogs with renal lymphosarcoma have lived for many months with chemotherapy. However, for most tumour situations the situation is regrettably hopeless at the present time.

Ureters

Although the ureters are vital to the flow of urine from the kidneys to the bladder, they seldom let the system down. Occasionally a kidney stone (urolith) becomes lodged in a ureter, and if the obstruction is not relieved quickly, hydronephrosis (i.e., a damming back of urine in the renal pelvis, with eventual destruction of the kidney if pressure is severe and prolonged) will develop in the associated kidney.

Rupture of the ureter with consequent leakage of urine into the peritoneal cavity can occur if a urolith lodges in one place and the ureteral wall ulcerates. External trauma leading to rupture of a ureter is possible but very rare.

Tumours of smooth muscle (leiomyomas) can occasionally arise in a ureter, leading to obstruction.

ECTOPIC URETERS

This is a congenital condition affecting mainly bitches, in which one or both ureters bypasses the bladder and empties into the urethra or vagina, less commonly into the uterus. The result is urinary incontinence and any young dog which suffers from genuine urinary incontinence, i.e. unconscious lack of control over urination, should be investigated for the condition. Certain breeds, including West Highland White Terriers, Fox Terriers, Miniature and Toy Poodles, Labrador Retrievers and Siberian Huskies, have a higher than normal risk of being affected.

Clinical features

The puppy is usually normal in every respect except that it dribbles urine frequently, as well as urinating normally. There is often a wet patch where the dog lies and larger volumes of urine may be passively passed on rising. The rear end is wet and smells of urine.

Diagnosis

This can be difficult and requires careful radiographic assessment following infusion of contrast medium into the vagina or intravenously.

Treatment

Surgical repositioning of the ureters into the bladder is essential if both are ectopic, but success is not guaranteed. Unilateral ectopia is often dealt with by removing the affected ureter and its associated kidney. The same procedure is required if reimplantation of a ureter into the bladder is unsuccessful.

Diseases of the urinary bladder

The bladder is a highly resilient organ, capable of considerable expansion and contraction as it fills slowly with urine and then empties relatively quickly. However, it is also a very vulnerable organ, open to trauma (see bladder rupture, page 194), infection (see cystitis, pages 200–202) and the presence of uroliths (page 213).

One of the most distressing and socially unacceptable conditions involving the bladder is urinary incontinence. There are a number of diseases which lead to incontinence, in addition to the problem of ectopic ureters (page 210). However, it is important that a distinction is made between true incontinence and uncontrolled conscious urination. The latter can occur in immature puppies not fully house-trained, undisciplined adult animals, frightened, cowed, over-excited puppies and dogs, and in animals which produce excessive volumes of urine (polyuria) due to underlying diseases, such as chronic renal failure, diabetes mellitus, diabetes insipidus, Cushing's syndrome, pyometra and certain liver diseases. True incontinence is said to occur when the animal passes urine in an uncontrolled and usually unconscious manner. This means that the animal is usually wet with urine and leaves a patch of urine wherever it lies for any length of time. Among the causes of true incontinence are:

(a) *Persistent urachus*
In the unborn foetus, a tube called the urachus runs from the bladder to the umbilicus and carries fluid waste to the placenta, where unwanted metabolites are absorbed by the dam's circulation and excreted in her urine. By birth the urethra is already in use and the urachus has closed, withering to a fibrous remnant. Very occasionally the urachus remains open and an affected puppy will be constantly wet at the umbilicus and along the ventral body wall. Although the abnormality can be corrected surgically when the puppy is old enough to withstand anaesthesia, breeders are often unwilling to put up with the social nuisance for so long and affected puppies are often put to sleep soon after a diagnosis has been made.

(b) *Acquired structural defects*
These can present as several problems, including fistulas (abnormal

permanent ways) linking the urethra with the rectum or the vagina in females, and those linking a ureter to the vagina, which can be a rare sequel to spaying. Adhesions of the bladder to another abdominal structure are not uncommon, usually to the uterine stump following spaying, or to the intestine after previous bladder or intestinal surgery. The bladder can be small or have a short neck, in which case it may lie in the pelvic canal (an intra-pelvic bladder). Associated sphincter problems, together with external pressure, lead to incontinence. Careful veterinary investigation is required to elucidate these problems and nowadays surgical correction of some of these conditions is successful.

(c) Outflow problems

Tumours in the neck of the bladder can interfere with the sphincter valve control, but often will earlier cause difficulty in urination. Stricture of the bladder neck, enlargement of the prostate gland and diseases of the urethra can all lead to incontinence, due to an increase in pressure within the bladder, which overcomes outlet (sphincter) resistance. These are all serious problems, but some, for example prostatic hyperplasia – a benign enlargement of the prostate gland – can be treated medically and others, for example uroliths in the urethra, can be dealt with surgically or by dietary management.

(d) Hormone imbalances

Spayed bitches and older castrated male dogs can suffer from incontinence due to the loss of hormones secreted by the ovaries and testes respectively. In many cases, hormone replacement therapy using oestrogen in bitches and testosterone in dogs will control the problem, although continuing courses of treatment are usually required. Care is needed to ensure a balance between controlling the incontinence and the development of undesirable side-effects. Overdosage of oestrogen will make a bitch become attractive to male dogs, while in the male, testosterone can lead to aggressive or hypersexual behaviour.

(e) Nerve control problems

Diseases affecting any level of the nervous system, from the brain, through the spinal cord to nerves supplying the bladder, can give rise to urinary incontinence. Such conditions include tumours of the nervous system or in related structures, traumatic injuries to nerves, intervertebral disc protrusions, infections of the nervous system and degenerative nerve diseases. If the sensory nerve supply from the bladder stretch receptors, or the motor nerves controlling the contraction of bladder wall muscles, are reduced or absent, then the bladder will not be voluntarily emptied. Thus it overfills, with involuntary passage of urine whenever the pressure within the bladder exceeds the urethral resistance. This condition is known as urinary retention with overflow. This form of urinary incontinence can be helped temporarily by the insertion of indwelling catheters, but these predispose to bladder infection; or twice daily manual expression of the bladder. However, a careful diagnostic and prognostic assessment is necessary before any more lasting treatment can be considered.

UROLITHIASIS

Because dogs produce concentrated (hypertonic) urine, water reabsorbed in the kidney tubules leaves urine supersaturated in respect of a number of salts and crystals are frequently present in urine samples. If crystals are allowed to accumulate in the renal pelvis or bladder, either because of difficulty in urination or decreased frequency of opportunity to urinate, then stones may begin to form. In dogs, they can be composed of any of five substances, and the composition and approximate rate of occurrence is given in Table 15 overleaf.

For crystals and stones to form, some or all of the following factors are involved:

1. A sufficiently high urine concentration of stone-forming constituents.
2. An adequate time in the urinary tract, i.e., the longer the time, the greater the chance.
3. A urine pH favourable to crystallisation (see Table 15).
4. A centre or nidus on which they can form – this can be a plug of cellular debris, a clump of bacteria or foreign material such as a suture.
5. For struvite uroliths, pre-existing urinary tract infection.

Clinical features

Uncommonly, stones may develop in the kidneys and cause obstruction to the outflow of urine from the renal pelvis, or they can become lodged in a ureter, leading to hydronephrosis. More usually they form in the bladder and affected dogs frequently have recurrent episodes of cystitis during the early stages. This is especially true of struvite stone formation. Once uroliths are present, and there can be from one stone up to several hundred in the bladder, urination is usually more frequent, often involves a degree of discomfort or pain, and the urine contains visible or invisible blood. Males may choose to squat to urinate.

Large stones stay in the bladder and act as an abrasive on the bladder wall, causing chronic cystitis until they are removed. Small stones, especially in males, may pass out of the bladder, and lodge at any point in the urethra. Common sites are the ischial arch, where the urethra curves round the back of the pelvis, and on the bladder side of the bone in the penis (os penis). Dogs with partial urethral obstruction have varying degrees of difficulty in passing urine, from simply taking longer to urinate

Table 15: Canine urolithiasis

Composition of stone	Occurrence
Struvite (magnesium phosphate plus small amounts of calcium and urate)	Up to 95% of all uroliths in the bitch and immature male; up to 75% of all uroliths in adult males.
Calcium oxalate (with small amounts of phosphate)	Up to 20% of all uroliths in adult males.
Ammonium urate (often with small amounts of phosphate and oxalate)	Up to 7% of all uroliths, especially in dogs with chronic liver disease and male Dalmatians.
Cystine	Up to 3% of uroliths in adult male dogs.
Silicate (made of silicon dioxide)	Up to 3% of uroliths in male dogs. German Shepherd Dogs especially, but reason unknown.

to passing urine, often blood-stained, in small spurts, usually from a squatting position and wearing a pained facial expression. In this situation dogs seldom empty their bladder, which increases the opportunity for further crystals and stones to form. If total urethral obstruction occurs, no urine is passed and the bladder becomes very distended, with potentially disastrous consequences, namely acute renal failure and possibly bladder rupture unless the obstruction is rapidly relieved.

Diagnosis

The clinical signs should arouse suspicion of urolithiasis, but other conditions have to be considered. These include tumours of the bladder and other hind-end locations such as prostatic disease in males and vaginal problems in bitches. Large bladder stones can sometimes be felt through the abdominal wall. Many calculi are visible on routine abdominal X-ray pictures and those which are not can be demonstrated by means of contrast media infused into the bladder via the urethra. The position and composition of calculi have to be taken into account in order that appropriate treatment can be given. For this reason it is important that urine should be examined for pH and the presence of crystals and bacteria. The predominant crystal type often helps in identifying the nature of the stone. If possible a stone should be obtained for accurate analysis; small ones can often be recovered from urine samples.

edisposing/causal factors	Treatment
creased dietary protein, magnesium d phosphorus; bacterial infection, eutral or alkaline urine.	Dietary management to control predisposing factors (e.g. Hill's Canine s/d diet). Maintain on Canine c/d diet to prevent recurrence. *Or* surgical removal.
creases dietary calcium, sodium, alate; vitamins D and C. Increased obilisation of body calcium; renal sease. Acid urine.	Surgical removal. Avoid recurrence with dietary management – a kidney disease diet. Alkalize urine.
creased dietary protein; inability of er to handle ammonia. Neutral to kaline urine.	Low-protein diet (e.g. Hill's Canine u/d diet). Allopurinol to prevent formation of uric acid.
herited defect in cystine reabsorption, x-linked in males. Acid urine.	Surgical removal. D-penicillamine. Alkalize urine.
obably a high dietary intake of icate. Acid urine.	Surgical removal. Avoid dietary plant protein/soil eating. Add salt to diet.

Treatment

Traditionally, treatment for urolithiasis has been almost entirely surgical, requiring either flushing techniques or more radical opening of the urethra and bladder. However, in recent years, with improved understanding of the nature and formation of calculi, a number of non-invasive regimes have been proposed involving the use of certain drugs and specially formulated diets. The latter are designed to provide much reduced dietary intake of the major constituents involved in the commonly encountered struvite stones (magnesium, ammonium and phosphate) as well as promoting the formation of acid urine. In combination with long-term antibiotic treatment for co-existing infection, dietary management of struvite stones is successful in many cases for both the dissolution of existing stones and prevention of new ones. Details of the various treatments available are given in Table 15.

HAEMATURIA

The presence of blood in urine has been mentioned already in relation to infection, tumours and trauma involving the kidneys and urinary tract. Haematuria is either visible as blood-stained or dark-coloured urine, or is occult, that is, red blood cells are present in the urine but in insufficient numbers to discolour it. Dip-stick tests for blood in urine are sensitive to the presence of occult blood. Pigments other than blood may also discolour urine, as follows:

1. Haemoglobin
If red blood cells are damaged or broken down (haemolysis) then haemoglobin is released, and if large amounts appear in urine, haemoglobinuria will be observed as very dark red-coloured urine. True haemoglobinuria results from haemolysis in the circulatory system, while false haemoglobinuria occurs following haemorrhage and haemolysis within the kidneys or urinary tract. In the latter case, empty red blood cells will also be seen in microscopic examination of the dark red urine.

2. Myoglobin
The sudden breakdown of excessive amounts of muscle, resulting in the release of large quantities of myoglobin – the oxygen-carrying pigment of muscle and closely related to haemoglobin in the blood – may lead to deep red-coloured myoglobinuria. It is potentially toxic to the kidneys and can cause nephrosis and acute renal failure in some cases. Myoglobinuria occurs in dogs subjected to sudden hard work, e.g., Greyhounds when racing, and in dogs suffering from acute muscle diseases, such as myositis.

3. Bilirubin
This is a breakdown product of haemoglobin and is normally excreted by liver, and much of it is eliminated via the kidneys, so it is present in small amounts in normal dog urine. Excessive amounts of bilirubin may circulate in the blood in cases of severe haemolysis and liver disease (often leading to jaundice) and when passed into the urine cause it to become a deep brown or khaki colour. Occasionally marked bilirubinuria can be confused with haematuria.

False haematuria
Blood appearing at the prepuce or vagina may not be of urinary tract origin. In males, prostatic and testicular diseases (prostatitis, prostatic tumours, orchitis) and trauma to the penis may lead to urethral haemorrhage. In addition, foreign bodies, trauma, infection and tumours in the prepuce (sheath) can also lead to blood appearing at the prepuce. In the bitch, vaginitis, oestrus, abortion, impending parturition, post-parturient bleeding and pyometra can all lead to vulval bleeding. All these conditions must be distinguished from true haematuria. The fact that blood from these sources may appear at times other than urination, and possibly with associated history, clinical or behavioural features, helps in their differentiation.

True haematuria

This requires investigation as to the site and reason for the haemorrhage. At the outset general haemorrhagic conditions, such as Warfarin poisoning (see Chapter 27), inherited blood-clotting defects and platelet deficiencies (see Chapter 9, page 141), need to be considered and ruled out. Thereafter, specific clinical features of kidney disease or lower urinary tract problems may lead to suspicion as to the level of the urinary tract involved and the possible cause. One condition which has been encountered in recent years, mainly in larger adult dogs, involves chronic haematuria arising from one or both kidneys, without other clinical signs. The disease has been called non-traumatic renal haematuria, but the cause of the condition is unknown. It is usually diagnosed on the basis of all other haematuric conditions being ruled out. Radiographic examination of the kidneys and bladder may reveal the presence of blood clots, but the shape and size of both kidneys and bladder are normal. Confirmation of the diagnosis is made at exploratory surgery, when the kidneys are examined externally, and if apparently normal, the ureters are cannulated upwards from the bladder. Urine coming down the cannulae can soon be recognised as containing blood. If the condition is unilateral, it is usual to remove the affected kidney. If bilateral then the dog has to live with the condition, which may resolve itself spontaneously in time.

Prostatic disease

The prostate is the only accessory sexual gland in the dog and it is a bilobed structure encircling the urethra just beyond the bladder neck, situated in the pelvic canal. A small amount of prostatic tissue is also present in the urethral wall. The gland produces seminal fluid which serves as a vehicle and life support medium for sperm produced in the testes.

In middle-aged and older dogs a number of diseases can affect the prostate. These lead to varying degrees of gland enlargement, usually resulting in the entry of the gland into the abdominal cavity over the brim of the pubic bone at the front of the pelvis. The effects of prostatic enlargement are to exert pressure downwards on the bladder and upwards to the rectum. Relatively few dogs with prostatic disease develop the common human male problems of dysuria and urinary incontinence but the passage of urine may be delayed and straining to pass urine and faeces may occur. Haematuria, especially towards the end of urination, is common. Continued straining due to prostatic enlargement may contribute to the development of perineal hernias (see Chapter 30 Ruptures and Hernias, page 517).

The diagnosis of prostatic disease rests on the appearance of clinical signs and is confirmed by means of rectal and abdominal palpation, X-ray pictures of the lateral posterior abdomen, gland washings via a urethral catheter, and biopsy techniques. More recently, ultrasound examination is proving very helpful.

There are three major types of prostatic disease:

(a) Benign prostatic hyperplasia. This is the commonest condition and up to 80 per cent of adult dogs over 5 years have some degree of prostatic hyperplasia. In many cases it is caused by a relative excess of androgen (male hormone). In addition cyst formation can arise and this is potentially more serious as it predisposes to the establishment of infection in the gland.

The condition is often sub-clinical and therefore undetected, but may be accompanied by haematuria (blood in the urine) and straining to defecate. The latter results in reluctance to attempt defecation in some dogs leading to constipation.

(b) Prostatic inflammation. This often arises additionally to hyperplasia, following infection by bacteria which commonly invade the urinary tract (see Urinary tract infections, page 200). Inflammation can be acute or chronic, with or without the formation of discrete abscesses, which may be single or multiple, small or large, closed or open (i.e., the pus may be locked in if closed or flow into the urethra if open).

The clinical signs depend partly on the severity of the infection and whether it is acute or chronic. Usually the dog is fevered, dull, reluctant to eat, and in abdominal pain. Straining, accompanied by obvious pain, occurs at attempts to urinate and defecate. Urine is often bloody and may also contain creamy-white pus. In severe cases the dog may have difficulty rising, stand with back arched and move with a stiff, guarded gait.

(c) Prostatic tumours. These are relatively uncommon in dogs compared with man. When they do occur, adenocarcinomas are the most likely type of tumour. These can spread to distant sites, such as bones. The clinical presentation is very similar to that seen in severe prostatic inflammation, and secondary infection of prostatic tumours is to be expected. In addition, nearby lymph nodes may also be enlarged and these can contribute to defecation difficulties. Urinary tract obstruction can also occur as a result of the pressure on ureters of prostatic tumours and associated lymph nodes.

Treatment

At present, there are few options for treating prostatic disease in the dog. In most cases, especially in hyperplasia, hormonal manipulation is the first choice. Successful cures are often achieved either by administration of oestrogens (female hormone), in tablet form or by injection, or castration. Oestrogens can be administered either in tablet form or by injection. Continued use of oestrogen can be a disadvantage for two reasons: firstly, the dog may become feminised and attract the attention of other male dogs; secondly, and more importantly, the consistency of the prostate gland substance may become much firmer and organised, preventing size reduction if castration is later carried out.

Whenever infection is present, whether due to prostatic inflammation or tumour, antibiotics are used. However, it is difficult to achieve high levels of many antibiotics in the prostate and a careful choice of antibiotic is necessary, together with a prolonged course of treatment. In cases of chronic prostatitis this can be for as long as eight weeks.

In addition to cysts associated with benign hyperplasia dogs can occasionally develop large paraprostatic cysts from embryonic duct remnants. Surgical drainage of large abscesses and cysts may be necessary and various techniques have been developed to achieve maximum and prolonged drainage. Pre-operative and continuing antibiotic therapy is also necessary.

Partial or total surgical removal of the prostate gland in the dog is both difficult and potentially dangerous. It is seldom carried out and is not recommended by most veterinary surgeons unless there are very special reasons for doing so.

13

THE NERVOUS SYSTEM

There are many circumstances during the normal functioning of the body when some action is initiated at a site remote from where the action is actually required. The 'message' is transmitted either by a humoral (chemical) mechanism or by a nervous (electrical) impulse.

The humoral mechanisms usually involve chemical secretions called hormones, produced by endocrine glands, and transported in the blood to their target site. Insulin is a good example of a humoral messenger; it is produced and released by the islet cells of the pancreas in response to an increase in glucose in the blood, e.g., after a meal. The insulin then controls the metabolism and utilisation of glucose by the body.

This chapter is concerned with the complex system of communication elaborated by the nervous system. Despite extensive research over centuries there are many aspects of the functioning of the nervous system that are still not fully understood. For example, it is clear that much voluntary, or conscious, activity originates in the part of the brain called the cerebral cortex, although the actual thought processes that comprise that origin remain a mystery.

The nervous system consists of a central neuraxis (i.e., the brain and spinal cord)* and a network of peripheral nerves that penetrate and supply the tissues of the body. The role of the nervous system in innervating the muscles of locomotion causing them either to contract or relax, is well known. Less familiar are the innervation of glandular tissue, promoting or inhibiting secretion and the regulation of blood vessel diameter.

The functional unit of the nervous system is the neuron, or nerve cell. Structurally a neuron is unlike any other cell in the body; it comprises a cell body, containing the nucleus and a number of processes or nerve fibres that either contact other cells or bear receptors for the detection of stimuli. Most nerve cell bodies are either within the central nervous system or

---

*There is a glossary of terms at the end of this chapter, page 235.

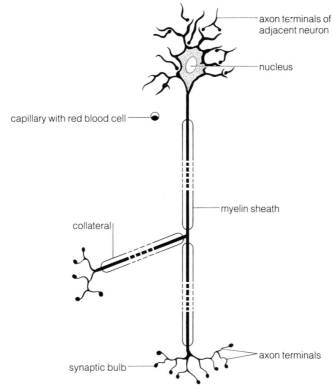

axon terminals of
adjacent neuron

nucleus

capillary with red blood cell

myelin sheath

collateral

synaptic bulb

axon terminals

Figure 103   A typical nerve cell

accumulated into ganglia very close to the brain or spinal cord. This means that some neurons are very long cells indeed; a touch receptor in the hindpaw of a dog has its cell body near the lumbosacral spinal cord, so its nerve fibre could be at least one metre long in a Great Dane.

The peripheral nerve fibres are called afferent (sensory) fibres if they conduct impulses towards the central nervous system, or efferent (motor) fibres if they conduct impulses away from the CNS.

The impulse conducted by a nerve fibre resembles an electrical current, although it is really a chemical change that is propagated along the nerve fibre. The impulse can be transmitted from one nerve cell to another, so that nervous activity can be generated over a large network of cells, or passed through a relay of nerve cells within a specific pathway.

Typically, a nerve cell has many processes. There are numerous dendrites that carry impulses towards the cell body and a single axon that carries an impulse away from the cell body towards several branching axon terminals. The axon terminals each end at a small swelling or synaptic bulb. This is part of the specialised structure called a synapse, through

Figure 104
Diagram of a synapse

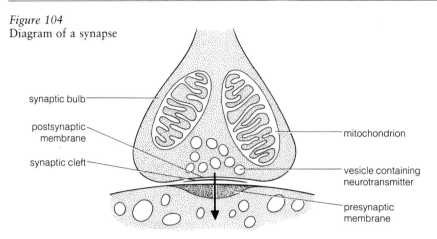

synaptic bulb

postsynaptic membrane

synaptic cleft

mitochondrion

vesicle containing neurotransmitter

presynaptic membrane

which the transmission of an impulse from one nerve cell to another must take place. The axon terminals may form synapses either with cell bodies or dendrites. Within the synaptic bulbs are small vesicles containing transmitter substance. During synaptic transmission the transmitter substance is released into the gap, or synaptic cleft, between the synaptic bulb and the postsynaptic membrane of the adjacent neuron. The transmitter substance is either excitatory or inhibitory, influencing the electrical activity of the postsynaptic cell accordingly. In fact, many excitatory stimuli may be necessary before a cell is sufficiently excited to propagate the impulse along its axon. The level of excitation at which a nerve cell does fire is known as the threshold. In the convulsive activity of epilepsy the thresholds of neurons are lower than normal so that premature electrical discharges occur.

The speed at which an impulse travels along a nerve fibre is known as the conduction velocity, and is related to the diameter of the nerve fibre and whether it possesses a myelin sheath. Large-diameter fibres conduct impulses more quickly than smaller ones. The myelin sheath that surrounds some nerve fibres consists of a spiral of lipid-protein produced by Schwann cells in the peripheral nervous system, and oligodendroglia cells in the neuraxis. Myelinated axons have a faster conduction velocity than unmyelinated axons. As an approximate guide, the conduction velocity (in metres per second) of myelinated fibres is given by multiplying the diameter of the nerve in microns by a factor of 6. The largest myelinated fibres are those conveying sensory information about muscle contraction (muscle proprioception) to the brain; these fibres have a diameter of 20 microns and so conduct impulses at 120 metres per second, or 270 miles per hour. In disease processes in which myelin either does not form properly, or becomes degenerated, conduction velocity is slowed and nerve function severely affected.

The central nervous system consists of the brain and spinal cord. They are both developed from a single neural tube extending along the dorsal midline of the embryo. Sometimes, during development in the mother's uterus, the formation of the neurons is adversely affected by some influence, e.g., genetic, viral, toxic. The result may be failure of the neural tube to fuse in the midline (spina bifida) or failure to close the entry to the tube in the head (anencephalus). There are many other possible anomalies.

The brain and spinal cord are both well protected by bone. The brain is entirely encased by the skull and the spinal cord lies along the canal extending through the chain of vertebrae. Sometimes these rigid surroundings are a disadvantage; if the brain suffers haemorrhage or swelling it cannot expand, so that a life-threatening rise in intracranial pressure occurs. Damage or distortion of the vertebrae or the intervertebral discs invariably involves the spinal cord and results in neurological deficits.

THE BRAIN

The brain is a very complex organ and includes the following important divisions:

> Cerebral cortex
> Thalamus
> Hypothalamus
> Pons
> Cerebellum
> Medulla oblongata

The *cerebral cortex* includes projection areas which receive sensory information such as vision, hearing, touch and pain, allowing these sensations to reach a conscious level (Fig. 105). In addition, there are large areas that can initiate motor (muscle) activity. In man, 85 per cent of the cerebral cortex is concerned with association. This is the complex function of processing information, comparing with previous experiences, selecting a suitable response and predicting the consequences. In dogs only 20 per cent of the cerebral cortex is concerned with association.

The cerebral cortex comprises two cerebral hemispheres and each of these possesses four lobes (Figs. 106, 107). The frontal lobe and the temporal lobe are important behavioural areas, contributing to the alertness, intelligence and temperament of the individual. Lesions in the temporal lobes of dogs are sometimes responsible for behavioural changes, e.g., aggression, hysteria, compulsive licking. Lesions anywhere in the cerebral cortex may cause epilepsy.

The *thalamus* is an important relay station for sensory information which arises at the periphery (e.g., vision, hearing, touch, pain) and is then projected from the thalamus to the cerebral cortex. In addition, the thalamus is part of the mechanism that monitors and regulates the motor activity initiated in the cerebral cortex. Lesions of the thalamus are rare in the domestic animals (Fig. 105).

The *hypothalamus* is a principal component of the autonomic nervous system within the neuraxis. It exerts a general integrating control over homeostasis (Fig. 105).

An important function of the hypothalamus lies in its control over the release of the pituitary hormones, themselves humoral messengers with a diversity of actions. Thirst, hunger and body temperature are all regulated

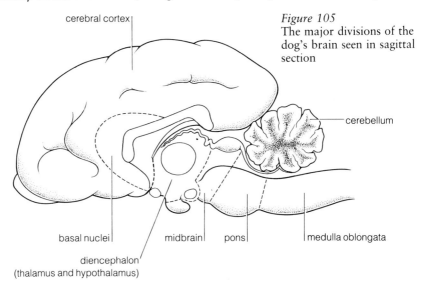

Figure 105
The major divisions of the dog's brain seen in sagittal section

cerebral cortex

cerebellum

basal nuclei   midbrain   pons   medulla oblongata

diencephalon
(thalamus and hypothalamus)

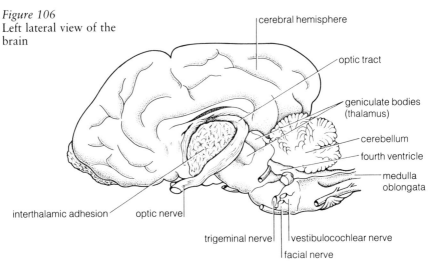

Figure 106
Left lateral view of the brain

cerebral hemisphere

optic tract

geniculate bodies
(thalamus)

cerebellum

fourth ventricle

medulla
oblongata

interthalamic adhesion   optic nerve

trigeminal nerve   vestibulocochlear nerve

facial nerve

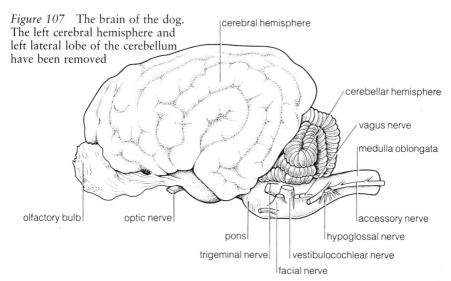

Figure 107 The brain of the dog. The left cerebral hemisphere and left lateral lobe of the cerebellum have been removed

cerebral hemisphere

cerebellar hemisphere

vagus nerve

medulla oblongata

olfactory bulb

optic nerve

accessory nerve

pons

hypoglossal nerve

trigeminal nerve

vestibulocochlear nerve

facial nerve

by specific centres within the hypothalamus. The emotions of rage and aggression also seem to originate in the hypothalamus, although they are normally inhibited by the hippocampus and the frontal lobe of the cerebral cortex. The rabies virus invades the hippocampus and removes this inhibition so that the powerful aggressive urges of the hypothalamus are allowed to prevail.

The *pons* is a prominent, saddle-shaped structure on the underneath of the brain (Figs. 105, 106). It provides a pathway for nerve fibres passing to the cerebellum from the higher centres. In addition, the pons includes a micturition centre for the higher centre control of urination.

The *cerebellum* is the co-ordinating centre of the brain. It has a complex tree-like appearance and lies towards the hind part of the brain (Figs. 105–107). The cerebellum receives information about intended muscle activity from other parts of the brain (e.g., the cerebral cortex) and compares it with information from stretch receptors in muscles and tendons. This function of the cerebellum represents a feedback mechanism for muscle activity, ensuring precision of movement. Lesions of the cerebellum invariably result in clinical signs of clumsiness, tremors and exaggerated movements.

The *medulla oblongata* is the most caudal part of the brainstem and is continuous with the spinal cord through the foramen magnum of the skull (Figs. 105–107). The medulla contains a number of important accumulations of neurons, called centres (e.g., respiratory centre, cardiac centre), which have special roles in the control of specific body functions. A number of cranial nerves also have their origins within the medulla in areas of grey matter called nuclei. The medulla also provides a roadway for many tracts passing to or from the spinal cord.

THE SPINAL CORD

The spinal cord of the dog is between half and one centimetre in diameter. It extends from the foramen magnum to the level of the seventh lumbar vertebra (Fig. 108). In cross-section the central region of grey matter and the outer region of white matter are clearly visible (Fig. 109). The grey matter consists of neuron cell bodies, whilst the white matter is made up of axons ascending or descending through the cord. The term 'white matter' refers to the prevalence of the white myelin in these areas. Throughout the length of the spinal cord pairs of spinal nerves leave the cord at intervals corresponding to the vertebrae. These spinal nerves each arise by a dorsal and a ventral root and give origin to the peripheral nerves, which ramify through the tissues.

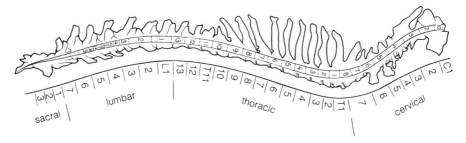

Figure 108   Sagittal section of the spine of the dog showing the relationship of the spinal cord segments to the vertebrae

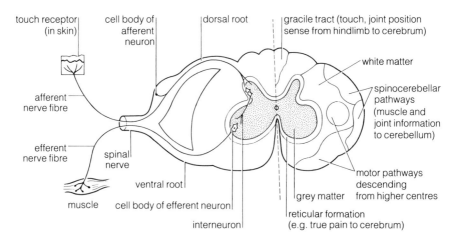

Figure 109   Transverse section of spinal cord. The left side shows a simple reflex arc. The right side shows the position of some of the ascending and descending tracts

THE PERIPHERAL NERVES

The peripheral nerves are the bundles of axons that extend from the body organs and tissues to the spinal cord. Most of these nerves are mixed, i.e., they contain both efferent and afferent nerve fibres. The efferent fibres mainly supply innervation to the muscles, whilst the afferent fibres carry information about modalities such as pain, touch, temperature and tendon stretching. When important peripheral nerves like the radial nerve in the forelimb or the sciatic nerve in the hindlimb are damaged, there is a paralysis of the muscles that they supply. In addition, many peripheral nerves supply areas of skin with a variety of pain and touch receptors so that damage to these nerves results in desensitisation, or analgesia.

THE MENINGES

Both the brain and spinal cord are enclosed in three thin membranous layers, collectively called the meninges. The innermost layer, the pia mater, is adherent to the nervous tissue. The sub-arachnoid space separates the pia mater from the middle layer, the arachnoid mater. The outermost layer, the dura mater, is the toughest of the meninges and is separated from its bony surroundings by the epidural space, which is fat-filled, around the spinal cord.

The sub-arachnoid space contains a watery liquid, cerebrospinal fluid, and is continuous with the cavities of the brain, the ventricles.

Neurological disease in dogs

It is beyond the scope of this chapter to discuss every neurological disease that may affect dogs. It is of more practical value to describe the common signs of neurological disease and to consider their likely origin and significance. Certain conditions, however, do provide good examples of the types of neurological disorder that occur in this species and accordingly some specific diseases are discussed at the end of this section.

PARESIS/PARALYSIS

A complete absence of voluntary motor activity of muscles is called paralysis, whereas a weakness of muscle use is known as paresis. In either case there is a disturbance of the innervation of the affected muscles somewhere between the initiation of motor activity in the brain and the terminal connection of the nerve fibres to the muscle.

When the lesion involves the peripheral nerve itself, the muscles become flaccid and may even begin to lose volume after about seven days. This

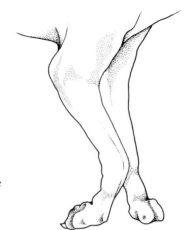

Figure 110 Characteristic stance of a dog suffering from radial paralysis of the right forelimb

type of disorder is known as a lower motor neuron (LMN) syndrome. Another characteristic of LMN disease is the loss of spinal reflex activity, e.g., the patellar reflex. Radial paralysis is a frequent sequel to a road traffic accident in dogs. This is a disorder in which the nerve is damaged, often at its roots; the dog is unable to bear weight on the limb and tends to stand with the forepaw knuckled over (Fig. 110). Radial paralysis is a potentially serious condition, since the damage may be too severe for reparation of the nerve to occur.

Damage to the spinal cord above the level of the lumbosacral outflow to the hindlimb often results in an upper motor neuron (UMN) syndrome. In this case muscle tone tends to be increased and the spinal reflexes are exaggerated. Intervertebral disc protrusions at the level of the twelfth thoracic to fourth lumbar vertebrae frequently result in a UMN syndrome of the hindlimbs. In these circumstances it may be necessary to surgically relieve the pressure on the spinal cord, although conservative treatment may yield good results. The choice between a surgical and a non-surgical approach depends on a number of factors, e.g., in a patient in which pain sensation has been lost from the limbs, surgery should commence within four to six hours of the onset of signs if there is to be any hope of recovery.

ATAXIA

A clumsy, unco-ordinated gait is called ataxia. Stumbling when turning corners, involuntary knuckling of the paws and swaying of the hindquarters are all signs of ataxia. This disorder results from a disturbance of the spinocerebellar pathways conducting information about the stretching of muscles and tendons. The spinocerebellar nerve fibres within the spinal cord are large and possess a lot of myelin; they are thus very vulnerable to damage if their blood supply is reduced. In 'Wobbler' syndrome in some breeds of dogs the distortion of the vertebral canal by displaced cervical vertebrae results in a compression of the blood vessels supplying the spinal cord at that level so that ataxia is an early sign of this condition.

Ataxia may also be a feature of disease of the cerebellum. Congenital deficits in cerebellar neuron metabolism may occur in young dogs of a number of breeds; the clinical signs are of a slowly progressive cerebellar ataxia.

SEIZURES OR FITS

A seizure is a short-lived episode of abnormal motor or behavioural activity. The term epilepsy refers to any condition in which seizures are recurrent. The most familiar type of seizure is the one in which there is a brief loss of consciousness and convulsive muscle activity, often accompanied by salivation and involuntary defaecation and urination. Such an episode is often called a grand mal seizure and is the physical manifestation of a generalised premature discharge of neurons of the forebrain. Sometimes the abnormal electrical activity is restricted to a discrete focus of neurons so that the bizarre physical or behavioural activity is only related to the part of the brain in which the focus is situated. Seizure foci induce partial seizures, although sometimes these undergo secondary generalisation.

Most partial seizures result from acquired foci so that the recognition of localising signs as evidence of a seizure focus is an important part of the diagnostic routine. Generalised seizures may be congenital in origin, due to a diffuse lesion, e.g., encephalitis (inflammation of the brain), or secondary to disease elsewhere in the body, e.g., renal or cardiac conditions.

A high proportion of cases of generalised seizures show no physical, haematological or biochemical abnormalities. These cases are labelled as idiopathic epilepsy because their true cause is not determined. Although idiopathic epilepsy has been definitely shown to have an inherited basis in only a few breeds, e.g., German Shepherd and Keeshond, inheritance is suspected in many others, e.g., Irish Setter, Beagle, Golden Retriever, etc.

The management and treatment of the seizure case depends on a clear understanding of the potential difficulties. Anticonvulsant drugs must be carefully chosen for a minimum of side-effects, maximum effectiveness and low cost. Anticonvulsant therapy should not be commenced in any dog that has suffered only one or two isolated seizures. The dosing regime aims to maintain a fairly consistent therapeutic blood level of the drug; wide excursions in concentration may actually induce seizures. Many epileptic dogs can be adequately controlled on an appropriate anticonvulsant therapy, and in a proportion of cases it is even possible to gradually withdraw therapy after effecting a 'pharmacological cure'.

It is important that any underlying cause of seizures should be identified and treated appropriately. It is worth remembering that idiopathic epilepsy generally shows an onset at one to three years of age, and that seizure activity is very rarely the first sign of the existence of a brain tumour.

VESTIBULAR SIGNS

The vestibular apparatus is concerned with maintaining the balanced posture of the individual. The peripheral components comprise the structures of the inner ear, e.g., the semicircular canals, whilst the central connections are within the medulla oblongata. The characteristic signs of vestibular disease are loss of balance, leaning to one side, head tilt and nystagmus (rapid eye movement). Sometimes the loss of balance is so severe that the dog compulsively rolls over and over. If these signs are accompanied by ataxia and/or paresis, the lesion involves the brainstem. Signs of peripheral vestibular disease may result from the extension of inflammation from the external and middle ears.

A vestibular syndrome of very rapid onset (hours) can occur in any breed of dog, usually middle to old-aged. This condition is often misdiagnosed as a 'stroke'. At post mortem in some of these cases no evidence of a vascular accident has been found. Most cases of this idiopathic vestibular syndrome show good recovery within 72 hours.

An idiopathic vestibular syndrome affecting litters of puppies at five to six weeks of age (e.g., Dobermann, German Shepherd) is recognised. The severity of the signs varies between individuals and many show hearing deficits. Most of these puppies, however, are very much improved by 12 weeks, when a slight head tilt may be the only residual sign.

VISUAL DEFICITS

A thorough examination of the eyes of any dog suffering from neurological disease can provide very important diagnostic information. There are a number of reflexes that depend on an intact visual pathway and functional efferent pathways to the muscles of the eyelids, the orbit and the iris. Tests which elicit these reflexes can be used to localise the lesion to the eyes, the optic nerves, the thalamus, the cerebral cortex, the brainstem or the specific cranial nerves representing the efferent pathways.

Sudden bilateral blindness in the dog is usually due to optic neuritis, an inflammatory reaction of the optic nerves. The cause is not clear, but the response to corticosteroid therapy is often dramatic.

COMA

The main centre for consciousness in the brain is located in the reticular formation of the midbrain. When this region becomes compressed or suffers direct traumatic damage the dog suffers an altered state of consciousness, from depression to coma.

Traumatic damage to the cerebrum may result in haemorrhage and accumulation of fluid and when this occurs the intracranial pressure rises and the cerebrum is forced to expand back towards the cerebellum and midbrain. The result is a gradual compression of the midbrain with consequent development of coma. The neurons which innervate the constrictor muscle of the iris are also located in the midbrain, so that the onset of coma is often accompanied by progressively dilating pupils.

Specific neurological conditions

The various conditions that may affect the nervous system of the dog can be classified according to the pathological process by which they develop. In the following selection of conditions an example of each type of process has been chosen.

CANINE DISTEMPER

The virus of canine distemper commonly causes inflammation of the brain (encephalitis) and/or the spinal cord (myelitis)*. Several distinct clinical syndromes are now recognised as due to infection with distemper virus.

In young dogs distemper is characterised by systemic signs of vomiting, coughing and an oculonasal discharge. The neurological signs that develop are varied and reflect a multifocal distribution of the inflammation. Paresis, ataxia, disorientation, depression and seizures provide the usual evidence of central nervous system involvement. Typically, affected dogs develop rhythmical muscle spasms in either the face or the limbs.

Mature dogs between the ages of 4 and 8 years may develop a more chronic form of encephalitis through infection with canine distemper virus. Even vaccinated dogs may develop this form of distemper. The slowly progressive neurological signs are not preceded by the systemic signs seen in younger animals. Paresis, paralysis and ataxia are the usual signs of this disease and seizures and muscle spasms do not occur. The inflammation is usually restricted to the cerebellum and adjacent brainstem, and does not involve the cerebral cortex. Often this disease becomes clinically static.

---

* Myelitis: inflammation of the spinal cord should not be confused with myelitis referring to inflammation of bone marrow as in osteomyelitis.

So-called old-dog encephalitis has been attributed to infection with canine distemper virus. This is a slowly progressive inflammatory disease of the brain in dogs over six years of age. In contrast to the distemper encephalitis of mature dogs, described above, the lesions of old-dog encephalitis involve the cerebral cortex. The clinical signs of this disease are visual impairment, depression, circling, head-pressing and aimless wandering. There are no systemic signs.

MYELOPATHY IN THE GERMAN SHEPHERD DOG

A number of degenerative diseases of the nervous system have been described in dogs. Chronic degenerative radiculomyelopathy (CDRM) in the aged German Shepherd is a good example, although the disease has now been recorded in a number of other large breeds. Affected dogs are usually over eight years of age and show a slowly progressive (over several months) hindlimb ataxia and paresis. An early sign is knuckling of the hindpaws, especially when turning corners. Pathologically the lesions are restricted to the thoracic spinal cord and dorsal nerve roots; both grey and white matter undergo degeneration. An hereditary basis for this disease is suspected, although the aetiology is obviously complicated. The prognosis for dogs affected with CDRM is poor since they gradually become completely paraplegic. A whole variety of so-called treatments has been recommended, e.g., steroids, vitamins, strychnine, blackcurrant seed oil, but none of these has any influence on the pathological process, although they may improve a concurrent arthritis.

Degenerative diseases of the nervous system may also involve the peripheral nerves; progressive axonopathy, an inherited disease in the Boxer, is an example.

FIBROCARTILAGINOUS EMBOLISM

Although true stroke is a very rare occurrence in dogs, there are other examples of diseases that disturb the blood supply to nervous tissue. Fibrocartilaginous embolism (FCE) is a syndrome of acute obstruction of the blood supply to a segment of spinal cord. Affected dogs are usually mature individuals of the large breeds, although there is a high incidence amongst Miniature Schnauzers. Typically there is an acute (minutes to hours) onset of ataxia, paresis or total paralysis on one side. The condition is not usually painful and shows stabilisation after about 24 hours. Most cases make a functional recovery within 7–14 days; if no improvement is seen in this time the prognosis is very poor. The cause of FCE is thought to be the sudden obstruction of spinal cord blood vessels by fragments of intervertebral disc.

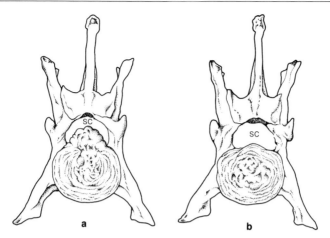

Figure 111 Diagram to show two types of intervertebral disc protrusion, (a) sudden explosive prolapse, (b) gradual bulging of the disc. The spinal cord lies within the canal at sc

INTERVERTEBRAL DISC DISEASE

Between the bodies of successive vertebrae are small discs of cartilaginous material. The very centre of each disc consists of a jelly-like substance that undergoes degeneration and sometimes calcification as part of the normal ageing process. In some breeds, e.g., Dachshund and Pekingese, this degeneration occurs at an early age (eight months to two years), whereas in most other breeds the changes occur at 8–10 years. The loss of elasticity of the discs makes them liable to rupture, when they become extruded into the spinal canal and compress the spinal cord.

Disc protrusions are of two types: (a) a sudden explosive prolapse of disc material, or (b) a slower bulging of the disc (Fig. 111). Both types are examples of trauma to the central nervous system. The commonest site for a disc protrusion is at the thoracolumbar junction, but cervical disc protrusions occur frequently. The clinical signs of disc protrusions include varying degrees of paresis, paralysis, loss or exaggeration of reflexes and incidence of local pain.

The assessment of a case of intervertebral disc protrusion, and the choice of therapy, conservative or surgical, takes account of a number of factors. A complete loss of pain sensation below the lesion is a very bad prognostic sign and indicates a need for urgent decompression.

NEOPLASIA

Many different types of tumour of the nervous system and meninges of the dog have been recorded. Primary tumours of the nervous system in the dog are found more frequently in the brain than in the spinal cord and peripheral nerves. The clinical signs reflect the location of the tumour within the nervous system. Affected animals are usually over five years of age, but certain tumours can occur in dogs under one year of age.

STORAGE DISEASES

A number of storage diseases are now recognised in dogs. These are conditions in which there is an inherited deficit of an intracellular enzyme so that a normal metabolic substance cannot be broken down. As a result the substance accumulates in the cells and seriously disrupts their function. Neurons are particularly vulnerable to this disturbance since they can neither divide nor discard the unwanted substance.

The neurological signs of storage diseases are various, although ataxia, tremor and visual deficits are common. The signs are not apparent until the puppy is about three months of age, since it takes that long for the substance to accumulate.

BOTULISM

This is an example of toxicity of the nervous system. The bacterium *Clostridium botulinum* produces a very potent toxin which blocks transmission of impulses from nerves to muscles. Dogs may become affected by ingesting dead seabirds or other carrion. There is a rapid onset (hours to two days) of a generalised flaccid paralysis. Most dogs will recover from botulism with appropriate treatment and attentive nursing.

GLOSSARY OF TERMS

analgesia   elimination or absence of pain sensation.

axon   long or short process of a nerve cell, conducting impulses away from the cell body

cervical vertebrae   the bones of the axial skeleton (spine) of the neck.

corticosteroids   a family of drugs including the naturally produced hormones of the cortex of the adrenal gland.

encephalitis   inflammation of the brain.

dendrite   long or short process of a nerve cell, conducting impulses from the periphery towards the nerve cell body.

homeostasis   the maintenance of physiological stability within the body.

meningitis   inflammation of the meninges, three layers of thin membranous tissue that surround the brain and spinal cord.

micturition   process by which the urinary bladder is emptied.

modality   sensation, e.g., touch, pain.

myelin   compound consisting of fat and protein that surrounds some nerve fibres within both the central and peripheral nervous systems.

myelitis   inflammation of the spinal cord.

neuraxis   the brain and spinal cord.

neuritis   inflammation of a peripheral nerve.

paralysis   complete loss of voluntary movement.

paresis   a deficit of voluntary movement seen as a muscle weakness.

pituitary gland   an important endocrine gland on the ventral surface of the brain; it secretes a whole variety of hormones and largely controls the function of the other endocrine glands of the body.

projection areas   discrete areas of the cerebral cortex with specific functions, e.g., primary motor cortex, visual cortex.

proprioception   position sense.

synapse   the point of communication between nerve cells.

thoracolumbar vertebrae   the bones of the axial skeleton (spine) located in the chest and abdomen.

14

THE ENDOCRINE SYSTEM

The many activities which take place within the body of a dog need to be regulated and co-ordinated. Obviously the nervous system (Chapter 13) plays a major role, but the endocrine system is also essential in achieving proper control and integration of body functions. The endocrine system consists of a number of glands (endocrine glands) whose secretions, known as hormones, are discharged directly into the blood. They tend to act in a similar way to chemical catalysts in changing the rate at which reactions proceed in the body, and most of them act at a number of different sites. As a result, disorders of hormone production often produce a variety of clinical signs.

There are seven major endocrine glands (Fig. 112). These are the pituitary, thyroid, parathyroid and adrenal glands and also the pancreas, ovaries and testicles. Although other organs, such as the stomach, kidney and liver, also produce hormones they are not regarded *primarily* as endocrine glands. The last three endocrine glands named above also have other major functions; the pancreas produces pancreatic juice required in

Figure 112 Locations of the major endocrine glands of the dog

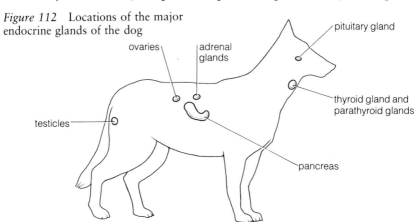

the digestion of food (Chapter 8), the ovaries produce eggs and the testicles produce sperm – both, of course, required for reproduction. The role of the ovaries in producing the female hormones oestrogen and progesterone, and that of the testicles in producing the male sex hormone testosterone, is bound up with the subject of reproduction and is therefore best dealt with under that heading (Chapter 11). The other major endocrine glands, and their hormones, are dealt with in this chapter.

Pituitary gland

This is a small oval organ connected to the underside of the brain by a short stalk (Fig. 113, overleaf). It is subdivided into an anterior lobe and a posterior lobe, each of which produces more than one hormone.

The anterior lobe produces the growth hormone (responsible for the regulation of growth), the thyroid stimulating hormone (TSH, which controls the production of thyroid hormone by the thyroid gland), the adrenocorticotrophic hormone (ACTH, which regulates hormone production from the outer layer [cortex] of the adrenal glands), and also hormones which control the activities of the ovaries and the testicles (referred to as gonadotrophic hormones). It also synthesises hormones regulating lactation (luteotrophic hormone or prolactin) and pigmentation in the skin (melanocyte-stimulating hormone).

Thus the anterior lobe of the pituitary gland exerts a major influence over the functioning of other endocrine glands.

The posterior lobe of the pituitary releases two hormones. One of them prevents the uncontrolled loss of water through the kidney (diuresis) that would otherwise occur. Accordingly it is known as antidiuretic hormone (ADH), which regulates the extent to which water is reabsorbed in the kidney after being filtered, so that it can be conserved in the blood rather than being lost in the urine. The second hormone, oxytocin, stimulates the contraction of smooth muscle, and in particular of the uterus at the time of giving birth.

The production and release of all these hormones is itself controlled by an adjacent part of the brain, the hypothalamus. In the case of many of the hormones a complex 'feed-back' mechanism operates to ensure that the output of the hormone closely matches the requirements for it, but unfortunately if the gland becomes diseased these mechanisms do not operate efficiently.

DISORDERS OF THE PITUITARY GLAND

Pituitary dwarfism

A lack of growth hormone during the normal growth phase of development results in an animal which is stunted, though perfectly proportioned,

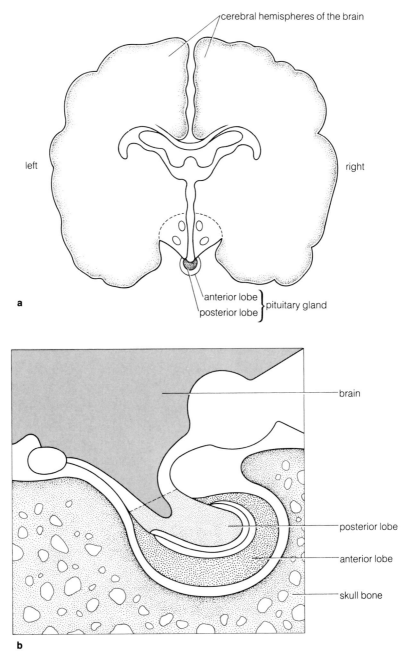

Figure 113 The pituitary gland
(a) Section across the brain to show the pituitary gland on its lower surface
(b) Section of the brain from front to back to show the division of the pituitary gland
   into lobes and its situation within a small cavity in the skull bone

and which retains for much longer than usual many of the puppy characteristics, e.g., a fluffy hair coat, a shrill bark and its first (milk, or deciduous) teeth. This is generally an inherited disorder, e.g., in the German Shepherd Dog and the Alaskan Malamute.

Usually a lack of growth hormone is associated with a lack of other hormones also, particularly thyroid hormone and the gonadotrophic hormones. Treatment, although possible, is usually expensive and disappointing.

Acromegaly

Excessive growth hormone production in adults results in this comparatively rare disorder. There is overgrowth of both soft and bony tissue, particularly around the head, which results in snoring, the impression of the skin being too large for the dog (causing folds on the head, neck and legs), exaggerated spaces between the teeth and a reduced tolerance of exercise. It is seen primarily in bitches, because progesterone (produced by the ovary in the dioestrus phase of the oestrous cycle, i.e., immediately after being in heat) and synthetic progesterones (i.e., progestagens, given to control oestrus) stimulate growth hormone production. The obvious treatment therefore is to spay the animal or discontinue the offending drug.

Diabetes insipidus

The kidneys are continually filtering water from the blood that passes through them, and then reabsorbing (i.e., putting back into the blood) a greater or lesser proportion of it in order to keep the water content of the blood plasma relatively constant. Efficient reabsorption requires an adequate level of antidiuretic hormone (ADH); the more ADH there is released, the more water is reabsorbed and the less urine there is formed. In diabetes insipidus the synthesis of ADH is deficient, so that a high proportion of the water filtered from the kidney is *not* reabsorbed but passes out as urine. The animal drinks a correspondingly large amount of water (polydipsia) to compensate for the increased loss in its urine (polyuria), and the large volume of urine produced over a long time span (e.g., overnight) often exceeds the capacity of the bladder, so that the animal is obliged to urinate. Tests may be required to distinguish this condition from others in which polyuria and polydipsia are a feature, but a major characteristic is that the urine is only marginally more concentrated than water. Successful treatment may be possible by injecting ADH or administering it as nasal drops.

Thyroid gland

The thyroid gland consists of two separate lobes which are situated in the neck on either side of the trachea (windpipe) just below the larynx (or

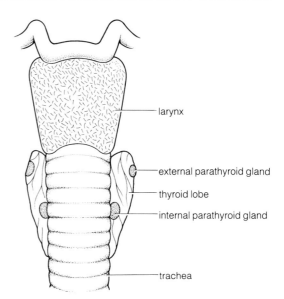

Figure 114 The lobes of the
thyroid gland and the
associated parathyroid glands.
The internal parathyroid
glands lie against the trachea
and are covered by the thyroid
lobes

larynx

external parathyroid gland

thyroid lobe

internal parathyroid gland

trachea

voicebox) (Fig. 114). Associated with each lobe is a pair of parathyroid
glands which functionally are quite independent of the thyroid gland.

The majority of cells, which are arranged in the walls of microscopic
spheres, termed follicles, are concerned with the production of two
metabolic hormones, thyroxine (otherwise known as T_4) and tri-
iodothyronine (T_3). Collectively these two hormones are often referred to
simply as thyroid hormone. As mentioned previously, the anterior pituitary
lobe produces thyroid stimulating hormone (TSH), which stimulates, and
helps to regulate, the output of thyroid hormone by the thyroid. These
thyroid hormones regulate the level of activity in all parts of the body, for
instance controlling the rate at which foodstuffs are utilised, the heart rate
and blood pressure, and the activity of the nervous system.

In between the follicles are larger cells (C cells), which produce a quite
separate hormone, calcitonin. Its effect is to lower the level of calcium in
the blood, so it is released after a meal to prevent the increased absorption
of calcium leading to an undesirably high blood level.

DISORDERS OF THE THYROID GLAND

The two major disorders in the dog are hypothyroidism and thyroid
cancer; the latter *may* lead to the overproduction of thyroid hormone.

Hypothyroidism

This is one of the more common hormonal disorders in the dog, especially
affecting large or medium-sized breeds (such as Retrievers, Setters,

Dobermanns and Boxers), and arises from deficient production of the metabolic hormones. Over 90 per cent of cases are due to a loss of three-quarters or more of the follicles due either to atrophy (wasting away), for reasons which are not precisely clear, or because the body has developed antibodies which attack and destroy its own thyroid cells. This is an example of an autoimmune disorder (see Chapter 20). These changes usually do not occur until the animal is middle-aged (i.e., four years old) or older, although in giant breeds they may arise from as young as two years of age.

Less than 10 per cent of cases of hypothyroidism are due to a lack of the stimulating hormone, TSH.

In the past much has been made of iodine deficiency as a cause of hypothyroidism, because iodine is an essential component of the hormone, but in modern developed countries iodine deficiency is unlikely to occur. This is because the population is not dependent on crops and livestock produced in a single area, which might have soils deficient in iodine, but consumes foods from a variety of sources, especially the sea. Fish and fish products (such as cod liver oil), and gelling agents derived from seaweed, are all rich in iodine, and commercial petfood rations have a very high iodine content. Goitre, which means an enlargement of the thyroid gland, was an accompaniment of severe iodine deficiency – an attempt on the part of the gland to acquire a greater share of what little iodine was available to the body. Today, goitre in the dog is almost invariably a consequence of tumour formation.

Congenital cases of hypothyroidism, known as cretins, *can* arise, but rarely do so nowadays; in the past they were associated with severe, long-standing iodine deficiency in their mother. In addition to the clinical signs of hypothyroidism mentioned later, cretins exhibit stunted physical development, i.e., are dwarfed but with a broad skull and short, thickened legs.

The signs of hypothyroidism are diverse, and the fact that they may be present in any combination causes hypothyroidism to mimic and be mistaken for many other diseases. The classic signs are those of lethargy, obesity and hair loss (alopecia); of these the sign that is most consistently present is lethargy, with animals spending most of their time sleeping. This is due to a combination of impassive behaviour produced by mental depression and the reduced ability to exercise as a result of muscle wasting. Obesity is a feature which can develop in affected animals, but it is clear that in the past its importance has been overestimated and many dogs of normal weight, and even thin animals, may be hypothyroid.

Alopecia (Fig. 115) is only one of a number of skin changes that can develop. Classically it is a bilaterally symmetrical, non-pruritic alopecia, meaning that the pattern of hair loss is more or less identical on both the right and left sides of the body and that the animal shows no signs of

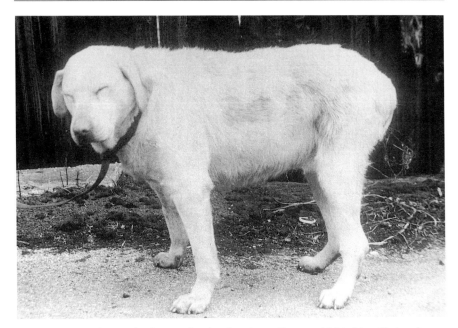

Figure 115 A drowsy-looking Labrador Retriever (9-year-old bitch) suffering from hypothyroidism. The coat is dry and sparse throughout, with obvious areas of hair loss on the trunk

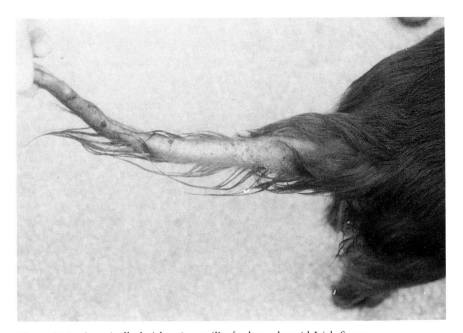

Figure 116 A typically hairless 'rat tail' of a hypothyroid Irish Setter

itching and scratching. This is an example of a typical endocrine alopecia, also seen in other disorders, e.g., Cushing's syndrome (described later), and where there is a deficiency or excess of oestrogen, the female sex hormone. In all these conditions, rather than a few hairs 'dying' at any one time and being replaced by new hairs growing from the same hair follicles, most of the hairs, particularly in certain areas, 'die' simultaneously, but still remain in the follicles because there is no new hair growth to push them out. These dry, brittle hairs tend to be shed most profusely from areas subjected to the greatest friction, usually the flanks and ventral abdomen as animals lie down, the back of the thighs and the tail as they sit, and around the neck if they wear a collar regularly. In some breeds, e.g., the Irish Setter, the loss of hair from the tail, giving a 'rat-tail', is particularly obvious (Fig. 116). Also, to confuse matters, in some breeds, such as the Boxer and the Irish Setter, the reduced rate of hair replacement can lead to a *thickening* of the coat, referred to as a 'carpet coat'.

Often there is excessive deposition of the dark pigment melanin in the skin, and the hair follicles become plugged with keratin, giving it a feel like fine sandpaper. The puffy thickening of the skin (myxoedema) can produce pronounced folds of skin on the neck and the forehead, the latter giving affected animals a worried, anxious expression. Hypothyroid dogs usually feel the cold more and much prefer to lie right up against fires and radiators, even in mild weather.

There is generalised muscle weakness, and muscle wasting can also involve the heart muscle producing typical changes, including slowing of the heart, which may be detected by electrocardiography (i.e., measuring the electrical signals from the heart). Hormone lack may also affect the peripheral nerves and be responsible for varying degrees of paralysis in certain individuals. Severe cases may show constipation, although diarrhoea and vomiting seem to be more frequent complications. In addition there may develop in hypothyroidism a variety of other changes, including eye lesions, mild anaemia, lack of libido (i.e., sex drive), abnormal lactation, infertility, an absence of oestrous cycles and, in extremely severe cases, a lower body temperature. Successful treatment requires an adequate level of thyroid hormone to be given each day to compensate for the deficiency in secretion.

Neoplasia (i.e., cancer) of the thyroid gland

This is the only common cause of goitre (an enlarged thyroid gland) in the dog (Fig. 117). Apart from causing mechanical pressure on structures in the neck, causing difficulty in swallowing, breathing and even barking, thyroid tumours are significant because they are almost invariably malignant. This means that they may invade, and damage, other structures in the neck and also spread to other areas of the body, principally the lungs.

Such tumours occur mainly in middle-aged and elderly dogs (especially

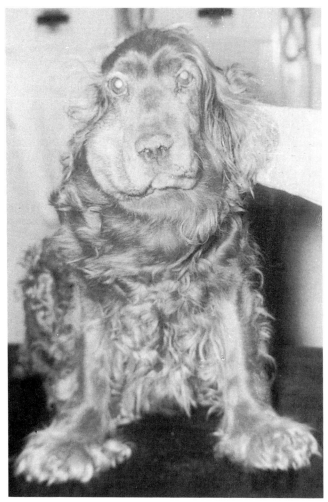

Figure 117   A 12-year-old Cocker Spaniel bitch with a large goitre in the neck caused by a malignant thyroid tumour (i.e., thyroid cancer)

Boxers), and in about 85 per cent of cases only one lobe is affected. In the majority of cases the amount of metabolic hormone produced remains within normal limits, but occasionally more than three-quarters of the functional cells may be obliterated and replaced by non-functional tumour cells, resulting in *hypo*thyroidism. Over-production of the hormone is also possible (occurring in up to 10 per cent of cases) and this causes signs of *hyper*thyroidism, i.e., weight loss despite an excessive appetite and increased thirst, diarrhoea and vomiting, a poor haircoat, restlessness, panting and weakness. If possible surgical removal is undertaken, although often it is not feasible.

Parathyroid glands

There are two pairs of parathyroid glands, each pair lying in association with one of the thyroid lobes (Fig. 114). The larger gland of each pair, ⅛–¼ in. (2–5 mm) long, is on the outer face of the thyroid lobe, and the smaller gland is on the inner surface, i.e., where the thyroid lobe lies against the trachea.

The glands produce a hormone – parathyroid hormone or parathormone – which enables fine adjustments to be made to the level of calcium in the blood to maintain that level within normal limits. Parathyroid hormone achieves this effect by increasing the release of calcium from bone, decreasing the excretion of calcium in the urine and increasing calcium absorption from the intestine. The glands are able to assess the calcium level in their blood supply and it is this which influences hormone output; in this instance the pituitary gland is not involved in regulation.

DISORDERS OF THE PARATHYROID GLANDS

Hyperparathyroidism

The increased production of parathyroid hormone, hyperparathyroidism, has four possible causes. Primary hyperparathyroidism, the uncontrolled oversecretion of the hormone by an abnormal gland, is a rare condition, usually due to a benign tumour, but which can result in very high calcium levels. Pseudohyperparathyroidism is more common. This is the excessive production of parathyroid hormone, or a substance which has exactly the same effect, by a malignant tumour located in some organ other than the parathyroid glands. Malignant tumours of the lymphoid tissue (lymphosarcomas) are particularly likely to act in this way. Surgical removal of the offending tumour is the preferred treatment, assuming that it is possible.

In the remaining two causes the increase in parathormone production is a response to a marked fall in the blood calcium level. One of these, renal secondary hyperparathyroidism is associated with kidney failure; the kidneys find themselves unable to efficiently eliminate phosphate from the blood, with the result that it accumulates and produces a reciprocal fall in the calcium level. In the other condition, nutritional secondary hyperparathyroidism, the problem is caused by feeding young dogs a diet containing large amounts of meat or offal, which is notorious for containing relatively far too much phosphate and far too little calcium. (The recommended dietary ratio of calcium:phosphate is approximately 1.2:1, whereas in horsemeat the ratio is 1:10 and in liver 1:50.) This disorder seems confined to an age range of 3–12 months, and is seen particularly around six months of age. The high phosphate content of the diet results in a high level in the blood and, again, a reciprocal fall in the calcium level.

In the last two conditions described the low blood calcium level stimulates increased parathyroid hormone output, which is often extremely successful in restoring the calcium level to within, or only just below, the normal range. Treatment requires correction of the underlying cause, and will often involve sophisticated veterinary diagnostic techniques.

In all four hyperparathyroid disorders the abnormally high level of parathyroid hormone causes excessive amounts of calcium to be removed from the bones, resulting in them becoming structurally much weaker. Often comparatively trivial accidents will result in severe fractures. Also the high level of calcium that occurs in primary and pseudo-hyperparathyroidism causes a variety of signs, including generalised muscle weakness, increased thirst, a loss of appetite, vomiting and depression; it may also result in calcium being deposited in soft tissues and increase the possibility of bladder stones (urinary calculi) forming.

Hypoparathyroidism

This denotes reduced output of parathyroid hormone. It is a much less common disorder which results from damage to the parathyroid glands, most frequently as the result of an autoimmune reaction in which the body has formed antibodies which attack the glands. The resultant fall in the blood calcium level increases the 'excitability' of nerve-muscle junctions and animals become liable to show muscular twitches, inco-ordination and weakness (especially when handled). This may progress to muscle tremors and convulsions, which can persist for long periods of time. The administration of calcium is necessary to control these signs.

Adrenal glands

Each of the two adrenal glands lies to the front of the inner aspect of the corresponding kidney in the upper part of the abdominal cavity (Fig. 118). Each gland has two separate hormone-synthesising components – an inner medulla (accounting for 10–20 per cent of the mass) surrounded by an outer cortex. The medulla produces adrenaline (and the related hormone noradrenaline), which is regarded as an 'emergency hormone' to allow the animal to respond to situations where it might need to flee or to fight. Adrenaline increases the rate at which the heart pumps blood around the body, releases glucose from the liver and muscle to provide an instant energy source and shunts blood from non-vital areas, such as the skin, to the heart and muscles, which would require more in an emergency.

Disorders of the medulla are unusual, but a functional adrenaline-secreting tumour (phaechromocytoma) occasionally arises, producing a variety of signs, including a tendency towards diabetes mellitus.

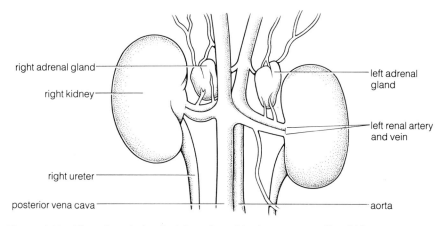

Figure 118 The adrenal glands, lying alongside the corresponding kidneys

However, the steroid secretions of the adrenal cortex are more important for day-to-day survival of the animal; two groups of steroid hormones are produced, the corticosteroids and the adrenal sex hormones. Small amounts of both male and female sex hormones are produced by the cortex regardless of the sex of the individual. It is, however, the corticosteroids which are essential for life, and hormones in this group have generally been classified as either glucocorticoids or mineralocorticoids. The most important glucocorticoid is cortisol (also known as hydrocortisone) and the main mineralocorticoid is aldosterone. Cortisol has widespread metabolic effects throughout the body, affecting the metabolism of most foodstuffs, and preventing or suppressing inflammation in the tissues. As mentioned previously, its output is regulated by the hormone ACTH, derived from the anterior lobe of the pituitary gland.

Aldosterone increases the reabsorption of salt and water in the kidneys, thereby helping to regulate the amounts of each in the body. Its production is not controlled by ACTH, and in fact regulation of its synthesis is achieved by a complex hormone system involving the kidney and the liver, which is known as the renin-angiotensin system.

DISORDERS OF THE ADRENAL CORTEX

Hyperadrenocorticism

This disorder, also known as Cushing's syndrome, the name of its human counterpart, is a common endocrine disorder of dogs from middle age onwards. It occurs particulary in small terriers, Poodles, Cavalier King Charles Spaniels and in Boxers. In the majority of cases (90 per cent) the disorder is attributable to the excessive output of the hormone ACTH from the anterior lobe of the pituitary, which stimulates the adrenal cortex to produce excessive amounts of cortisol. In the remaining natural cases the cause is a tumour of the adrenal cortex, usually in one gland only, which, quite uncontrolled, secretes large amounts of cortisol. In all these cases it is cortisol which is responsible for the many clinical signs which appear. However, the same effects can be produced by administration of a synthetic corticosteroid (particularly the more potent, long-acting preparations), especially when they are given for a long time in high dosage.

Whatever the cause, the clinical signs are similar, but as with other endocrine disorders and medical disorders generally, not all of the signs will appear in every case. The most consistent features are excessive urination and thirst (polyuria and polydipsia) and a good, or even excessive, appetite; a poor appetite is rare. Most animals are depressed, and gradually the abdomen becomes distended, giving a 'pot-belly' due in part to weak abdominal muscles (Fig. 119). Muscle wasting is also especially obvious around the head and posterior thighs; the latter can lead to trembling and difficulties in jumping or even walking (especially up and down stairs).

Almost all affected dogs show one or more skin changes. These include the loss of hair from the flanks, lower abdomen and thighs (Fig. 120), which, as with hypothyroidism, is a typical endocrine alopecia. By this we mean that it is identical on both sides of the body and not accompanied by itching. The skin is often paper thin and wrinkled due to reduced elasticity. At times calcium salts are deposited in the skin as plaques, eventually causing raw-looking erosions which can bleed or become infected. Successful treatment can be achieved with the use of a drug to suppress the activity of the adrenal cortex, but in the case of adrenal tumours, surgical removal (where possible) is more effective.

Hypoadrenocorticism

As a naturally occurring disease this affects young animals, and there is a deficient output of both cortisol and aldosterone (i.e., all corticosteroid production is diminished). The disorder is often given the name of its human counterpart, Addison's disease. In 90 per cent of cases it is again the result of an immune disorder causing wasting of the hormone-producing cells. Less commonly the cells may be destroyed by tumours or following chronic diseases. Likewise a complete lack of both types of hormone will follow surgical removal of both adrenal glands, which in the past has been performed as a treatment for Cushing's syndrome (although rarely nowadays).

A lack of cortisol production alone (i.e., with little or no reduction in aldosterone release) can follow excessive dosing with the adrenal-suppressant drug mitotane (in treating Cushing's syndrome), failure of the anterior lobe of the pituitary to produce ACTH or suddenly stopping a course of corticosteroid therapy. In the last-named instance one effect of

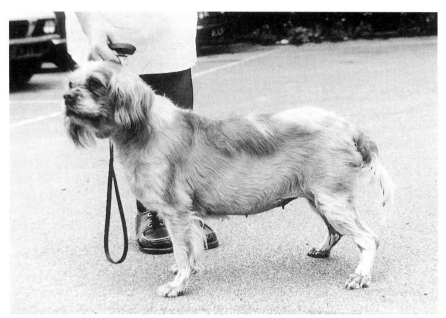

Figure 119   This 10-year-old Cavalier King Charles Spaniel bitch possesses the typical 'pot belly' of Cushing's syndrome (hyperadrenocorticism)

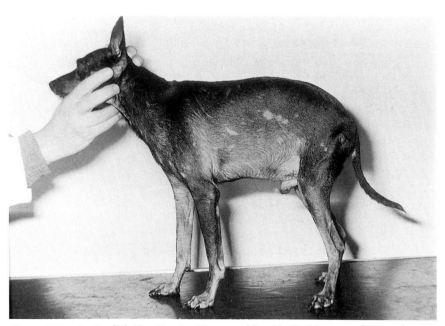

Figure 120   An English Toy Terrier (8 years old) with Cushing's syndrome, showing a generally sparse haircoat plus areas of complete hair loss

administering corticosteroid to an animal is that it reduces its own production of cortisol, and if the given supply is subsequently abruptly terminated it can take a little time for the adrenal glands to commence normal production again. In this 'lag' phase there will be a deficiency of glucocorticoids, since none is being administered and little, if any, is being naturally produced. This is the reason for insisting that corticosteroid therapy is always *gradually tailed off.*

At times the clinical signs may be sudden in onset, with severe shock and renal failure, referred to as an Addisonian crisis, but more usually signs develop progressively. In the majority of cases there is a loss of appetite, vomiting and/or depression and muscle weakness of fluctuating severity. Diarrhoea, weight loss and abdominal discomfort may also arise, and where there is also a deficiency of aldosterone these signs are intensified and animals show muscle trembling and an increased thirst.

Diagnosis can be a major problem, since signs are often vague and resemble disorders of the digestive tract or kidneys. Treatment involves supplying the hormone(s) of which there is a deficiency.

Pancreas

In the dog the pancreas is a V-shaped gland (Fig. 121) which lies in the upper part of the abdominal cavity, alongside the stomach and the duodenum (the first part of the small intestine). As described in Chapter 8,

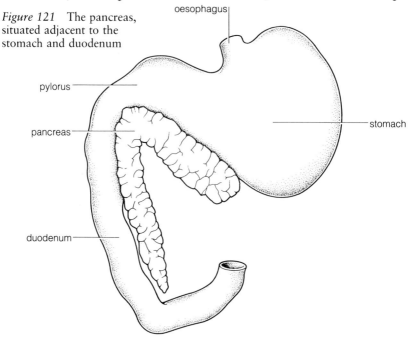

Figure 121 The pancreas, situated adjacent to the stomach and duodenum

oesophagus

pylorus

pancreas

stomach

duodenum

most of the cells of the pancreas (acinar cells) are concerned with the production of pancreatic juice containing enzymes for the digestion of food in the intestine. This secretion passes along the pancreatic ducts to enter the first part of the duodenum. However, scattered throughout the gland, like currants in a cake, are small clusters of cells known as the *islets of Langerhans*. These cells secrete hormones directly into the blood. The cells are of different types, the most important of which are *alpha* cells secreting *glucagon* and *beta* cells secreting *insulin*. To a large extent these hormones have opposite actions – the effect of glucagon is to raise the glucose level in the blood and that of insulin to lower it. Most of the endocrine disorders of the pancreas are the result of over- or under-production of insulin, rather than problems with glucagon production.

Insulin facilitates the use of glucose as an energy source by all body cells; furthermore it stimulates the conversion of glucose to glycogen by the muscles and liver to act as an energy store, and it also increases the synthesis of fats and proteins. The release of insulin is triggered by the presence within the digestive tract of glucose (the substance into which virtually all carbohydrates are converted during digestion) and by the appearance in the blood of increased amounts of absorbed foodstuffs after a meal, especially glucose.

ENDOCRINE DISORDERS OF THE PANCREAS

Diabetes mellitus

This is a complex disorder of carbohydrate, fat and protein metabolism caused by the inability to produce, or to utilise, adequate amounts of insulin. Two major types of diabetes mellitus are recognised. The most common type in the dog (Type I) is due to a deficiency of functional beta cells resulting in a deficiency of insulin (hypoinsulinism). It seems likely that, particularly in genetically-susceptible individuals, environmental factors such as drugs or infectious agents (especially viruses) stimulate the development of antibodies against the beta cells. As a result, beta cells are progressively destroyed until insufficient remain to produce adequate levels of insulin. Less commonly, destruction of the beta cells may be the result of tumours, injury or long-standing or recurrent inflammation. This is often regarded as the classical type of diabetes, i.e., where there is a lack of insulin.

However, in recent years it has become clear that diabetes mellitus can also develop when body cells fail to respond to insulin, i.e., when the body develops *insulin resistance*. In fact in these situations the body may be trying desperately to raise the level of insulin in order to achieve its normal effects, and if the level in the blood is measured it is found to be either within, or above, the normal limits. This type of diabetes mellitus (Type II) can result from *overeating* (because in obesity the number of receptor sites where insulin can act is reduced) or from an excess of other hormones. Two types of hormone known to interfere with the action of insulin are glucocorticoids (either cortisol produced naturally in Cushing's syndrome or cortisol-like drugs used in therapy) and growth hormone. In the bitch the production of growth hormone is stimulated in two unique ways, mentioned earlier in describing acromegaly.

Firstly, for a period of time after the end of each heat a bitch produces the hormone progesterone (whether she is pregnant or not), which has the effect of stimulating the output of growth hormone and which in turn blocks the effects of insulin. This may be sufficient to produce signs of diabetes mellitus for a while after each heat in some bitches, but generally they spontaneously recover, i.e., when the natural progesterone secretion stops, insulin becomes effective again.

Secondly, the drugs known as progestagens (progesterone-like substances), which are used to delay or suppress heat, act in the same way, but of course if they are being given continuously, the effects will also be continuous, i.e., the signs of diabetes mellitus will persist.

All of these situations are best dealt with as soon as they are recognised, i.e., animals with obesity should be dieted (when weight is lost the number of insulin receptor sites increases again), cases of Cushing's syndrome should be appropriately treated, dosage with corticosteroids or progestagens should cease and bitches showing diabetes mellitus after heat periods should be spayed. If nothing is done to correct the insulin resistance the beta cells eventually give up the struggle to put out more insulin, i.e., they become exhausted, and this will result in permanent Type I diabetes mellitus, i.e., hypoinsulinism.

The special problems in bitches in part account for why diabetes mellitus is three times as common in that sex as in males. Overall the disorder probably affects one dog in every 250 in Western countries. It is seen most often in dogs eight years old and over, although younger dogs can be affected, and in almost all surveys the Dachshund appears to be most at risk, though several other breeds, among them the Miniature Poodle, Scottish Terrier, Samoyed, King Charles Spaniel and Rottweiler, figure prominently.

Regardless of the type of diabetes the clinical signs are virtually identical in all cases. The inability to utilise or store glucose means that high levels accumulate in the blood, and so much is filtered out by the kidneys that it cannot all be reabsorbed (in normal dogs reabsorption is complete). Consequently some glucose is excreted in the urine and, since it needs to be in solution, takes more water with it. Thus there is increased urine production and a compensatory increase in thirst. There is also muscle wasting and weight loss, despite an increased appetite in most dogs. Around 25 per cent develop cataracts (opacity of the lenses in the eyes) and some show damage to small blood vessels and nerves.

Eventually, in an attempt to obtain a source of energy the body increases the breakdown of its fat stores, and fatty acids are released faster than they can be metabolised. Instead they are converted into three substances, referred to collectively as *ketones*, which accumulate in the blood, and their appearance causes a dramatic change in the clinical picture. Effectively the onset of ketosis marks the beginning of the end. Ketones are toxic to the brain and cause a loss of appetite, vomiting, marked dehydration and listlessness, progressing to coma and death. Unfortunately, usually half the cases of diabetes mellitus in the dog (whether Type I or Type II) show the presence of ketones in their urine on the first occasion when they are presented to a veterinary surgeon.

Treatment has to be by the injection of insulin, with the daily dose being adjusted according to the level of glucose present in the urine. Diabetics should have a relatively uneventful life, being fed the same type of diet (80 per cent easily digestible protein, low fat, 20 per cent carbohydrate) at the same times each day and having the same amount of exercise each day. The inadvertent administration of excess insulin leads to a severe fall in the blood level of glucose (hypoglycaemia), ultimately resulting in a coma. At the first signs of drowsiness, weakness or staggering, one or two tablespoonsful of glucose, honey or any sweet substance, should be administered by mouth. Most dogs will readily take this and the result is very dramatic, the dog becoming normal once more in a very short time.

Today diabetes is diagnosed frequently and many diabetic animals lead relatively normal lives with the help of a daily injection of insulin administered by the owner. If you suspect your dog may be a diabetic do not delay. Discuss the condition with your veterinary surgeon. Control in the majority of cases really is a lot easier than at first thought. After all, without the benefit of insulin your dog's days are limited.

Hyperinsulinism

In dogs (usually above six years old) tumours, generally malignant, of the pancreatic beta cells can arise which secrete excessive amounts of insulin quite unrelated to the animal's requirements. As a result the glucose level in the blood falls disastrously and the animal shows appropriate clinical signs. Initially there may just be restlessness and inco-ordination, but progressively there can occur collapse, twitching, uncontrolled barking and later even convulsions. Often these signs are intermittent and last only a short time; generally they develop following exercise or excitement, or they may appear 2–6 hours after feeding (because of the increased insulin output stimulated by a meal). Perhaps surprisingly, 20 per cent of such dogs show an increase in weight.

Although some drugs may help control the signs, permanent treatment is by removal of all or part of the pancreas. Depending on how much functional tissue remains the animal may subsequently need to be supplied with pancreatic enzymes and insulin to correct the resultant deficiencies.

15

THE SKIN

Skin disease is one of the commonest reasons for which dog owners seek veterinary advice. In an average small animal practice more than 20 per cent of all cases are dermatological and the majority of these patients are dogs.

Skin is the largest organ of the body and has many functions essential to life. It is the barrier between the animal and its environment and protects against physical and chemical damage. It inhibits infection with bacteria, fungi and viruses and prevents loss of important materials (especially water and mineral ions) from the body. The skin is involved in regulation of body temperature and blood pressure. It is elastic and flexible to allow movement and is responsible for nail production. Pigmentation protects against sunburn and the camouflage it affords helps prevent attack by predators. Skin is a reservoir for water, nutrients and mineral ions and is a site for Vitamin D synthesis.

Skin has two main structural components, a thin outer component, the epidermis, and a thicker inner component, the dermis (Fig. 122). The epidermis is divided into a number of layers (Fig. 123). It is a major barrier restricting loss of water and other materials from the body and preventing entry of infectious micro-organisms such as bacteria and fungi.

The dermis contains blood vessels, nerves, skin glands, hair follicles and connective tissue components, the latter mainly comprising collagen and elastic fibres, which confer mechanical strength and allow mobility. The main function of the dermis is to support and nourish the overlying epidermis and the hair follicles.

There are two types of skin glands in dogs. Contrary to popular opinion dogs have large numbers of sweat glands in their skin. They do not open directly on to the skin surface via pores as in man, but discharge sweat on to the skin surface through openings in the hair follicles. Sweat may have an important role in skin disinfection, but plays little part in temperature regulation in dogs – heat loss in the dog is effected mainly by panting.

Figure 122
Normal hairy skin

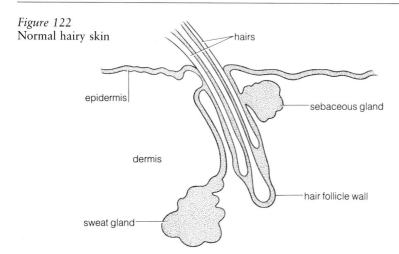

Figure 123
Epidermis

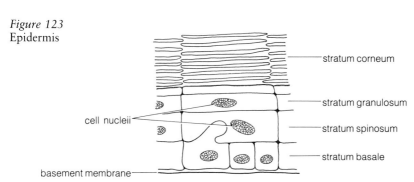

Sebaceous glands produce sebum, which is important in waterproofing the skin surface, maintaining skin pliability and resistance to infection. Hair follicles in the dog contain bundles of about a dozen hairs, each bundle comprising a large, long, rigid primary or guard hair and several secondary or undercoat hairs, which are thinner and more wool-like. Some breeds of dogs, such as Poodles and Bedlington Terriers, have few primary hairs and a predominantly woolly coat. Other breeds, such as Rottweilers, have a coat that is predominantly composed of primary hairs.

Diseases of the skin

Skin diseases are challenging yet frustrating for both owners and veterinary surgeons. The clinical manifestations of many different skin problems are very similar and may require a wide range of laboratory tests and trial therapy in order to reach a diagnosis. In some instances this may take several months, and is likely to be quite expensive. On rare occasions the underlying cause of an animal's skin problem is never discovered and life-long symptomatic therapy is required. Dermatological therapy depends heavily on medicated shampoos and treatments applied directly to the skin itself and consequently involves considerable investment of time and effort by the owners of affected dogs.

FLEA-RELATED DISEASE

Fleas are probably the most common cause of skin disease in dogs. The usual species of flea found on dogs is the cat flea (*Ctenocephalides felis*) (Plate 6). The life cycle of the flea varies between three weeks and two years depending on climatic conditions. The greater part of the life cycle (about 90 per cent) is spent off the host animal in the environment, with adult fleas jumping on to the host to obtain a blood meal. They may also feed on humans. Typically skin disease is seasonal, coinciding with a peak in flea activity in late summer and early autumn, although with the widespread use of central heating it has become an all-year-round problem.

It is likely that skin disease occurs as a result of an allergic reaction (see later) to flea saliva injected when the flea feeds, which leads to a sensation of itchiness (pruritus) and causes the dog to scratch and chew. The degree of pruritus varies. Some dogs may tolerate large numbers of fleas on the skin with few clinical signs whilst others may be extremely itchy (pruritic) for many days after just a single flea bite. Affected dogs may be generally itchy, but often are particularly so at the base of the tail and the posterior portion of the back. In multi-pet households cats are often symptomless carriers of fleas and introduce them into the house. Diagnosis is based on identification of fleas or flea dirt (excrement) in the coat, skin damage (lesions) in typical sites and response to a flea eradication programme. In some instances fleas and flea excrement may be absent on clinical examination. This usually occurs when few fleas are present in the environment but the dog is highly allergic to them. In these cases an effective flea-control programme (Table 16) is essential in providing a diagnosis. Veterinary surgeons will often initially recommend a strict flea eradication programme when confronted with an itchy dog in order to rule out this diagnosis at an early stage, even if no fleas have actually been seen.

SARCOPTIC MANGE (SCABIES)

Sarcoptic mange is a highly contagious, extremely pruritic skin condition caused by a microscopic mite (*Sarcoptes scabei* var. *canis*). The entire life cycle of the parasite occurs on or within the outer layer of the skin, the stratum corneum. Contagion is from direct contact, or indirectly via grooming instruments and other equipment. The parasite can survive off

Table 16   Guidelines for flea control

1. Treat all dogs and cats in the household regularly with residual insecticides such as sprays and dips. Observe any recommendations by the manufacturer regarding frequency of application and precautions for use. Powders and flea collars are of limited use. Shampoos have no residual action as they are rinsed off after application.
2. Treat the environment regularly (every four to eight weeks) with a residual environmental insecticide after thoroughly vacuum cleaning the house (house dust is a breeding site for fleas). Again note any manufacturer's recommendation for usage. A professional pest-control company may be needed to treat the environment in some cases.
3. Some flea-control products may have little activity against fleas. Consult a veterinary surgeon for advice in selecting suitable products.
4. Recommendations for flea control vary with time of year, geographical region, severity of problem and number and type of pets owned. Ideally, the particular flea-control programme used should be designed specifically for each individual case in consultation with a veterinary surgeon.

the host for two to three days, hence dogs may become infected from the environment. The disease is common among the fox population in Great Britain and can also transiently affect people.

Lesions in dogs mostly result from self-mutilation due to pruritus; severe skin damage may occur due to scratching and chewing. The disease can occur in any area of the body, but particularly affects the ear flaps and the elbows.

Diagnosis is difficult, often circumstantial. Diagnostic clues include intense pruritus and self-mutilation, spread to other dogs and people, presence of affected foxes in the locality and characteristic distribution of lesions. The diagnosis may be confirmed by microscopical examination of skin scrapings by a veterinary surgeon. The technique involves abrading the skin surface with a scalpel blade until slight bleeding is seen and microscopically examining the material collected on the blade. Adult and immature mites and parasite eggs may be present (Plate 1). However, in a high percentage of cases mites are not detected with this method and a therapeutic trial with an anti-parasitic shampoo is required to confirm the diagnosis.

Treatment is straightforward; an antiparasitic shampoo or dip, obtained from your veterinary surgeon, should be used at weekly intervals for about a month. Long-haired dogs should be clipped to allow penetration of antiparasitic agents into the skin. The *entire* skin surface of *all* dogs in the household should be treated. Affected humans recover spontaneously after treatment of in-contact canine cases. To prevent re-infestation of dogs a residual antiparasitic agent should be used to treat the environment, although the disease may recur if affected dogs or foxes are within the vicinity.

DEMODECTIC MANGE (DEMODICOSIS, FOLLICULAR MANGE)

Demodectic mange is a potentially serious disease caused by the microscopic mite *Demodex canis*. In contrast with sarcoptic mange the mites live in hair follicles rather than the stratum corneum. The entire life cycle takes place within the skin, and it has been shown that the disease is not contagious between dogs and cannot spread to man. Most dogs carry small numbers of *Demodex* mites, which they acquire as puppies when suckling. Normally the dog's immune system restricts the multiplication of the parasite within the skin and disease does not occur. A small percentage of dogs have an immunodeficiency or defect in their immune system and are unable to limit multiplication of the parasite and so develop lesions. Demodectic mange is usually seen in puppies and young adult dogs. Lesions commonly appear on the face and forelegs, although the disease can occur at any site.

Hair loss, scaling and reddening (erythema) of the skin is typically present but pruritus is mild or absent (Plate 7). The disease can be localised, affecting a few areas, or generalised, involving large areas of the body surface. Many cases of localised demodicosis resolve spontaneously at around one year of age, but in some instances no such 'self-cure' occurs and the disease generalises and becomes life-threatening.

Diagnosis can be confirmed by microscopical examination of the skin scrapings. Large numbers of mites are often present (Plate 5). Treatment can be difficult, expensive and time-consuming except in those cases where 'self-cure' occurs. Insecticidal dips that penetrate deeply into hair follicles are used. Such products are only available from veterinary surgeons. Multiple treatments up to three times weekly (depending on choice of insecticide) are required for about 10 to 12 weeks and there is no guarantee that this will cure the condition. Even today euthanasia may be necessary on humane grounds in a few cases.

It is likely that the immunodeficiency involved in this condition is hereditary and therefore owners should not breed from recovered animals, even if the disease was present in the localised form.

CHEYLETIELLOSIS (*CHEYLETIELLA* MITE INFESTATION, 'WALKING DANDRUFF')

Cheyletiellosis is another common canine mite infestation and is caused primarily by *Cheyletiella yasguri*, although other *Cheyletiella* species may be involved. The life cycle occurs entirely within scales and debris at the skin surface. The disease is contagious between dogs and other animals, and may transiently affect man. Most cases occur in puppies, especially those from pet shops, although skin disease due to another species called

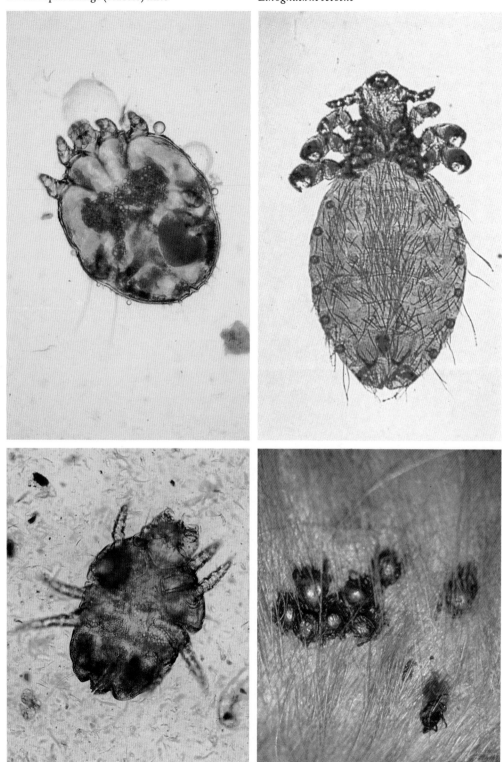

Plate 1   Photo micrograph of *Sarcoptes scabei* – the sarcoptic mange (scabies) mite

Plate 2   Photo micrograph of canine louse: *Linognathus setosus*

Plate 3   Photo micrograph of *Cheyletiella*

Plate 4   Collection of ticks on a dog

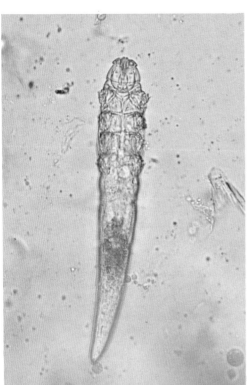

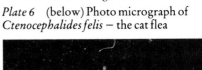

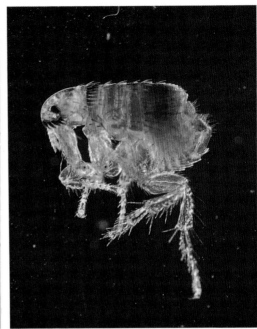

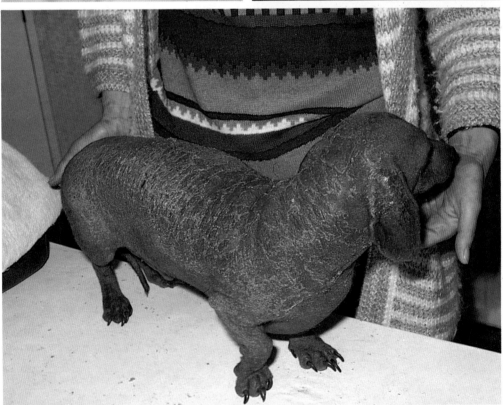

Plate 7 Dachshund with severe demodectic mange

Plate 9 (right) Entropion – inward turning of the lower eyelid

Plate 8 (below) Distichiasis – extra hairs on the upper eyelid

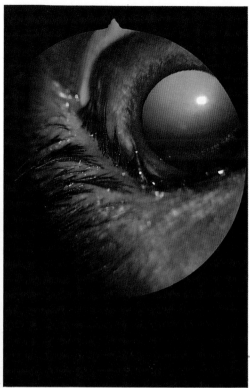

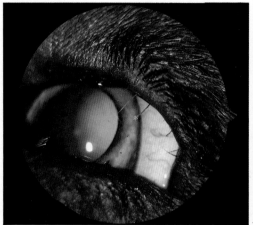

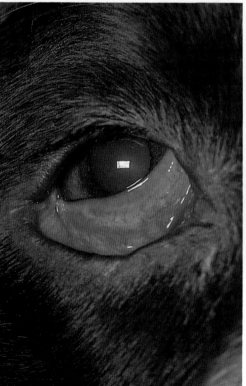

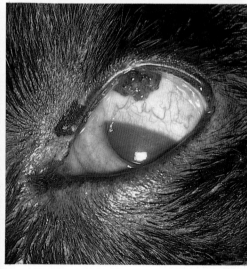

Plate 11 (above) Papillomatous tumour of the upper eyelid

Plate 10 (left) Ectropion — drooping of the lower eyelid

Plate 12 Prolapse of the tear gland of the third eyelid

Plate 13 Kinking of the third eyelid

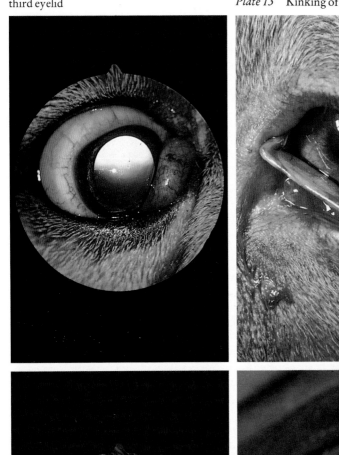

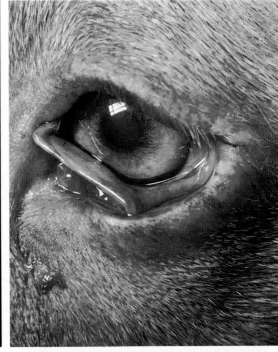

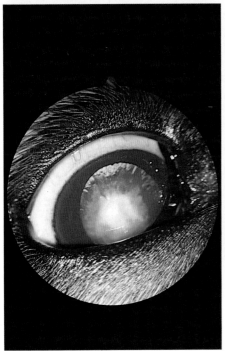

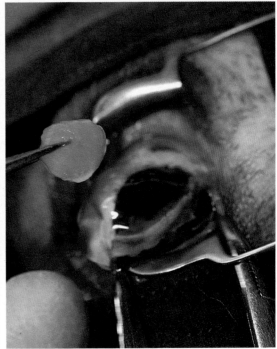

Plate 14 Cataract, occupying the central part of the lens

Plate 15 Lentectomy – the operation to remove cataract

Cheyletiella parasitivorax can be seen at any age following contact with infected rabbits. The condition is characterised by the presence of excessive surface scaling (dandruff) with variable pruritus. Diagnosis is based on detection of mites on microscopical examination of skin scrapings and surface scales (Plate 3). Samples of drandruff may be obtained by collecting material from brushing the coat or by applying adhesive tape to the skin surface. Using a magnifying lens adult mites may occasionally be seen moving through specimens of scales ('walking dandruff').

Treatment with three applications of antiparasitic shampoo at weekly intervals and environmental decontamination is curative. In-contact pets should also be treated.

EAR MITE INFESTATION

Ear mites (*Otodectes cynotis*) are one of the major causes of otitis externa in the dog (see Chapter 17). They are just visible to the naked eye as white dots and are usually confined to the ear canal, although they can spread on to the skin surface to cause dermatitis. Typically the disease is characterised by inflammation and a thick, waxy discharge from the ears. Head shaking and ear scratching may also be present. The disease is contagious between dogs and cats. Diagnosis is based on observation of the mites on examination of the ear canal using an auroscope. Treatment of all cats and dogs in the household with antiparasitic eardrops for at least three weeks is usually effective.

HARVEST MITE INFESTATION

Occasionally immature stages of the harvest mite, *Trombicula autumnalis*, will attack the feet of dogs. The condition is seen usually in late summer and autumn in dogs exercised in rural areas, especially if the soil is chalky. Man, cats and other species are also susceptible. In dogs infestation leads to severe pruritus of the feet, and on examination the mites will be seen with the naked eye as bright orange dots, especially between the toes and on the lower parts of the legs. Treatment with antiparasitic shampoos is curative and prevention is by avoidance of grassland during the appropriate season.

TICKS

Ticks are grey, bean-shaped parasites, 5 to 10 mm (¼–½ in.) long, which infest animals in order to obtain a blood meal. They can affect dogs as well as all other domestic animals, and man. In the UK the common tick is *Ixodes ricinus*, the sheep tick, although *Ixodes hexagonus*, the hedgehog tick, is also found in dogs. The incidence of tick-related disease depends on climate, season and geographic location. Feeding ticks are particularly prevalent in south-west England and on the west coast of Scotland, especially in the spring and autumn. In most instances the sole problem is the presence of the tick itself on the skin (Plate 4). In more severe cases irritation at the site of the tick bite leads to self-trauma and, if many ticks are feeding for a long period, blood loss anaemia may result. In addition ticks may transmit infectious diseases between animals. Fortunately, tick-borne diseases and anaemia are uncommon in dogs in the UK. However, tick-borne diseases are not uncommon throughout the rest of the world.

1.   *Canine Ehrlichiosis* occurs worldwide but not in the United Kingdom. It is caused by *Ehrlichia canis* which is a rickettsial agent and is transmitted by the brown dog tick, *Rhipicephalus sanguineus*.
2.   *Rocky Mountain fever*. This is another rickettsial disease which can occur in many small mammals, dogs and humans. In dogs it is called tick fever and is transmitted by *Dermacentor* species of ticks.
3.   *Tick paralysis*, another tick-borne disease is due to a neurotoxin secreted by the tick and not to an infectious agent carried by it. Dogs are most commonly affected although it can also occur in man. Various species of ticks have been implicated and it is usually the female tick that produces the neurotoxin. It does not occur in the UK but is fairly widespread in Australia, North America and South Africa. Species of *Dermacentor* and *Ixodes* ticks are responsible.
4.   *Babesiosis* is due to the protozoan *Babesia* spp. These diseases are transmitted by blood-sucking ticks. They have not been recorded in dogs in the UK although they occur in both North and South America.

Treatment is by manual removal after killing the tick with a parasitical agent. Care must be taken to remove the entire parasite as mouth parts left embedded within the skin may lead to infection. Traditionally surgical spirit, dry-cleaning fluid or nail varnish remover, on a piece of cotton wool have been used to loosen the mouth parts of the tick before it is pulled off. Lighted cigarettes have sometimes been employed, but none of these methods can really be recommended. Insecticidal shampoos or sprays should be employed and the ticks pulled off when dead. If in doubt, consult your veterinary surgeon.

LICE INFESTATION

Two species of lice can infest dogs in the UK: *Trichodectes canis*, the biting louse, and *Linognathus setosus*, the sucking louse (Plate 2). Clinical signs of lice infestation vary. Some individuals may be symptomless, whereas others may be pruritic. Lice are host specific, hence dog lice will not spread to man or other non-canine pets. Diagnosis is based on identification of lice within the coat and eggs attached to hairs.

Lice are easier to control than fleas as they live and breed on the host and are susceptible to most insecticidal shampoos.

ALLERGIC SKIN DISEASE

Allergic skin diseases are among the most common, difficult and frustrating conditions to diagnose and treat in veterinary medicine. Allergic or, more correctly, hypersensitivity reactions occur when the immune system makes an exaggerated response to a foreign substance leading to tissue damage. In dogs four major groups of foreign materials, or allergens, are involved: flea saliva, food constituents, inhaled particles (dust and pollens) and contact allergies. Canine allergic reactions usually lead to skin damage via complex and, in many instances, incompletely understood mechanisms, resulting in inflammation and pruritus. Animals are not born with allergies but develop them after repeated exposure to an allergen. Consequently dogs may develop food allergy dermatitis having been fed the same diet for many years. Dogs may become allergic to more than one substance, which can make diagnosis and treatment difficult. Furthermore, dogs may develop *new* allergies after previous ones have been identified and controlled.

Inhalant allergy (atopy)

After flea allergy, inhalant allergy, or atopy, is probably the commonest allergic skin disease in the dog. When an affected individual inhales dust, pollens and moulds an allergic response occurs. The disease is similar to human asthma or hay-fever, except that the target tissue is the skin, not the respiratory tract. The disease can affect any breed, particularly terriers, labradors and setters. There is often a history of related individuals also being affected, suggesting a genetic basis to the problem. Symptoms usually begin at one to three years of age and may initially be seasonal, for example, associated with high pollen counts in the summer just like human hay-fever. However, the condition may develop into a perennial problem. Affected individuals are itchy and may rub and scratch their faces, particularly around the eyes and ears, and lick or chew their feet. The armpits (axillae), groin and the inside of the thighs may also be affected. Diagnosis is based on the presence of the features discussed above and by ruling out other causes of pruritus. In around 80 per cent of cases the diagnosis can be confirmed by intradermal allergy testing. This complicated procedure involves the injection of small volumes of a range of liquid allergens into the skin. In atopic dogs one or more of these will elicit an allergic response at the site of injection. These tests are currently only performed by veterinary surgeons specialising in dermatology. Treatment is difficult. In rare instances the dog can be isolated from the offending allergens, although this is seldom practical as allergic dogs are frequently hypersensitive to more than one substance. Anti-inflammatory drugs including glucocorticoids (steroids) anti-histamines and essential fatty acids are used to reduce inflammation, irritation and pruritus. However, antihistamines and essential fatty acids will not improve all dogs and glucocorticoids may induce serious side-effects. Some dermatology specialists use multiple injections of allergens in an attempt to desensitise or to hyposensitise an animal, but this is expensive and may only be of value in 60 per cent of cases.

Dietary allergy

The prevalence of food allergy in the canine population is a subject of much debate. However, it is the easiest of the allergic diseases to investigate and treat and therefore most veterinary surgeons suggest a dietary change at some stage in the management of the itchy dog. Dogs can become allergic to a wide range of foods, although dairy and beef products, together with gluten from wheat, are amongst the commonest offenders. Clinical signs vary, but pruritus is a common feature, especially affecting the face and around the anus. Some dogs may have a history of gastrointestinal disturbances (see Chapter 8).

Diagnosis is based on a two- to four-week dietary trial, with a home-cooked diet fed to the exclusion of all other foods. The diet should be boiled rice or potato with a source of protein *to which the animal has not been previously exposed*, for example, fresh or frozen fish, chicken or lamb. Only water should be given to drink. This diet must be strictly adhered to. *No other foods should be fed during the trial*. If the condition improves, the dog should be challenged with the original diet to determine whether a relapse occurs, thus confirming the diagnosis. Treatment is based on feeding a diet that does not induce skin disease. Commercial tinned, balanced low-allergy (hypoallergenic) diets are available and are convenient for the maintenance of some cases, but may contain ingredients to which the dog is hypersensitive. Alternatively, additional sources of food can be added sequentially to the test diet until a balanced, non-allergic, home-cooked diet has been formulated. Some dogs may eventually develop hypersensitivity to their new diet and hence the problem may recur. Considerable dedication is required in long-term management of dogs with dietary allergy.

Contact allergic dermatitis

This condition is seen uncommonly in dogs as their hair coat prevents substances from contacting the skin surface. The major clinical sign is pruritus at contact sites such as the feet, chin, scrotum, elbows and hocks. Many substances can induce contact allergy, including plant materials, disinfectants, wool, nylon and dyes, and sometimes shampoos, ointments and insecticides used in the treatment of skin disease. Contact allergy develops slowly and so a recent change of bedding or carpets is usually not significant. Diagnosis involves removing the suspected allergen from the environment for two weeks. If the condition improves, the diagnosis is confirmed by re-exposing the animal to the suspected material. Treatment involves avoiding the offending allergens. Contact *irritant* dermatitis is commonly seen in dogs and should be distinguished from contact *allergy*. Only a small percentage of dogs will have an allergic response to a contact allergen, whereas all dogs will have a skin reaction on exposure to an irritant such as concentrated disinfectant or detergent solutions. Clinical signs of contact irritation are similar to those of contact allergy and occur at similar body sites.

Urticaria (hives)

Occasionally single or multiple wheals or swellings of variable size appear suddenly in the skin of dogs. This is an allergic phenomenon; foods, drugs, vaccines and insect bites or stings have been implicated as the causal allergens. Treatment with anti-inflammatory drugs may be of value since itching can be a problem. In most instances the condition regresses rapidly and spontaneously. If possible the cause should be identified and removed from the dog's environment to prevent recurrence.

Drug hypersensitivity (drug allergy)

In rare instances dogs may develop allergic reactions to drugs given orally, by injection or applied topically to the skin surface. Many drugs are potential causes of this condition. Clinical signs are variable. If drug allergy occurs, then use of the offending drug has to be discontinued.

Flea allergic dermatitis

This is the commonest form of allergy in the dog and has been covered previously in detail (see page 256).

Other allergic skin diseases

In rare instances allergies other than those discussed here may occur. Hypersensitivity to internal parasites, skin parasites other than fleas, hormones, bacteria and fungi have all been reported.

BACTERIAL SKIN DISEASE (pyoderma)

Bacterial skin disease or pyodermas are common in small animal practice. They usually occur as a result of some other disease such as allergy altering the skin surface environment and allowing bacteria to multiply and hence aggravate the original condition. The usual bacteria involved is *Staphylococcus intermedius*, although other bacteria occasionally cause skin disease. Pyodermas have been classified according to depth of the infection within the skin (surface, superficial and deep) as more aggressive treatment is needed for the deeper and more severe forms.

Surface pyoderma

Two major forms of surface pyodermas are seen; acute moist dermatitis and skin-fold pyoderma.

1. *Acute moist dermatitis* (wet eczema, hot spot, summer eczema) Intense self-trauma as a result of flea allergy, anal sac disease, otitis externa or other irritant diseases may lead to acute moist dermatitis. The problem is particularly common in hot, humid weather, especially in long-haired dogs, as these factors will produce warm, humid conditions suitable for bacterial growth. The lesions appear suddenly and are initially very inflamed. They become moist and painful, with reddening and hair loss. They are usually located close to the original painful area, such as impacted anal sacs or the site of a flea bite.

Treatment involves identification and removal of the underlying cause, clipping of the surrounding hair to allow ventilation, cleansing and then the application of an antimicrobial cream with or without glucocorticoids (steroids).

2. *Skin-fold pyoderma* (intertrigo) Skin folds allow the surface of two adjacent areas of skin to lie in close contact with one another, preventing ventilation and creating a warm, humid environment in which bacteria can multiply. Certain breeds appear to be predisposed to this condition. Examples include: Spaniels (lip-fold pyoderma), Pekingese, Pugs and Bulldogs (facial-fold pyoderma) and Shar Peis or obese individuals of any breed (body-fold pyoderma).

Treatment is based on surgical removal of the anatomical defect or, in the case of obesity, on dietary control. In some instances antibacterial shampoo, to cleanse or dry the area, may be of value. However, surgical resection of the excess folds to correct the condition is preferable and often necessary to prevent recurrence.

Superficial pyoderma

Superificial bacterial infections may occur in the stratum corneum, when it is known as impetigo (see Fig. 123) or in the hair follicles, leading to folliculitis.

1. *Impetigo* Impetigo is a mild, transient disease of puppies affecting the skin of the axillae, abdomen and groin, especially around the penis and vulva. The lesions are small pustules or 'white heads'. Treatment with antibacterial shampoos will bring about a rapid resolution of lesions in most cases, but the advice of your veterinary surgeon should be sought.

2. *Superficial folliculitis* Superficial folliculitis can occur in any age of dog especially young adults. Breeds particularly predisposed to the condition

include German Shepherds and Retrievers. Pustules and tiny red spots (papules) are initially present, but self-trauma due to pruritus alters the clinical picture leading to redness (erythema) and open sores (excoriations). Chronic cases can show skin thickening and darkening of the surface of the skin (hyperpigmentation). In superficial pyoderma, circular areas of scaling surrounded by a ring of erythema and with central hyperpigmentation are not uncommonly seen. These areas are known as epidermal collarettes and are frequently a source of anxiety to owners, who consider that the dog may have ringworm. Any part of the body may be affected, but particularly the abdomen, the groin, the thighs and the axillae. It is very unusual for ringworm, which is a fungal skin disease, to be implicated in these lesions.

Many underlying diseases may lead to superficial pyoderma, including flea allergy, sarcoptic mange, atopy, food allergy and hormonal diseases such as hypothyroidism and Cushing's syndrome (see later). Diagnosis is difficult as such a wide range of underlying causes may be involved. Treatment involves correction of the initial cause, followed by antibiotic and antibacterial shampoo therapy for at least three weeks. In many instances the initiating disease may not be determined and pyoderma may become a chronic recurrent problem and may necessitate life-long therapy, which unfortunately occurs in many skin problems.

Deep pyoderma

This group of pyodermas are the most serious and potentially life-threatening and hence require the most aggressive treatment. Underlying causes include demodicosis, hormonal disease and immunodeficiency. Lesions can vary in their locations but are commonly found on feet, over joints (hocks and elbows) and on the chin and muzzle. A severely thickened, hyperpigmented skin with much scarring and which oozes pus on digital pressure is highly suggestive of deep pyoderma. A common example of deep pyoderma is an infected pressure sore of the elbow in one of the giant breeds such as the Great Dane or Irish Wolfhound.

Treatment is based on detection and correction of the underlying cause if possible. Antibiotic therapy and antibacterial shampoos may be required for months or even years. In the USA regular antiseptic 'Jacuzzi' or whirlpool baths are used as an adjunct to treatment.

HORMONAL SKIN DISEASE

Hormonal or endocrine diseases commonly affect the skin. Hormones, particularly thyroid hormone, sex hormones and glucocorticoids, can profoundly influence skin function via extremely complex and in most cases poorly understood mechanisms. Endocrine skin disease usually takes the form of non-pruritic bilaterally symmetrical hair loss or alopecia.

Alterations in skin pigmentation and thickness, and impaired resistance to both bacterial or fungal infections may also be a feature. These changes are due to major disturbances in skin function and require prolonged treatment.

The internal aspects of hormonal diseases are covered in Chapter 14. In this section only the dermatological manifestations of endocrine disease will be discussed.

Hypothyroidism

The clinical signs of skin disease associated with lack of circulating thyroid hormones (hypothyroidism) vary. Bilaterally symmetrical alopecia, hyperpigmentation, skin thickening and scaling, pyoderma, dull coat, puffy, swollen skin, cool skin and easy bruising have all been reported. However, some cases of hypothyroidism may show few or none of these signs. There is no classic diagnostic picture and so blood tests are needed to confirm this diagnosis.

Hyperadrenocorticism (Cushing's syndrome)

Excess production of glucocorticoids (steroids) from the adrenal glands will lead to naturally occurring Cushing's syndrome. However, prolonged, high-dose glucocorticoid therapy may also induce this disease in some individuals. A major use of these cortisone drugs in veterinary practice is the control of pruritus. Consequently specialist veterinary dermatologists may sometimes encounter patients with pruritic skin conditions (e.g., allergy) and concomitant drug-induced Cushing's syndrome.

Irrespective of the cause, the following skin changes may be seen in Cushing's syndrome: bilaterally symmetrical alopecia, hyperpigmentation, excessively thin (almost transparent) wrinkly skin and blackheads (comedomes). Pyoderma, easy bruising and poor wound healing may also be a feature. In about 40 per cent of cases solid lumps of calcium will be detected within the skin (calcinosis cutis). The clinical signs of Cushing's syndrome are more diagnostic than those of hypothyroidism, but blood testing is still needed to confirm the diagnosis and to distinguish between the natural and drug-induced forms of the disease. Inappropriate treatment of Cushing's syndrome without laboratory confirmation of the diagnosis may lead to serious side-effects.

Sex hormone-related skin diseases

Currently these diseases are poorly understood in veterinary medicine. Sex hormones can induce unpredictable skin responses. In bitches, for example, excess production of female sex hormones (particularly oestrogens) from the ovaries may lead to alopecia. Paradoxically, in spayed bitches a similarly distributed alopecia may also be seen *which is responsive to treatment with oestrogens*! Consequently interaction between sex hormones and the skin is a very active area of medical research.

1. *Hyperoestrogenism* (Type I ovarian imbalance) In some middle-aged bitches ovarian disease (tumours or cystic ovaries) leads to overproduction of oestrogens (hyperoestrogenism, see Chapter 11). This is also seen when bitches are treated with oestrogens to control other unrelated diseases such as urinary incontinence. This rare condition is associated with hair loss around the thighs and genital area; enlargement of nipples and vulva and oestrus cycle abnormalities. There are no reliable laboratory tests for this disease: spaying is both diagnostic and curative. In bitches receiving oestrogen therapy, alternative forms of therapy should be sought or discontinuation of treatment should be considered.

2. *Oestrogen-responsive alopecia* (Hypo-oestrogenism; Type II ovarian imbalance) This is a rare condition in which young *spayed* bitches exhibit alopecia with the distribution described for hyperoestrogenism, but the nipples and vulva remain immature. This condition responds to oestrogen therapy; however, treatment is not recommended as this is merely a cosmetic disease and long-term oestrogen therapy may induce serious side-effects.

3. *Castration-responsive alopecia* Certain testicular tumours (Sertoli cell tumours) may produce oestrogen in male dogs and lead to alopecia and signs of feminisation such as attractiveness to other male dogs and enlarged nipples. One testicle may be enlarged, but this is not a constant finding. No reliable blood tests are available and castration is curative. A much rarer form of alopecia is seen in male dogs with no other signs of disease and normal testicles. These dogs may also respond to castration, although it is not clear how or why this occurs.

4. *Testosterone-responsive alopecia* Alopecia responsive to male hormones (testosterones) may occasionally occur in male individuals. Affected dogs may be castrated or entire. Again the question of whether to treat arises: this is a cosmetic problem and treatment may cause medical and behavioural side-effects.

RINGWORM (DERMATOPHYTOSIS)

Ringworm, despite its name, is a fungal infection. It can affect the hairs, the stratum corneum and, rarely, the nails. The fungi involved are usually *Microsporum* or *Trichophyton* species. Ringworm is rare in dogs. Lesions are variable in appearance and can affect any part of the body. Areas of hair loss associated with greyish scaling and crusting are suggestive of ringworm. However, such lesions should not be confused with the epidermal collarettes of superficial pyoderma. Infection is from contact with affected individuals or indirectly from sharing collars or grooming equipment. Diagnosis is based on growing and identifying the fungus in the laboratory. Veterinary surgeons may shine special ultraviolet lamps (Wood's lamps) on to the animal's coat as a screening test, because around 60 per cent of *Microsporum* fungi glow or fluoresce in this light. However, it is not a reliable method of diagnosing ringworm as 40 per cent of *Microsporum* strains and 100 per cent of *Trichophyton* strains do not fluoresce. Spontaneous recovery usually occurs after six to eight weeks, but treatment with antifungal antibiotics and environmental decontamination is advised because infection of in-contact animals and people can occur. Occasionally recurrent cases that are resistant to treatment are seen; these animals generally have an associated defect in their immune response.

SKIN TUMOURS

Tumours are commonly seen in dog skin: 30 per cent of all canine tumours occur within the skin. They occur when cells start to multiply in an out-of-control fashion and are classified as benign, which are slow growing and have little or no tendency to spread within the body, or malignant, which tend to spread within the body and are more rapid growing. Malignant tumours are often known as cancers. It should be recognised that not all skin swellings are tumours; abscesses, cysts and certain other lesions may be present as 'lumps' in the skin. Furthermore, even if a tumour is present, it may not be a life-endangering problem. The majority of these problems are easily treated if veterinary advice is sought at an early stage in the disease. Early treatment is always worthwhile and may involve surgery as it is seldom possible to evaluate the nature of the lesions on inspection alone. Surgical removal is always warranted, although at some anatomical sites this is not feasible. If total removal of the tumour is not possible then a small piece of the lesion (biopsy) should be taken for diagnostic purposes.

The biopsy should be examined microscopically by a specialist histopathologist so that a definitive diagnosis can be made. In this way it is possible to determine whether the lesion is a tumour and, if so, whether it is benign or malignant. With this information, decisions can be made regarding undertaking further tests (for example X-rays) or instituting further therapy. In some instances treatment with anti-cancer drugs (chemotherapy), radiotherapy, or cryotherapy (treatment with intense cold) may be required. Unfortunately, some animals have to be put to sleep on humane grounds.

IMMUNE-MEDIATED OR AUTO-IMMUNE SKIN DISEASE

Immune-mediated skin disease is uncommon in veterinary dermatology. These diseases occur when the immune system attacks skin components and elicits damage in a manner similar to the rejection of transplanted organs in human patients (Chapter 20). The trigger factors for this inappropriate immune response are largely unknown, but genetic factors, viral infections, stress and exposure to sunlight have been implicated in some cases. Diagnosis is based on histopathological examination of biopsy specimens. Treatment is long-term, high-dose therapy with drugs that suppress the immune system, such as glucocorticoids (steroids) and chemotherapeutic (anti-cancer) drugs.

NUTRITIONAL SKIN DISEASE

Nutritional deficiencies or imbalances are uncommon in the UK due to the widespread feeding of commercial diets from reputable companies. However, poor-quality commercial foods and incorrectly formulated home-cooked diets may lead to dietary deficiencies. In addition, some dogs may have a partial inability to absorb or utilise nutrients in a normal diet and hence have an abnormally high requirement for these nutrients. Nutritional skin disease may occur months after an imbalanced or deficient diet is introduced. Dietary supplementation therapy may take a similar period before a response is seen.

1. *Zinc-responsive dermatosis* (Zinc deficiency) Skin disease responding to dietary zinc supplementation has been recognised in two forms. In the first, certain breeds of dog, especially Dobermanns, Great Danes, Huskies and Malamutes, were found to have an inability to utilise zinc from high-quality balanced diets. In the second form, the disease occurs in dogs fed dry, cereal-based foods. Certain constituents of cereal-based foods interfere with zinc absorption from the gut. In recent years this form of zinc deficiency has become uncommon as most cereal-based foods are now supplemented with zinc to compensate for this effect.

Crusting, scaling, alopecic areas appear on the face (especially around the eyes and lips) and over the joints of affected dogs. Diagnosis is based on detailed investigation of diet, skin biopsy and response to therapy. Treatment involves introducing a good-quality, commercial diet and, in those cases where impaired zinc utilisation is suspected, supplementation with zinc sulphate capsules. In most cases improvement is seen six to eight weeks after commencement of treatment.

2. *Fat deficiency* In recent years the significant role of fats, notably essential fatty acids, in canine skin disease has been recognised and is the subject of much clinical research today.

Fat deficiency can result from the inadequate fat content of a diet or inability to utilise or absorb fat, as may occur with some dogs with liver or pancreatic disease. Dogs with atopy (inhalant allergy) appear to have an impaired ability to handle essential fatty acids; this may aggravate the initial allergic problem. Prolonged storage of foods or exposure to high temperatures may lead to breakdown of fat (rancidity) if anti-oxidants have not been included in the formulation of the diet. Clinical signs may be vague and include poor coat quality, excessive scurf and, paradoxically, greasiness. Diagnosis is based on investigation of diet and response to therapy. These cases may be managed by improvement of the fat status of the diet, treatment of any underlying disease and in some cases supplementation with essential fatty acids.

Other dietary skin diseases

Protein, vitamin and mineral deficiencies or imbalances, although uncommon, may occur if poor-quality foods are fed. Consequently, diet should always be considered as a possible cause of skin disease.

CONGENITAL AND HEREDITARY DISEASE

In congenital skin disease lesions are present at *birth*. They may be inherited or may occur as a result of toxic and infectious problems. In contrast, animals with hereditary skin diseases do not necessarily show signs at *birth* but are *genetically programmed to develop disease later in life*. Congenital diseases are rare and include some quite bizarre problems. These include: dermatosporaxis or so-called India-rubber disease, in which the skin stretches excessively and is rather fragile. Another example is epitheliogenesis imperfecta, in which skin formation is incomplete and the animal is born with gaps or holes in the skin. These diseases may be serious and if a genetic basis to the condition is suspected, then affected individuals and their relatives should not be bred from.

Many skin diseases have a hereditary basis. Atopy, demodicosis and some tumours occur more frequently in certain breeds or lines, suggesting a genetic basis. It is therefore recommended that affected individuals should not be bred from. Unfortunately irresponsible dog breeders have on occasions disregarded this advice and so dogs from certain lines of some breeds frequently develop skin disease.

In some breeds hereditary skin disease is a desired objective of breeding programmes. A relatively innocuous example is the creation of hairless breeds such as the Chinese Crested and Mexican Hairless Dogs. Of greater concern are examples such as blue and fawn Dobermanns, which are beautiful puppies but inevitably develop extensive alopecia and secondary pyoderma as they mature and need lifelong therapy.

In specialist dermatology practice, less than 5 per cent of cases are in mongrel dogs, yet they represent a much higher percentage of the canine population. This suggests that in our pedigree breeds we are selectively breeding animals that are more likely to develop skin disease. Ideally, breeding stock should be selected on the basis of freedom from inherited disease rather than for future show-ring performance.

MISCELLANEOUS SKIN DISEASES

Lick granuloma (acral lick dermatitis) Some Labrador Retrievers, Dobermanns and other breeds constantly lick at an area around the wrist (carpal) joint, causing extensive skin damage and ulceration. This is often a behavioural problem (rather like human nail biting) and may be related to boredom or stress. Treatment is difficult, involving avoidance of factors inducing frustration and boredom. Various medical and surgical treatments have been described but many cases are difficult, if not impossible, to solve. Another similar psychogenic (behavioural) dermatosis is flank sucking, which is seen predominantly in Dobermanns.

Juvenile cellulitis (juvenile pyoderma, puppy strangles, puppy head gland disease). Puppies of many breeds (mostly Retrievers, Great Danes and Dachshunds) may develop swelling of the face, ears and neck, often before four weeks of age. The lesions may form abscesses and burst. Some puppies will appear quite ill in themselves. The cause is unknown, but treatment with antibiotics and high doses of glucocorticoids is usually curative.

GLOSSARY OF TERMS

Allergen a foreign substance eliciting allergy or hypersensitivity.
Allergic reaction an exaggerated response to a foreign material leading to tissue damage.
Alopecia loss of hair.
Auroscope instrument for examining the ear canal.
Dermatitis inflammation of the skin.
Dermis thick inner portion of the skin.
Epidermis thin outer portion of the skin.
Glucocorticoids anti-inflammatory drugs used to control pruritus and pain.
Hypoallergic diet a diet that does not elicit an allergic reaction in an individual with food allergy.
Hypersensitivity allergy.
Immuno-deficiency a defect in the immune system.
Lesions any deviation from normality in a tissue.
Pyoderma infection of the skin with pus-forming bacteria.
Pruritus itchiness.
Ringworm (dermatophytosis) a form of fungal infection of the skin.
Stratum corneum outer layer of the epidermis.

16

THE EYE

The disease problems which involve the dog's eye are many. This is a sad but true statement to have to make at the beginning of a chapter which deals with the eye and sight. Acquired disease is bad enough in terms of its effect on sight, but this tends to be equalled by the enormous amount of inherited eye disease present in today's pedigree dog. Inherited eye disease is avoidable. The first question a would-be dog owner should ask the breeder is 'are there any inherited eye problems present in this breed?' and if the answer is 'yes', then the next question should be 'do you have certificates to prove my puppy and her parents are free from that disease?' Prevention is always to be preferred to cure, and the existence of an official examination scheme run jointly by the British Veterinary Association and the Kennel Club means that today's pet owner should expect to buy a puppy with normal eyes and little or no threat of an inherited sight-destroying problem occurring later in life. It is easy to fall in love with six weeks of wriggling fur on four legs, but it is essential to know that you, your family and your pet will enjoy the relationship that is about to unfold. Disease always brings heartache, and awareness of specific breed problems is the only way you can be certain that the addition to your family will enjoy normal eyesight for the rest of his or her days.

Despite the variety of both acquired and inherited eye diseases, all are characterised by one of two clinical signs, and in some diseases both signs may be present together. These signs are discomfort or pain and loss of sight, and while the former will be obvious the latter may not be noticed until extensive impairment of sight or even total blindness has occurred. Acquired disease is usually the result of accident or infection, and by and large treatment is often possible for many of the problems seen. Many inherited diseases are silent in onset, and some may not occur until late in life. Treatment is not possible in many cases and avoidance is only possible where awareness exists.

Structure of the eye

The eye is an extremely complex, composite structure which, for the purpose of simple discussion, is best described as a camera constructed of living tissue (Fig. 124). Just as the camera is built around the task of producing a picture on film, the eye is built around a light-sensitive living 'film', the retina. The process of sight starts within the retina, light being converted by a complicated biochemical process known as phototransduction into a series of nerve impulses, which are transmitted to the vision centre (visual cortex) in the brain. Here the nerve impulses are converted into images, and sight occurs. The retina, then, is the *raison d'être* for the eye to exist and take on its fascinating appearance and delicate structure. The amount of light entering the camera can be adjusted by a diaphragm, and the object focused upon the film by a lens system. The same process occurs within the eye, the amount of light entering being regulated by movements of the eyelids and pupil, and focusing being achieved by the combined action of the transparent front of the eye, the cornea and the lens. This process of focusing or accommodation is not as developed in the dog as it is in the human being – developmentally, awareness rather than accurate definition has been the requirement. Despite the size of the lens in the dog's eye it is known that it is responsible for only some 40 per cent of the accommodation that occurs.

The box or case of the camera is called the sclera of the eye, and this is covered by a delicate mucous membrane, the conjunctiva. The structure that regulates the size of the pupil is the iris, and this is the coloured part of the eye. In essence it is simply a disc of muscle with a hole in the centre. In reality it is a lot more than that, being mainly responsible for the

Figure 124 The dog's eye, in vertical section

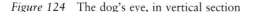

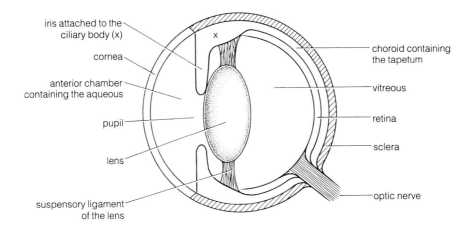

iris attached to the ciliary body (x)

cornea

anterior chamber containing the aqueous

pupil

lens

suspensory ligament of the lens

choroid containing the tapetum

vitreous

retina

sclera

optic nerve

appearance of the eye and the expression within the eye. Some iris colours are even dictated by the Kennel Club's Breed Standards, and competitions may be lost or won on the 'depth of colour' or the 'expression of the eye'. The lens is supported behind the iris by a structure known as the ciliary body, and the accommodative facility or focusing ability is dictated by the amount and type of muscle present within this structure. The ciliary body has another important function in that it produces a fluid known as the aqueous, and this fluid is responsible for feeding the lens and the cornea. Constant production of aqueous is required to do this, and constant drainage of this fluid back through the ciliary body helps to sustain the nutritional cycle and maintain the optically correct shape of the eye. Disease of the ciliary body, which prevents drainage of the aqueous, results in glaucoma, a painful blinding disease that is as difficult to treat in human beings as it is in the dog. The space behind the lens and in front of the retina is filled with a transparent jelly, the vitreous, and the retina is fed in part by a tissue interposed between itself and the sclera, the choroid. The nerve impulses generated in the retina pass back to the brain in the optic nerve. The two nerves meet at the base of the skull with some of their fibres crossing from one side to the other. Thus some messages produced by the left eye are seen on the right side of the brain, and vice versa. The use of the two eyes in unison is called binocular vision and this facility takes approximately six weeks to develop in the puppy. Binocular vision helps the dog to judge distances and appreciate depth.

The eye is physically protected by the depression in the skull in which it is suspended, the orbit, and by the outer eyelids and a third eyelid. The orbit is shallow in breeds like the Pug and the Pekingese, and in these breeds the eye can literally fall out of the orbit between the eyelids with very little provocation. Taking these animals by the scruff of the neck is to be avoided at all costs! The eyelids (palpebrae) are basically movable folds of skin containing muscle. They are lined with the same conjunctival mucous membrane that covers the sclera. The third eyelid (membrana nictitans) is a movable shield of cartilage also covered in conjunctiva. When danger threatens the eye, the eyelids close and the eyeball is pulled back into the orbit, an action which releases the third eyelid to slide over the surface of the cornea. The old-fashioned name for the third eyelid is the haw, and its free edge can be seen at the point where the eyelids meet on the side of the nose. A large gland (the nictitans gland) built into the base of the third eyelid helps to secrete the tear film that keeps the exposed front of the eye moist. Most of this fluid, though, is produced by the tear or lacrimal gland, which is situated above the eye, beneath the upper eyelid. Disturbance of the tear film can lead to a drying out of the corneal and conjunctival surfaces, and inflammation, together with ulceration and pigmentation of the cornea, can severely affect sight if the condition remains untreated.

The type of eyesight developed in the dog has been dictated throughout evolution by a need for constant awareness of the environment: an awareness that senses potential danger and helps find food – in a word, survival. As such there are some interesting developmental features. By and large throughout dogdom the eyes are at the side of the skull to allow a very large field of vision. Specific adaptation to a 24-hour type of vision is seen within the retina. This structure consists of two types of light-sensitive cells (photoreceptors), the rods and the cones. The cones are used in bright light and are responsible for colour vision, while the rods work in low levels of illumination. The dog's retina consists primarily of the rod photoreceptors: thus night vision is very good, but colour vision has suffered at the expense of this awareness modification. In addition, a mirror-like structure called the tapetum has been built into the choroid along the visual axis to reflect light passing through the overlying retina back into the eye. This allows the retina to make use of the same light signal twice over and increase the size of the nerve impulse passing back to the brain. Elsewhere the retina is darkly pigmented, the pigment being a protective device to help absorb scattered light.

Diseases of the eye

The acquired disease problems seen most commonly in the dog are eyelid and corneal wounds, inflammation of the conjunctiva (conjunctivitis) and cornea (keratitis) due to a variety of causes, inflammation of the iris and ciliary body (uveitis), opacity of the lens (cataract) and degeneration of the retina. Very little first-aid treatment for traumatic damage or acute onset disease is possible, and professional help should be obtained as soon as possible. The list of inherited eye diseases is a long one (Table 16, overleaf) and all parts of the eye extending from the eyelids to the optic nerve are involved.

THE EYELIDS

Protection of the eye and movement of the tear film by blinking are the two functions of the eyelids. Thus the anatomical relationship between the edge of the eyelid and the cornea must be harmonious. Distortion of the eyelid following damage or inflammation and distortion due to congenital looseness or tightness of the eyelid aperture cause inflammation of the conjunctiva and the cornea.

Blepharitis

Painful inflammation and/or infection of the eyelid. The condition may be due to trauma, allergy or infection of the glandular tissues found within the eyelid. Very little first-aid treatment is possible and the veterinary surgeon will use anti-inflammatory and antibiotic treatment.

Table 17   The inherited eye diseases which occur in the dog in the United Kingdom

Part of eye involved	The conditions
Eyelid	Entropion Ectropion Combined entropion/ectropion – diamond eye Distichiasis
Tear system	Keratoconjunctivitis sicca – dry eye Abnormality of the lacrimal puncta Epiphora
Cornea	Corneal dystrophy Pannus Ulceration/erosion
Iris	Persistent pupillary membrane (PPM)
Lens	Cataract (HC) Luxation (LL)
Retina	Retinal dysplasia (RD) Collie eye anomaly (CEA) Generalised progressive retinal atrophy (PRA) Central progressive retinal atrophy (CPRA)
Glaucoma	Closed angle Open angle
Microphthalmos	Persistent pupillary membrane (PPM) Cataract Retinal dysplasia (RD)

Distichiasis

An inherited condition which is particularly significant in the Miniature Long Haired Dachshund, the Pekingese and the Cocker Spaniel. Sometimes the condition is referred to as a double row of eyelashes, for extra hairs arise from the edge of the eyelid to rub against the corneal surface (Plate 8). The effects are variable and mild irritation to corneal ulceration will be seen. Treatment is extremely difficult and invariably involves surgery to remove the hair roots permanently. Plucking out the offending hairs is useful, but requires the maximum co-operation of the patient. Of course it is followed by hair regrowth, and many surgical techniques have been invented to remove the roots. Even then success is difficult to achieve, and your pet may have to suffer this condition throughout its life.

Entropion

Primarily an inherited condition which involves several breeds, but particularly the Chow Chow and Shar Pei. It is due to an excess of eyelid tissue, or a small eye, or both, the result being that a varying amount of hair-covered eyelid can turn in to rub directly against the cornea or conjunctiva, or both (Plate 9). It is usually extremely painful, and the damage caused to the cornea can render the eye blind. Most dogs are affected by six months of age and in some the signs of the problem (excessive blinking and a wet face) may be seen within the first month of life. Occasionally the condition is self-correcting as the puppy grows, but in the vast majority of affected dogs surgery is necessary to turn the eyelid away from the surface of the eye. Usually such surgery is successful, but it is much better that, as with the other inherited eyelid defects, dog breeders try to avoid producing this condition in their stock.

Ectropion

Primarily an inherited condition in which the lower eyelid droops away from the eyeball to expose the third eyelid and the conjunctiva (Plate 10). It is seen classically in the Bloodhound and the St Bernard. Exposure of the delicate mucous membrane causes conjunctivitis. Unfortunately the defect has arisen as a direct result of the breed standard, and prevention necessitates breeding away from this desired feature towards a much more sensibly shaped eye. For those patients with ectropion, correction is possible by complicated surgery in which the eyelid is lifted and shortened. Occasionally further surgery may be necessary to change completely the shape of the eyelids.

Trichiasis

A condition which can be inherited or acquired, and in which hair arising on the surface of the eyelid grows towards the eye, not away from it. Contact between the eyeball and the hair causes irritation and keratitis, and surgery to evert the eyelid is required to produce the cure.

Tumours

Both benign and malignant tumours can grow within eyelid tissue, and most involve the skin or the glandular parts of the eyelid (Plate 11). Fortunately the vast majority do not spread to the rest of the body, and the associated problems are irritation of the corneal surface due to contact and the effect on sight when the tumour is large. Early surgery is usually very effective.

Wounds

Torn eyelids must be repaired as soon as possible, for delay can result in distortion. First-aid measures include cleansing the wound using warm salt

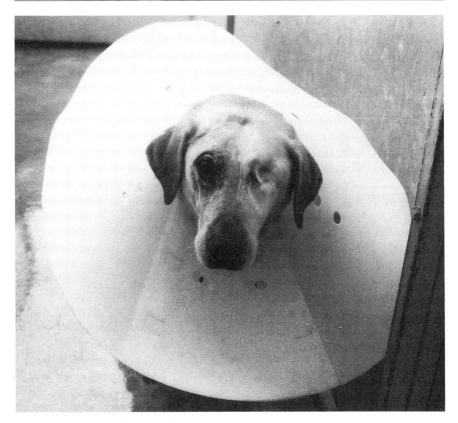

Figure 125 An Elizabethan collar

water and preventing the dog causing more damage by rubbing. One simple way of protecting a damaged eyelid or eyeball until professional attention is available is to use a plastic bucket. Remove the handle, cut a hole big enough to accommodate the dog's neck in the bottom, and slit the side from the rim to the hole. The bucket can then be sprung open so that the dog's head can be put inside with its neck passing through the hole: lace the side up with string. A more professional model called an Elizabethan Collar is available and veterinary surgeons will often dispense these where there is danger of self-trauma exacerbating the disease problem (Fig. 125).

THE CONJUNCTIVA

Inflammation of the conjunctiva (conjunctivitis) is a very common problem, occurring in its own right as the result of the presence of foreign body material, virus infection, trauma and allergy, or accompanying other

eye and eyelid diseases. The normal conjunctiva lining the eyelids and covering the third eyelid is pink, while the conjunctiva covering the sclera is white. When inflammation is present these membranes turn red, but this redness is much more easily recognised in the tissue which covers the sclera. There will be irritation and even pain, much winking and blinking and the discharge
may vary from excessive tears to thick mucoid and mucopurulent material. Other than clearing the eyelids of discharge, first-aid treatment is impossible, and professional help must be sought before permanent damage occurs.

THE THIRD EYELID

This structure can be involved in any conjunctivitis, but damage, distortion and tumour formation can also occur. Damage is usually sustained as the result of an encounter with a cat, the surface of the third eyelid being clawed as it covers the cornea. Surgical repair may be necessary, and antibiotics will be used to prevent infection.

The distortions which are seen are prominence, kinking (Plate 13) and prolapse of the tear-producing gland (Plate 12). Prominence of the third eyelid may indicate the presence of another disease problem, but kinking and the gland prolapse, sometimes called 'cherry eye', both require surgical attention.

THE NASOLACRIMAL SYSTEM

The tear film is produced mainly by the lacrimal and nictitans glands, but several other smaller glands in the eyelid and the conjunctiva are also involved. Tears are constantly produced to keep the corneal and conjunctival surfaces moist. There is some evaporation, but most of the tear film is drained off the surface of the eye into the nose by the narrow nasolacrimal duct. Disease of the lacrimal and nictitans glands produces dryness of the eye (keratoconjunctivitis sicca), and either medical or surgical treatment is required to prevent corneal and conjunctival damage. In those dogs in which medical treatment is not successful, an operation to divert saliva from the mouth to the cornea has been spectacularly successful. The eye is kept moist by the saliva at all times, and at meal times the patient literally cries into his food!

Disease of the nasolacrimal duct system causes an overflow of tears on to the face (Fig. 126). Now, painful conditions cause excessive tear production, and the first problem the veterinary surgeon has when he is faced with a dog with a wet face is to decide if this is a pain or a plumbing problem. If it is the latter he will then investigate the nasolacrimal duct, but it should be remembered that for several breeds like the Pekingese and

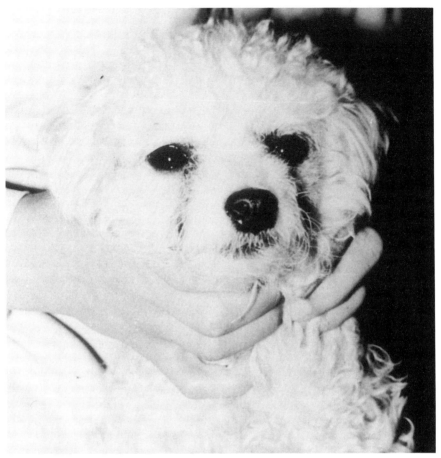

Figure 126 Epiphora – overflow of tears onto the face

the Cavalier King Charles Spaniel, the nasal drainage of tears is difficult and a wet face is very much the norm.

THE CORNEA

Inflammation of the cornea, keratitis, is quite a common condition in the dog, but the causes are several. Trauma, auto-immunity in which the dog makes antibodies against his corneal tissues, and infection all have a part to play, but the threat to any patient with keratitis is an impairment or loss of sight due to scar formation and pigmentation. Ulceration of the cornea is always a potentially serious condition, for deep ulcers can result in the eyeball bursting open. Corneal wounds also are always associated with potentially serious complications, and for these reasons any dog experiencing pain, excessive winking and blinking and producing an excess of tears should be seen immediately by a veterinary surgeon. Keratitis can be treated very effectively and even corneal ulceration does not hold the horrors that it used to do. Today's medicines and surgical techniques offer excellent chances of recovery, but speed of referral is essential. Again, first-aid measures are few and far between and professional help must be sought.

Some corneal diseases are inherited. Keratoconjunctivitis sicca is seen in the West Highland White Terrier, pannus, a type of keratitis, occurs in the German Shepherd Dog and corneal dystrophy, a condition in which fat appears as an opaque patch in the corneal tissues, involves several breeds, including the Cavalier King Charles Spaniel, the Rough Collie and the Siberian Husky.

THE UVEAL TRACT

The iris, ciliary body and choroid are jointly referred to as the uveal tract. Inflammation of these structures is uveitis, which is a sight-threatening disease. The causes are several, but in the absence of certainty of a particular cause, symptomatic treatment can often be very effective. Uveitis is usually very painful: the pupil becomes very small (miosis), the cornea may become milky with fluid retention (oedema) and the scleral and conjunctival blood vessels become engorged (hyperaemia). The danger to sight lies in the fact that the eye fills with exudate and the iris may become stuck on to the lens (posterior synechia), cataract may develop and the drainage of aqueous may be impaired and cause a glaucoma. Uveitis is an emergency disease situation, and immediate professional help is required.

THE LENS

Two disease problems beset the dog's lens. In some terrier breeds, today notably the Jack Russell Terrier, the lens will dislocate from its normal position behind the iris. This is called lens luxation and it occurs because the lens moorings to the ciliary body are inherently weak. When they snap the lens is free to move. If the lens moves into the pupil or comes to rest in front of the iris, then aqueous circulation is not possible and its drainage through the ciliary body stops. This causes the fluid pressure inside the eye to rise, and glaucoma occurs. This is an extremely painful condition and pressure-induced damage of the optic nerve can render the eye blind in just a few hours. Emergency surgery is necessary, the removal of the lens allowing the aqueous to circulate freely once again.

The other disease problem is cataract (Plate 14). Any opacity of the lens is called a cataract, and obviously only the larger cataracts have an effect on vision. Some cataract is acquired as the result of trauma, uveitis or diseases such as diabetes, but in the dog most of the cataract seen is inherited. Several breeds of dog are involved (Table 18, overleaf) and it is

Table 18   Hereditary cataract in dog breeds in the United Kingdom

Afghan Hound	
American Cocker Spaniel	
Boston Terrier	two types
Chesapeake Bay Retriever	
German Shepherd Dog	
Golden Retriever	two types
Labrador Retriever	
Miniature Schnauzer	two types
Siberian Husky	
Staffordshire Bull Terrier	two types
Standard Poodle	
Welsh Springer Spaniel	

Probable hereditary cataract

Cavalier King Charles Spaniel	two types
English Cocker Spaniel	
Lancashire Heeler	
Large Munsterlander	
Old English Sheepdog	two types
West Highland White Terrier	

one of the conditions to enquire about if you want to own one of these breeds. Treatment is only by the surgical removal of the lens and this is not simple surgery (Plate 15). Most patients go into the operating theatre with a 70 to 80 per cent chance of seeing again, but the outcome is far from certain. It is another situation where prevention is better than cure, and the BVA/KC eye disease certification scheme offers breeders an excellent chance to make certain that they are producing puppies from disease-free stock.

THE RETINA

Disease of the retina always carries the serious possibility that sight may be affected, or the patient rendered blind. Inflammation of the retina is usually caused by an inflammation of the underlying choroid, and often the reasons for that inflammation remain unknown. Distemper, toxoplasmosis, viral hepatitis and leptospirosis are all possible causes, but it is an area where symptomatic treatment is usually applied.

Several inherited retinal diseases occur in the dog, and as treatment is not possible, control based on routine annual eye examinations in those breeds susceptible has become absolutely essential.

Collie eye anomaly

Collie eye anomaly (CEA) is the commonest canine eye disease in the

Table 19 Progressive retinal atrophy in dog breeds in the United Kingdom

Breed	Type of PRA
Border Collie	Central
Briard	Central
Cardigan Welsh Corgi	Central & generalised
Dachshund (Miniature Long Haired)	Generalised
Elkhound	Generalised
English Cocker Spaniel	Central & generalised
English Springer Spaniel	Central & generalised
Golden Retriever	Central
Irish Setter	Generalised
Labrador Retriever	Central & generalised
Poodle (Miniature & Toy)	Generalised
Rough & Smooth Collies	Central & generalised
Schnauzer (Miniature)	Generalised
Shetland Sheepdog	Central
Tibetan Spaniel	Generalised
Tibetan Terrier	Generalised

United Kingdom. Its incidence in the Rough and Smooth Collie breeds and the Shetland Sheepdog is very high, and recently it has made an appearance in the Border Collie. It is a disease complex which includes abnormal development of the choroid, 'holes' (colobomas) in the optic nerve and congenital non-attachment of the retina. Fortunately blindness only occurs in approximately 6 per cent of affected eyes, but the way in which the condition is inherited means that dogs with normal eyes can produce affected offspring. Because it is present at birth whole litters can be examined for the disease and affected puppies discovered before they enter breeding programmes.

Progressive retinal atrophy

Progressive retinal atrophy (PRA) is a term used to describe a number of inherited retinal degenerations involving several breeds (Table 19). The group is broadly divided into two, generalised PRA and central PRA. In the former, blindness at night time (nyctalopia) is an early indication of the presence of the disease, but eventually the dog is rendered totally blind. Cataract is a common secondary feature of the disease. In central PRA night blindness is not a feature and though vision is severely affected, the dog may not become totally blind. In both groups of PRA there is degeneration of the photoreceptors, but in the generalised form this degeneration is the inherited defect, whereas in central PRA rod and cone degeneration follows an inherited defect elsewhere in the retina. Just as with hereditary cataract the level of awareness to the presence of PRA shown by the breeding community is high, but the success of disease control schemes again depends upon wholesale participation, the pooling of results and pedigree analysis. There is a long way to go, and only by asking about the PRA status of the puppy's parents can the prospective dog owner be as certain as possible that his new charge will not develop this disease.

Retinal dysplasia

Retinal dysplasia (RD) is a congenital defect which in its simplest form is seen as a multiple folding of the retina, while the most severe type is non-attachment of the retina to the underlying choroid. The effect on sight varies accordingly, ranging from no apparent defect to total blindness. Over the years RD has been described in several breeds, but of late the condition has made a dramatic appearance in the working strains of the English Springer Spaniel.

GLAUCOMA

Glaucoma is a disease process in which the internal fluid pressure of the eye rises above its normal upper limit. It is due to the fact that the aqueous cannot escape from the front chamber of the eye through the ciliary body quickly enough. Primary glaucoma is due to an inherited defect of the ciliary body, whereas secondary glaucoma occurs as the result of another eye disease causing ciliary body damage. In an acute situation there is a sudden rise in the fluid pressure, the patient is in pain and the eye is rendered blind because of pressure on the optic nerve. In a chronic situation a small rise in fluid pressure gradually destroys sight by slowly destroying the optic nerve. Speed is the essence in terms of treating glaucoma, but whereas the acute situation is easily recognised, in dogs the chronic situation is only diagnosed when a vision problem prompts the owner to seek veterinary advice for his pet. Basset Hounds, English Cocker Spaniels, Welsh Springer Spaniels and Siberian Huskies suffer from primary acute glaucoma, whereas primary chronic glaucoma is seen in the Elkhound in this country. Secondary acute glaucoma due to lens luxation is the commonest type of glaucoma in dogs in the UK and glaucoma following trauma or uveitis may be dramatic or chronic in onset.

Treatment involves reducing the fluid pressure to normal as quickly as possible. Where there is little disease or damage to the ciliary body, drugs might be able to achieve this, but elsewhere surgery to produce a new route of aqueous exit is necessary.

PROLAPSE OF THE EYE

In the brachycephalic breeds such as the Pekingese it is relatively easy for the eye to be traumatically prolapsed out of the orbit through the aperture

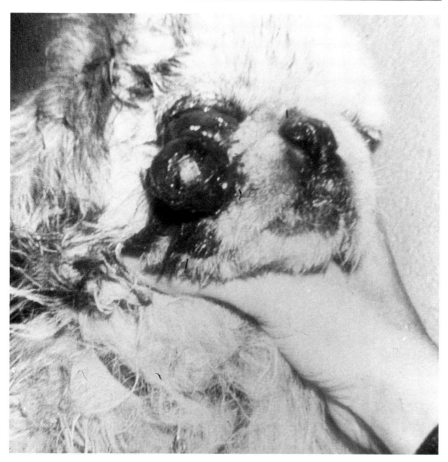

Figure 127   Prolapse of the eyeball

between the lids (Fig. 127). This happens in other breeds too, but, because of the deeper orbit, it takes much more force to do this and as such damage to the eye is usually greater. Eyeball prolapse is always a serious problem, the stretch often seriously damaging the optic nerve. First aid means the use of a saline-soaked pad to protect the eye from further damage while veterinary attention is being found. Your veterinary surgeon will then replace the eye under a general anaesthetic, but the outcome is not always certain. Muscle damage causes a squint, and the eye may be blind due to damage to the optic nerve.

CONCLUSION

It will be realised that all eye disease is of potentially serious consequence. Acute onset problems must always be seen as potential emergencies requiring speedy diagnosis and prompt treatment. First-aid care is very limited and is restricted to cleansing wounds, preventing self-trauma and relieving pain. The threat to sight is always present, and the reader has only to close his own eyes to realise the handicap of blindness. The fact that blind dogs do cope extremely well with their disability is no substitute for prompt treatment. It is a sad reflection that a percentage of all puppies born will lose their sight, many as a result of inherited disease which is not treatable. It is precisely for this reason that the BVA/KC eye examination scheme exists and its very existence demands full subscription. Dog breeders should be aware of the inherited problems that are present within their breeds and, further, they should be familiar with the eye examination scheme. It is the responsibility of today's breeder to ensure that his stock is sound, and ignorance of the disease conditions and the preventative measures that are possible is no longer a tenable excuse. For his part the would-be dog owner should be aware that the inherited eye diseases affect several breeds, and should ask the right questions at the time of purchase to ensure that his puppy will be as normal as possible throughout the whole of its life.

17

THE EAR

Browse through any illustrated publication on the many breeds of dog around in the United Kingdom, and the considerable variation in appearance of what is one species is amazing. There are flop ears, prick ears, semi-pricked ears, big ears, little ears – all variations upon the basic theme. The shape of the ear and its carriage give character and lend an important sense of expression to the dog's features. Appearance is a breed characteristic, and the Kennel Club's Breed Standards carefully prescribe appearance down to the last millimetre of detail. However, the ear that we see is just the ear flap (the pinna), and it is only a part of a very complex organ of special sense that is associated with both hearing and balance. Hearing is well developed in the dog, this capability having evolved as part of a general awareness system related to survival. The ear collects and transmits sound waves from the environment to a hearing centre (the acoustic radiations) in the brain. Like most structures of complexity it is subject to disease and disorder. Such problems may cause discomfort, pain, possible impairment or loss of hearing and, on occasion, loss of balance. Even the mildest signs of ear disease should prompt you to seek professional advice. Head shaking, excessive ear scratching, the presence of a smell or the sight of waxy discharge all suggest a possible problem. Ear disease is very common, in fact it is one of the commonest reasons for keeping your veterinary surgeon busy. 'Practice makes perfect' is an old adage, and ear disease is well understood and well treated by the professionals. 'Do-it-yourself' medicine is to be avoided at all costs – pouring solutions or puffing powders into the ear by the inexperienced often exacerbates the problem with more discomfort for the dog, and simply represents time lost. Complicated ear disease can be very difficult to treat, and early referral to your veterinary surgeon represents the best you can do for your pet.

Structure of the ear

An understanding of ear disease necessitates some knowledge of the underlying structure of the ear (Fig. 128).

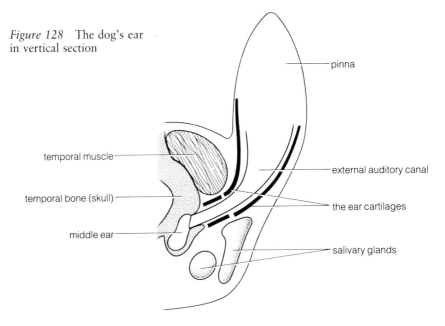

Figure 128 The dog's ear
in vertical section

pinna

temporal muscle

external auditory canal

temporal bone (skull)

the ear cartilages

middle ear

salivary glands

For the sake of description, the ear is divided into three main parts; the external, the middle and the internal ears. The external ear consists of the (pinna) and the ear canal (the external auditory canal). The middle ear is housed within a large skull bone, the temporal bone, and it consists of the ear drum (tympanic membrane) and three small bones (the auditory ossicles). The inner ear is also housed within the temporal bone, and it is divided into two specialised systems which deal with hearing and balance.

THE EXTERNAL EAR

The pinna is made of cartilage and covered with skin on both sides. Movement is effected by small muscles, but this activity is restricted mainly to the prick-eared and semi-prick-eared breeds. Here the pinna helps to pick up and locate the direction of sound, but in the floppy-eared breeds no such function is possible. Rather the opposite, in fact, for the pinna actually contributes significantly to the amount of ear disease seen in these breeds. Thus more disease is seen in breeds like the Basset Hound and many of the several Spaniel types, and the reasons will be explained a little later in this chapter.

The external auditory canal is also made of cartilage and lined with modified skin (integument). The canal can be divided into two parts, a long vertical portion which is directed towards the heavens, and a short horizontal part which ends at the level of the ear drum. The lining integument contains many glands of two types which jointly produce the ear wax (cerumen). Wax is essential in that it covers the integument to protect it from fluids and particulate foreign body material.

THE MIDDLE EAR

This part of the ear is found within the tympanic cavity of the temporal bone of the skull (Fig. 129). It is divided from the external ear by the tympanic membrane and is in contact with the inner ear through two membrane-covered holes or windows, the vestibular or oval window and the cochlear or round window. The air vibrations are picked up from the ear drum by the chain of three small bones, the auditory ossicles. The malleus is the largest ossicle and it is attached to the ear drum. It transmits vibrations to the second ossicle, the incus, which is in contact with the third ossicle, the stapes. This is the smallest bone in the dog's body, measuring just 2 mm (¹⁄₁₂ in.) in length, and it makes contact with the inner ear via the oval or vestibular window. Thus sounds waves collected by the pinna and conducted to the ear drum by the ear canal are transmitted by the ossicles as vibrations to the inner ear.

The ossicles are found within the roof of the middle ear: the lowest part of the middle ear (hypotympanicum) opens into the throat (pharynx) by a short canal known as the Eustachian or auditory tube. The presence of this

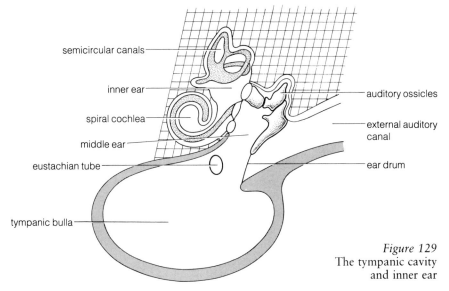

semicircular canals

inner ear

spiral cochlea

middle ear

eustachian tube

tympanic bulla

auditory ossicles

external auditory canal

ear drum

Figure 129
The tympanic cavity
and inner ear

canal means that pressure can always be equalised on both sides of the ear drum, and this delicate structure is not ruptured when the environmental pressure increases. We have all experienced a tightness in both ears when a plane takes off or a train passes through a long tunnel at speed, and know the relief that swallowing or chewing brings. This is the Eustachian tube at work. Most disease of the middle ear occurs as an extension of disease from the ear canal through a ruptured ear drum. This is referred to as descending middle ear disease, but occasionally infection can pass from the throat up the Eustachian tube into the middle ear. This type of disease is called ascending middle ear disease.

The hypotympanicum is expanded into a large bubble of bone that is eggshell thick, and this swelling on the base of the skull is known as the tympanic bulla. In middle ear disease the bulla can fill with pus, and treatment can involve surgery to open it up and drain the infection, a kind of abscess in bone.

THE INNER EAR

This is the most complicated part of the ear and consists of many fluid-filled channels and sacs. It can be divided into three parts, the cochlea, the vestibule and the semicircular canals. The cochlea is so called because it looks like a snail's shell, and it is within its structure that the vibrations transmitted by the ossicles are converted into nerve impulses by the organ of Corti. These impulses pass via the cochlear nerve to the auditory centre within the brain and result in hearing. The vestibule and the semicircular canals are concerned with maintaining balance, this process being based on the movement of a fluid called perilymph within the cavities that make up their structure.

Disease of the inner ear may cause deafness, loss of balance, or both. In the dog it is a relatively rare occurrence, the most common defects being deafness in newborn puppies due to a failure of the cochlea to develop properly and deafness in old age due to degeneration of the organ of Corti.

Diseases of the ear

Otitis is a broad term used for diseases of the ear. Strictly speaking it means inflammation of the ear, and in essence all the problems seen are due to inflammation or have an inflammatory component. Otitis externa is disease of the external ear, otitis media, the middle ear, and otitis interna, the inner ear.

OTITIS EXTERNA

This disease occurs commonly in the dog. The picture is not always a simple one, for the causes of otitis externa can be several (Fig. 130). A

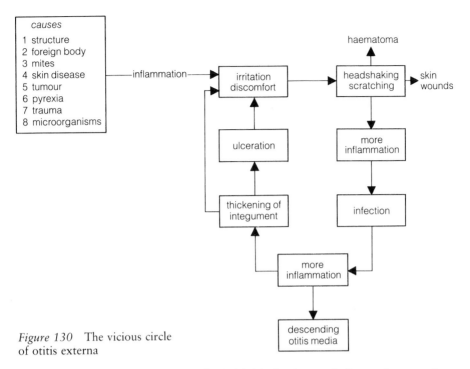

Figure 130 The vicious circle of otitis externa

vicious circle of change occurs, the initial irritation and discomfort causing more inflammation which predisposes to infection with bacterial and fungal micro-organisms. More inflammation is the result, with thickening and possible ulceration of the integument creating yet more inflammation and discomfort. Head shaking can rupture small blood vessels between the cartilage and integument of the pinna, and a large blood-filled swelling (haematoma) will require veterinary attention in order to prevent a cauliflower ear deformity developing. Violent scratching can damage the skin around the ear, and contribute to inflammation of the integument.

There are several factors involved in the initial stages of otitis externa and their differential diagnosis is the important step in treatment.

Structure of the normal ear

It is true to say that the shape and conformation of the external ear is perhaps the most important factor in the initiation of otitis externa. The basic design pattern can be wrong. Why is this? Accumulation of wax within the canal causes inflammation, but what anatomical defects help this to happen? Wax is produced continuously by the integument, and as such must be lost continually. Drainage up the vertical part of the canal is difficult at the best of times (it goes against all the laws of plumbing) and narrow canals that contain a lot of hair make it all the more difficult.

Aeration of the canal is an essential part of the process. The sticky wax becomes dry and crumbly and it is lost by muscle activity around the canal and head movements. Adequate aeration is impossible in the presence of a floppy pinna, which hangs over the entrance of the canal and effectively seals it off from the environment. Thus the increased incidence of otitis externa in our friends the spaniels and Basset Hound.

Where conformation is the underlying problem it is obvious that medical treatment can be of no permanent effect. Each and every time there is a flare-up there can be irreversible damage to the canal, making it less likely that medical treatment will succeed the next time. Thickening of the integument occurs, and as a result the canal lumen gets smaller, so that in chronic disease the lumen may barely exist at all. It is for this reason that your veterinary surgeon may suggest surgery as the means of cure. Obviously the size of the canal cannot be increased or a floppy pinna turned into an upright structure. What can be done though is that the outer wall of the vertical portion of the canal can be removed (Fig. 131). This functionally reduces the canal to just the short horizontal portion and increases aeration and drainage quite considerably. The operation is known as lateral wall resection, or aural resection, but it must be completed before the integument lining the horizontal portion of the canal becomes thickened. Several other modifications of this technique are possible, but all attempt to do the same thing – break the vicious circle of recurrent inflammation.

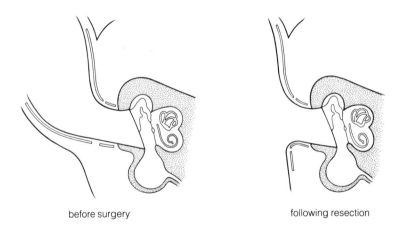

before surgery   following resection

Figure 131   The operation of aural resection

Foreign bodies

The presence of water, soap, grass awns and 'malevolent' foreign bodies will all induce otitis externa. There is usually violent head shaking and frantic ear scratching and rubbing, but with the passage of time this picture slides into one of chronic inflammation. Obviously it is essential that physical foreign bodies are removed as soon as possible, and a general anaesthetic may very well be required to get the job completed without further pain for the dog. Dogs with grass awns in the ear canal are often in a great deal of discomfort or pain and the hairs on the awns tend to dig into the integument and prevent their easy removal.

Mites

Infestation with the ear mite *Otodectes cynotis* is called otocariasis, and it occurs in dogs from time to time. It is a much more common condition in the cat, and in fact the cat probably acts as a reservoir of infestation for the dog. The mites are of pin-head size, white, and they do not like light. Thus they hide right down inside the canal, and their presence will only be revealed by an auriscopic examination. The auriscope is a long illuminated cone that is placed inside the canal to allow the veterinary surgeon to see what is going on. When the ear is painful a general anaesthetic may be required to allow the examination to be completed.

Adult cats seem to be able to tolerate large numbers of mites in their ears, and as such they may not show signs of infestation. It is different in the dog, and just a few mites can cause intense irritation and subsequent inflammation probably due to allergic reaction to the saliva or faeces of the mite. Fortunately treatment is relatively simple, the repeated use of an acaricidal agent ensuring a rapid return to normality.

Skin disease

The lining integument is modified skin, and as such it can be involved as part of a generalised skin problem. Inflammation due to an allergic response may be part of a widespread problem or simply a local reaction.

Tumour

The presence of benign and cancer growths is fortunately an uncommon cause of otitis externa. The integument, its glands and the cartilage can all be involved, and treatment invariably involving surgery depends upon the type of tumour present.

Pyrexia

It is possible for the integument to become inflamed when the dog is running a high temperature due to a systemic infection. Treatment of the underlying infection will require the use of antibiotics, but the otitis may persist if local treatment is not used as well.

Trauma

The term 'trauma' involves several factors which can lead to damage and inflammation of the integument. Self-trauma, in an attempt to relieve irritation by scratching, can exacerbate the problem. 'Owneritis' is a common factor, with the over-anxious owner zealously attempting to clean the ear canals and damaging the integument in doing so, or leaving water, soap or other cleansing agents within the canal. Ear cleansing is only necessary when disease is present, and treating that disease is very much the responsibility of your veterinary surgeon.

Micro-organisms

Otitis externa is complicated by the presence of bacterial or fungal germs. It is unlikely that any of these micro-organisms cause disease, but they can make use of an existing inflammation, multiply and possibly exert a harmful effect. Indeed, some bacteria can invade the inflamed integument and cause serious problems because of their resistance to antibiotic treatment. Breaking the vicious circle of otitis externa before an infection gains the upper hand is important but this requires speedy referral to and treatment by your veterinary surgeon. Undoubtedly rupture of the ear drum occurs in otitis externa, and some bacteria may actually be involved in this. The spread of bacterial infection into the middle ear represents the most serious complication of otitis externa.

OTITIS MEDIA

Most disease of the middle ear is due to a spread of inflammation and infection from the external ear through a ruptured ear drum. Seldom are there problems relating to hearing or loss of balance, but they can occur. There is some difficulty in assessing hearing deficiencies in the presence of a ruptured ear drum and otitis media, for the dog is able to hear across the bones of his skull, and provided the cochlea of the inner ear is intact, hearing will be possible. Occasionally ascending otitis media occurs, the pressure of infected material building up within the tympanic cavity and causing rupture of the ear drum. The presenting feature is pain, with discharge from the ear occurring some days later. However, most patients with otitis media have a long history of otitis externa, and the only common sign is one of chronic discharge from the ear. The ear canal may be closed if the integument has thickened a lot, and it is possible for the discharge from the middle ear to form an abscess elsewhere on the face near the ear. When this bursts, discharge will continually be lost from the hole that has been produced. The dog is in considerable discomfort and even pain when otitis media is present, and the jaw joint on the skull may also be involved, which causes pain during chewing. Otitis media is one of the most difficult disease problems to treat, for medical therapy is virtually useless. Recently surgery in which the whole of the diseased ear canal and that part of the middle ear known as the tympanic bulla are removed became possible and this currently offers the best chance of

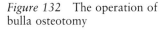

Figure 132 The operation of bulla osteotomy

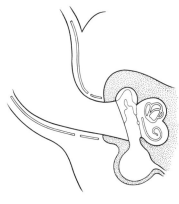
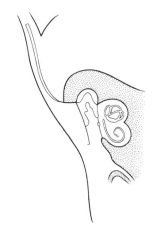

before surgery   following ablation and osteotomy

successful treatment for this difficult problem (Fig. 132). This technique involves major surgery that is not without risk and success cannot be guaranteed. It is much better that a simple otitis externa is cured rather than an otitis media be allowed to develop. Attention to the early signs of scratching and head shaking is amply rewarded, particularly in those breeds in which ear conformation predisposes them to otitis externa.

Occasionally otitis media is due to the growth of a tumour near or involving the tympanic cavity. Treatment depends upon early diagnosis and the type of tumour present.

OTITIS INTERNA

Inflammation and infection of the inner ear occurs usually as an extension of middle ear disease, but occasionally may be caused by disease involving the brain. Treatment relates to treatment of the middle ear disease, and occasionally spontaneous recovery may be assisted by antibiotic therapy. When hearing is lost it seldom returns, but, given time, the dog may be able to compensate for a loss of balance.

CONCLUSION

The simple message for the pet owner is that serious ear disease can be prevented by vigilance and prompt attention. Avoid the temptation to clean that smelly ear yourself, and seek professional help. Most otitis externa can be cured, and otitis media as a complication to otitis externa should not occur. Be aware of the fact that the floppy pinna predisposes to inflammation of the ear canal, and that simple resection surgery exists to counteract the effects of the floppy pinna and the narrow canal.

18

THE NOSE

What's in a nose? Well, apart from being the site of one of the dog's most specialised senses, smell, the shape of the nose divides dogdom into two. On one side of the division there are the dogs with long (dolichocephalic) and medium-sized (mesaticephalic) noses and on the other side dogs with the dramatically short or snub nose (brachycephalic). It is quite amazing that skull shape should vary so considerably within the same species: simple comparison of the Afghan Hound with the Pekingese demonstrates the two extremes explicitly. From a veterinary viewpoint it is interesting that the size of the nose tends to dictate the type of disease that may be present. The brachycephalic, for example, suffering from difficult breathing apparently remains relatively immune to the rigours of fungal infection and nasal cancer.

Structure of the nose

The nose can be divided into two parts, the rhinarium and the nasal cavity proper. The rhinarium is the black moist part at the end of the dog's nose. It is made of cartilage and is covered with a modified type of secreting skin. When either the dog's body temperature or the environmental temperature is high, then the rhinarium may be dry and warm. Having a dry nose, therefore, is not always a sign of illness, but it can be a useful layman's guide, particularly if the dog is listless and off its food. At rest, air passes through the rhinarium via the nostrils (nares). These are slit-like channels which directly communicate with the nasal cavity. During breathing in (inspiration), the nostrils are opened wide (dilated) by muscle action to allow the air to enter with ease. The sucking force for inspiration is generated by the diaphragm and the muscles of the chest wall; the chest cavity simply enlarges under their action during inspiration. Dilation of the nostrils occurs in both the dolichocephalic and mesaticephalic breeds, but is not a feature of the brachycephalic nose. In these breeds the nostrils are often semi-closed, and during inspiration they simply close completely. This makes deep inspiration through the nose impossible, and so many brachycephalic dogs must mouth-breathe simply to survive. Even at rest it is difficult for these dogs to nose-breathe, since the narrow nostrils coupled with a very small congested nasal cavity set up considerable resistance to the inflow of air. Thus the tongue-lolling 'grin' of the Pekingese or Pug is more than an expression of excitement, it is a manifestation of survival. But the breathing difficulties do not stop with the nose. An overlong soft palate can block the voice box (larynx) and even cause its collapse in these breeds.

The nasal cavity is a bony shell that is divided in the midline into two separate chambers. The midline dividing wall (nasal septum) is constructed of bone and cartilage, and normally there is no communication between the two chambers. The bony front part of the nasal septum is the home of a specialised 'scent' organ, the vomero-nasal or Jacobson's organ. Two ducts connect this organ to the mouth and 'lip curling' probably allows air to be drawn into its structure. Kin recognition and sexual attraction are the hypothesised functions of the structure.

The size and shape of the nasal chamber varies considerably between the brachycephalic and the longer-nosed breeds. Each chamber is subdivided into a series of longitudinally running air conducting passages by a number of mucous membrane-covered cartilage and bony tubes (Fig. 133). These tubes are collectively called the turbinates, and their scroll-like meshwork arrangement means that when air is drawn through the nasal cavity it is effectively broken up into lots of small currents. This allows the air to be adequately warmed, filtered and moistened before it passes into the throat and down into the lungs. Filtration and moistening require that the mucous membrane covering the turbinates is kept moist constantly as a result of very active glandular activity. When this mucous membrane is inflamed it overproduces mucus and this blocks up the fine turbinate

Figure 133   The dog's nasal cavity, in longitudinal section

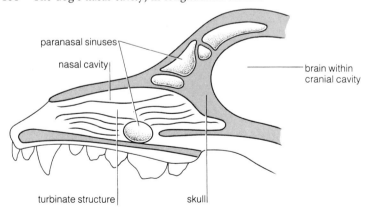

passageways. Olfactory function in the dog is highly developed and loss of appetite (anorexia) may be caused by a loss of the ability to smell food when nasal discharge is present. Cleaning the nose in the anorexic patient with nasal disease is sound nursing advice.

The paranasal sinuses are simply extension cavities of the nasal cavity (Fig. 133). Most are of no anatomical or clinical significance, but the large paired frontal sinuses are considerable structures in the dog which can become involved in disease of the turbinate structure. It is possible for infection and tumour growth to invade the frontal sinus from the nasal cavity, but true sinusitis probably does not exist. An important glandular structure, the lateral nasal gland, is found near the opening of each maxillary sinus. In the dog cooling by evaporation is a feature of heat exchange from the lungs and respiratory passageways. Panting to lose excess heat can result in a drying out of the respiratory mucous membranes and the lateral nasal gland helps to offset this problem. It has been calculated that when the environmental temperature is very high this gland can increase its rate of secretion by a factor of 40.

The problem of difficult breathing in the brachycephalic breeds is well recognised, and that which is something of an amusing snort or snore can become an emergency when hot weather causes excessive panting. Nasal diseases of the longer-nosed breeds tend to be restricted to inflammation (rhinitis), infection and tumour formation, but by and large they represent an extremely difficult area for veterinary treatment. Persistent sneezing, nasal discharge (rhinorrhoea) and haemorrhage (rhinorrhagia) are the warning signs, and these may be accompanied by mouth breathing and gagging or retching. While cure is possible on occasion it remains a sad comment that chronic inflammation and tumour formation remain resistant to the very best of veterinary endeavour.

Diseases of the nose

Difficult breathing (dyspnoea) in the brachycephalic breeds can be helped by surgery to modify the shape of the nostril and shorten the soft palate. Other features of what is known as the brachycephalic airway obstructive syndrome (BAOS) are impossible to treat, although the effects of distortion of the larynx can be relieved by the drastic surgery of tracheostomy, by which the dog is allowed to breathe through a hole in his windpipe. If ever there was a need to rethink the basic design of the dog, then it can never be more dramatically demonstrated than by the brachycephalic dog that dies of asphyxia.

Other disease problems of the nose tend to be just as dramatic in presentation. Owners are usually very aware that a nasal problem exists, for sneezing and discharge are very obvious features with considerable

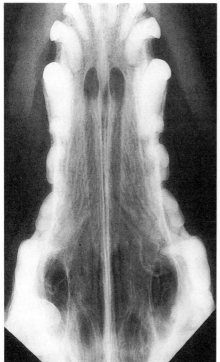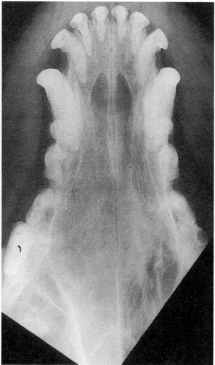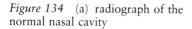

Figure 134 (a) radiograph of the normal nasal cavity

(b) radiograph of a nasal cavity containing a tumour

antisocial implications. Paroxysms of sneezing can cause nose bleeds (epistaxis), while the breakdown of the turbinate structure by some infections or tumour may be indicated by blood-tinged discharge or epistaxis. Discharge may be missed if the patient is a nostril licker, and occasionally most of the discharge may be swallowed: here gagging and retching may be the presenting features. Following a superficial examination when disease of the rhinarium, non-patency of the airways and distortion of the skull may be picked up, your veterinary surgeon may want to anaesthetise your dog to allow X-ray and endoscopic examinations of the nasal chamber to be completed. X-ray examinations are most important and can be most helpful in diagnosis (Fig. 134). In an endoscopic examination the inside of the nasal cavity is examined using an illuminated rigid tube or a flexible fibrescope, and this can be most helpful. In addition nasal discharge and blood samples will be taken, and even an exploratory operation to open the nose (rhinotomy) may be performed to arrive at a diagnosis.

So what are the conditions that give rise to nasal discharge and sneezing?

ULCERATION OF THE RHINARIUM

In this disease the dog produces rogue antibodies which attack the tissues of the rhinarium. Ulceration and haemorrhage may occur and eventually the nostrils may collapse and the airway is lost. This is a condition seen most commonly in the German Shepherd Dog, and control rather than cure is possible if attention is sought early in the process.

FOREIGN BODIES

All manner of foreign bodies ranging from grass seeds to bones can gain entrance to the nasal cavity. Initially there is violent sneezing in an attempt to dislodge the foreign body, but with time a chronic, often infected discharge makes its appearance. Early diagnosis means early removal, before the turbinate tissues are damaged permanently.

DENTAL DISEASE

Occasionally abscesses at the roots of teeth can break out into the nose, but given the amount of dental disease in the dog this is an extremely unusual occurrence. Loss of the large canine tooth in the older dog will sometimes allow a tract to develop between the mouth and the nasal cavity, and this can result in food and fluid passing into the nose to set up inflammatory disease.

DEFECTS OF THE HARD AND SOFT PALATES

The hard palate is the roof of the mouth. The soft palate is a sheet of muscle covered with mucous membrane which extends back from the hard palate into the throat. It closes off the openings into the nose from the throat, an important function when food is taken in from the ground. In man, eating is in the vertical position, and we have no need of a soft palate. The blob of tissue that you see at the back of your throat is called the uvula, and this is the primate remnant of the dog's soft palate. So both the hard and soft palates divide the nose from the throat, and if there is a defect of either, food and fluid passes into the nasal cavity to cause disease. Such defects are either accidental (the result of trauma) or congenital (present at birth) (Fig. 135), but both types can usually be repaired. The congenital defects become apparent because the affected puppy cannot produce negative pressure in his mouth when he sucks at the teat, and any milk that is eventually drawn out tends to come back down the nose.

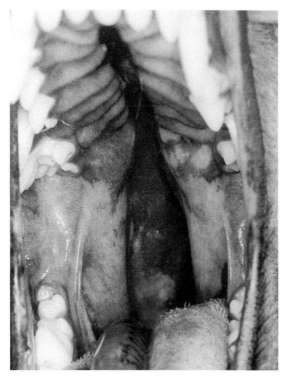

Figure 135 A midline cleft of the hard and soft palates

RHINITIS ASSOCIATED WITH INFECTION

The infections that cause rhinitis in dogs in the United Kingdom are viruses, bacteria, fungi and one parasite. Parasitic infection is uncommon, but a specific worm, *Linguatula serrata*, can live inside the nasal cavity. It is most often seen in kennels, and treatment is difficult, invariably requiring surgery to remove the parasite.

The viral infections which cause rhinitis are several, but canine distemper virus is the one that is universally known. Very often with viral infections the rhinitis produced is quite mild, and it is the secondary contamination with bacteria that causes all the trouble. However, recently a very severe viral rhinitis started to appear in the Irish Wolfhound, and although bacteria were also involved, it was believed that a herpes virus was responsible for the disease. Puppies picked up the infection from their mothers' birth canal during the birth process, and the effects were often serious. Fortunately the problem seems to have taken a back seat of late, and it may have been that a hereditary factor relating to immunity was responsible.

Lots of bacteria can be involved in rhinitis, but most of them are secondary invaders which have simply taken the opportunity to move into what, for them, is a very desirable environment of inflammation. The nasal cavity is always 'dirty' in terms of the bacteria present, and although antibiotic substances are used in the treatment of rhinitis, veterinary surgeons have to work hard to identify the underlying cause of the inflammation.

Infection of the turbinate tissues with a fungus, *Aspergillus fumigatus*, is a very important cause of rhinitis in the young dog. The fungal spores are all around us, and are constantly being breathed into the nasal cavity. Disease occurs where there is some damage already to the turbinate structure, or where the dog's immune system cannot destroy the fungus. Treatment is possible, but it is a very difficult problem to handle. The dog's nasal cavity must be washed out on a daily basis for seven to ten days using an antifungal preparation, and those of you who have had swimming pool or sea water in your nose will know just how uncomfortable the treatment will be. Newer treatments are easier to complete, but their worth has yet to be proved. Cure is not possible if the dog is immunologically deficient and cannot protect itself from re-infection, but there is no way of determining this fact before treatment commences.

TUMOURS

Both benign tumours and cancer can grow inside the nasal cavity. Benign tumours can be removed, but cancerous growths recur usually within about three months following surgery. The cancers usually affect the older dog and are several, with bone, cartilage and glandular tissues all being sites of origin. The turbinate structure is usually destroyed, and considerable haemorrhage may occur during this process. Fortunately pain is not usually a feature, and despite the discharge the patient may be able to live a relatively normal life until the facial bones become involved. When suffering occurs, then euthanasia is the only humane course open.

CONCLUSION

In summary the diseases of the nose are dramatic in appearance and difficult to treat. Early diagnosis can be helpful in terms of treatment, but knowledge of the condition helps the owner understand why treatment is difficult or impossible. First-aid help is often limited to the cleansing of nasal discharge and unfortunately veterinary surgeons cannot offer much more for some patients in what is a very depressing area of disease all round.

19

THE LOCOMOTOR SYSTEM

The locomotor system comprises the bones, tendons, ligaments and muscles. The bones form the skeleton (Fig. 136), whose function is to support the soft tissues of the body and protect them from damage. The bones also act as levers, to which the muscles, tendons and ligaments are attached.

A typical long bone is composed of two expanded ends, the epiphyses, and a central portion, the diaphysis. The latter consists of an outer cylinder of dense, compact bone called cortical bone, and an inner area that contains bone marrow. This central area is often referred to as the medullary cavity. The epiphyses consist of a more open, softer type of bone called cancellous bone.

Figure 136   Skeleton of a dog

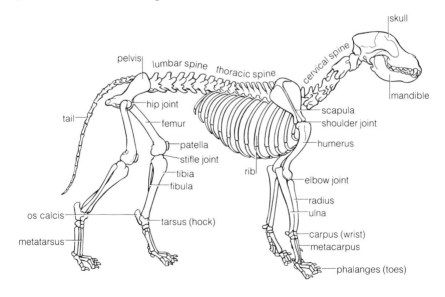

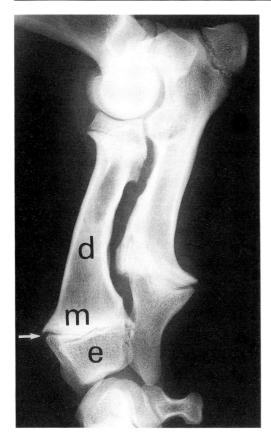

Figure 137 Radiograph of a skeletally immature Basset Hound. The growth plate, or physis, is arrowed
d – diaphysis
m – metaphysis
e – epiphysis

Figure 138 Diagram of a stifle joint

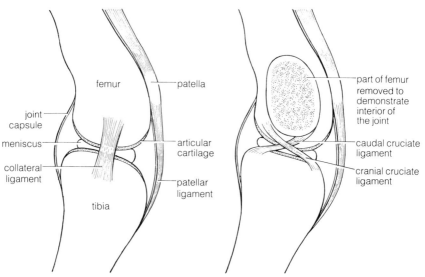

Bone is generally produced by a process called endochondral ossification. This entails the transformation of a cartilaginous template into bone. Long bones grow from a special area of cartilage at either end of the bone called the growth plate. This area is situated between the epiphysis and diaphysis, adjacent to the metaphysis (Fig. 137).

A joint is any connection between two or more bones or cartilage. Most joints are synovial joints, that is they contain a small amount of fluid called synovial fluid. This helps to lubricate the joint and nourish the articular cartilage that covers the ends of the bone (Fig. 138). Synovial fluid is produced by the synovial membrane, which is closely attached to the outer fibrous layer of the joint capsule. This joint capsule attaches to the periphery of the articular surfaces and the periosteum of the bones.

Fibrous thickenings called ligaments strengthen the joint capsule. These attach to the bones on either side of the joint to restrict excessive movement. Most joints have two collateral ligaments, the notable exceptions being the hip and shoulder joints. The carpus and tarsus have additional ligaments that join the multiple small bones that comprise these joints, while the stifle has two additional ligaments, the cranial and caudal cruciate ligaments, that cross within the joint. These prevent the tibia moving excessively on the femur and are important structures in maintaining stability of the stifle joint.

Skeletal muscles are composed of contractile, striated muscle fibres. The muscles contract by these fibres becoming shorter and thicker. Muscles have a rich blood supply and their activity is controlled by nerves that ramify in the bulk of their tissue. They are attached to the periosteum of the bone, either directly or via tendons.

Tendons are composed mainly of parallel bundles of collagen, a fibrous protein. They may be flat, such as the flexor tendons of the toes, or they may be round, like the triceps tendon that attaches the triceps muscles to the point of the elbow. All tendons have two major functions; they must possess great tensile strength and they must glide freely through the surrounding tissues to ensure easy movement of the joints which they control.

Diseases of bone

METABOLIC DISEASE

These conditions are generally seen in the growing puppy and result in defective bone production. Deficiency diseases are now uncommon since most owners feed proprietary diets that contain adequate nutrients in the correct proportions; indeed, most dietary problems are now the result of oversupplementation rather that undersupplementation!

RICKETS

In rickets the cartilage cells of the growth plates fail to mineralise properly so that the growth plates become thickened and weaker than normal. In addition, there is a generalised under-mineralisation of the skeleton, so that bending and pathological fractures of the limbs or spine may occur. Lameness is variable, but can be severe, particularly when such fractures are present.

Rickets is now a rare condition, since most puppies are fed adequate amounts of calcium, phosphorus and vitamin D. The calcium to phosphorus ratio of the diet should be 1.2–1.4 by weight, and the closer the diet is to this optimum ratio the less requirement there is for vitamin D. Suggested levels of vitamin D are 20 iu/kg body weight for growth and 7 iu/kg body weight for maintenance.

The condition is characterised radiographically by widened, irregular growth plates and 'mushrooming' of the metaphyses. The cortices of the long bones appear less dense in severe cases, reflecting their loss of mineral.

Treatment is directed towards correcting the dietary imbalance and limiting the puppy's exercise until its bones become stronger.

JUVENILE OSTEOPOROSIS

This is more properly called secondary nutritional hyperparathyroidism, since it is the result of oversecretion of parathyroid hormone in response to low calcium or high phosphorus levels in the diet. Parathyroid hormone encourages calcium to be withdrawn from the bones to maintain the blood level of calcium. This causes weakening of the skeleton. In contrast to rickets, the growth plates are not affected. The condition is usually seen in puppies of 3–5 months of age fed diets high in meat or meat by-products, with little added milk or cereal. It may also occur in puppies with a malabsorption problem.

Puppies are generally depressed and unwilling to move. Lameness and pain are evident and there may be limb deformities associated with folding fractures. The puppies may show hind limb weakness or paralysis if they have fractures of the spine.

Radiographically the bones have less density than normal and thin cortices. There may be pathological fractures of the limbs or spine. Dietary correction and cage rest are generally successful in reversing the bone changes, although folding fractures often result in permanent limb deformities. The bones remain fragile for several weeks after the diet has been corrected and exercise should be reintroduced gradually. Puppies with severe neurological problems may require euthanasia.

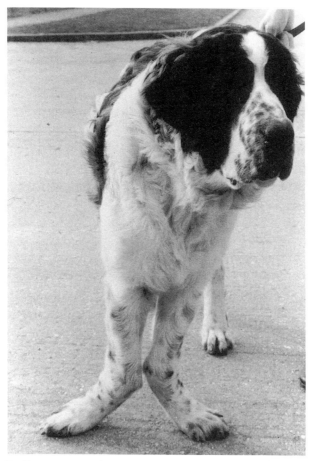

Figure 139 Radius curvus syndrome (carpal valgus) in a St. Bernard. Note the lateral deviation of both forefeet

OSTEOCHONDROSIS

Osteochondrosis commonly affects the cartilage of joints but may also affect the cartilage of the growth plates. It is caused by the interaction of a number of factors. There is a genetic predisposition and the condition is seen particularly in puppies which grow rapidly. Dietary oversupplementation, especially with calcium, has also been demonstrated to be an important factor.

Osteochondrosis may slow bone growth and cause the limb to become distorted or deviated. A typical example is the radius curvus or carpal valgus syndrome (Fig. 139). This occurs when the growth plate of the distal ulna is affected and the ulna fails to grow as quickly as it should. As a result the ulna impedes radial growth and causes the radium to bow. The first noticeable sign is a lateral deviation of the lower limb, followed by external rotation of the foot. The condition is generally seen in those larger breeds of dog and may involve one or both forelimbs. Trauma to the distal ulnar growth plate may also cause this type of angular limb deformity.

Treatment of radius curvus depends upon the age of the puppy. Those that are under six months of age should be treated surgically, to encourage the leg to straighten while the puppy continues to grow. This involves removing a section of the ulna, to eliminate its restraining influence, and placing a metal staple across the radial growth plate. The gap created in the ulna heals without the need for any support, and provided the deformity is not excessive, a reasonably straight limb can be expected. However, it is imperative that surgery is undertaken as soon as possible, in order to take advantage of all the remaining growth potential.

Older puppies also require surgery, but this has to be deferred until they are skeletally mature. In these cases, there is insufficient time left for the limb to straighten during growth and the leg must be straightened when the puppy is 10 to 12 months old. This is done by removing a suitably sized wedge of bone from the radius. Since this is the major weight-bearing bone of the foreleg the operated area must be repaired with a bone plate or other fixation device. The surgery is more complex and has to be delayed until growth has ceased in order to know how large a wedge is required to straighten the leg.

SECONDARY RENAL HYPERPARATHYROIDISM

This condition is often called 'rubber jaw' since the bones of the lower jaw become demineralised. The condition is caused by chronic kidney failure. The failing kidneys are unable to excrete the usual amount of phosphate in the urine and the blood calcium levels are temporarily lowered. As a consequence, the parathyroid glands are stimulated and the mandibles lose their calcium and become soft and distorted. There is no specific treatment other than treating the kidney disease. It is generally a condition of the older dog, although it is occasionally encountered in puppies with congenital kidney problems.

UNCLASSIFIED DISEASES OF BONE

These conditions have well-recognised clinical and radiographic signs, but their causes are poorly understood.

Metaphyseal osteopathy

This may be called hypertrophic osteodystrophy or skeletal scurvy. Clinical signs generally become apparent between three and seven months of age and the condition usually affects the large and giant breed dogs. The metaphyses of the long bones are hot, swollen and painful and the puppy is depressed, reluctant to move and has an elevated temperature. The swellings are bilaterally symmetrical and commonly involve the metaphyses of the distal radius and ulna and/or the distal tibia. The signs spontaneously regress in 7 to 10 days, only to recur a few weeks later. Thus the lameness is episodic, but, as the puppy reaches skeletal maturity, the interval between each bout of lameness lengthens and the severity of each attack diminishes. The growth plates are rarely affected and provided the pain can be controlled during the active phases the prognosis is favourable.

Radiographically there are changes which appear similar to those of skeletal scurvy in children. Thus it was thought that the condition was caused by a deficiency of vitamin C, as it is in man. It is now believed that *over-supplementation* with vitamins or minerals is responsible and any dietary excesses must be corrected. Extra vitamin C should not be given as it may increase the blood calcium levels and exacerbate the problem. Rest, good nursing and the provision of adequate analgesia are essential in the management of this condition.

Panosteitis

This condition affects many of the larger breeds of dogs but particularly the German Shepherd dog. Clinical signs are generally seen between the ages of 5 and 18 months, but occasionally dogs may be several years old before the condition becomes apparent. Affected animals are intermittently lame, with the lameness shifting from one leg to another. The pain is often severe enough to cause the dog to carry its limb and to have an elevated temperature. Sometimes more than one limb is affected at the same time. The shifting lameness commonly lasts for up to nine months but sometimes persists for much longer.

Analgesics and restricted exercise are indicated when the dog is lame. Since the condition is self-limiting the long-term prognosis is good.

Craniomandibular osteopathy

This is a condition seen mainly in the terrier breeds, notably the West Highland white, Scottish and Cairn terriers, although it is occasionally seen in larger dogs such as the Dobermann. It is characterised by symmetrical bony swellings of the lower jaw and/or the base of the skull (Fig. 140). Signs become apparent between the ages of 3 and 8 months and affected puppies are reluctant to eat. They have difficulty in opening their jaws and often drool saliva.

The condition is self-limiting and the bony swellings cease growing as skeletal maturity is reached around 9 to 10 months. Treatment comprises analgesics to control the pain and soft food to encourage the puppy to eat.

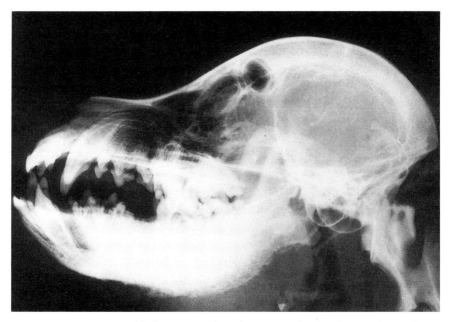

Figure 140 Craniomandibular osteopathy. There is much irregular new bone along the lower jaw

The swellings generally remain as hard, painless masses on the jaw or skull but cause no problems unless they involve the joints of the jaw.

Hypertrophic osteopathy

This is commonly called Marie's Disease. It is characterised by bilaterally symmetrical swellings of the feet, made up of bony deposits on the toes and an associated soft tissue reaction. It occurs in response to the presence of a mass, which is generally a tumour, in the chest or abdomen. Affected dogs are usually middle-aged or older. They have a stilted gait due to their swollen feet and painful toes.

Treatment is not usually attempted due to the existence of the tumour elsewhere, although in rare instances it is possible to remove the primary mass. If this is successful, the swellings of the feet subside.

Bone cysts

Bone cysts may be single or multiple. They appear initially as painless swellings, but they may weaken the bone and cause it to fracture. Large cysts should be opened surgically and packed with a bone graft taken from another part of the skeleton. The leg is supported post-operatively until the defect in the bone heals.

Neoplastic diseases – bone tumours

(see Chapter 28 Cancer in the Dog)

Tumours involving bone are generally malignant. The majority are osteosarcomas, but occasionally other types are seen. Benign tumours such as osteomas are rare.

Osteosarcomas occur mainly in the middle-aged and older dogs. The larger breeds are more commonly affected and the tumours occur particularly at the ends of the long bones (Fig. 141). The first signs are pain and lameness with or without a localised swelling of the limb. The lameness is progressive as the bone is destroyed. Pathological fractures may occur through the weakened area of bone.

Figure 141 Osteosarcoma of the tibia with marked bone destruction

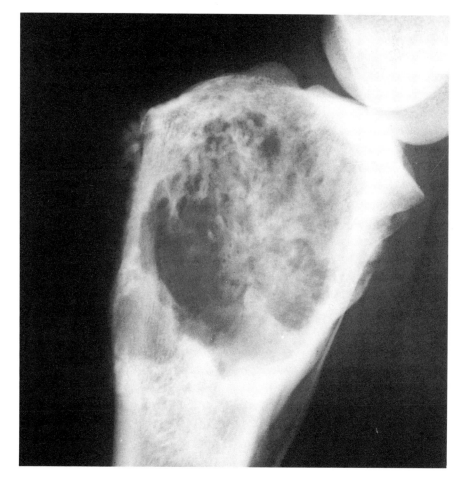

The radiographic changes are generally sufficiently typical to confirm the diagnosis of a malignant bone tumour. If there is doubt it is necessary to take a biopsy, i.e., a small portion of the mass, in order to examine it microscopically.

Osteosarcomas metastasise to the lungs and therefore tend to be difficult to treat. Amputation of the limb will remove the primary tumour and the pain associated with it, but will not prevent the spread of secondary metastases. It is possible to treat selected cases with radiotherapy or chemotherapy, but such treatment is palliative rather than curative. In exceptional cases it is possible to remove the tumour surgically, replace the excised portion of bone with a bone graft and treat the dog with cytotoxic drugs that kill the remaining cancer cells. Such cases are unusual and the treatment is expensive

Infectious diseases

Bone infections in the dog are not common except when associated with open wounds or fractures that have overlying defects in the skin. Infection of the bone is called osteomyelitis and it is a difficult condition to treat. In severe cases the dog is unwell and often has a fever. The affected area is hot, swollen and painful and there may be a discharge from the wound. Treatment comprises antibiotic therapy for at least one month. If possible a swab should be taken of the infected bone to identify the type of bacteria responsible and to ensure the chosen antibiotic is appropriate.

Less severe cases of osteomyelitis do not show generalised signs, but are characterised by the presence of discharging openings (sinuses) in the skin. Lameness is variable, but frequently there is localised scarring around the sinus as it heals and then re-forms. These sinuses will persist until all the underlying dead bone is removed, along with any metal implants that may have been used to repair the fracture.

Fractures

A fracture is defined as the disruption of the continuity of a bone. It may be *complete*, when the two ends of the fractured bone are separate, or *incomplete*. Most fractures are complete, but occasionally young puppies suffer a greenstick fracture, where one side of the bone bends but remains intact while the other side buckles. This is an example of an incomplete fracture.

Complete fractures are generally classified by the direction and number of fracture lines (Fig. 142). They are further classified as *open* (compound) or *closed* (simple). A closed fracture is one where there is no communica-

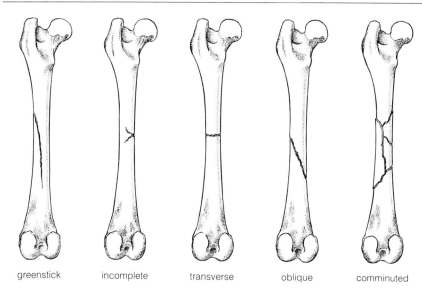

| greenstick | incomplete | transverse | oblique | comminuted |

Figure 142   Types of fractures

tion between the skin and the fracture, while an open one has a breach in the skin associated with the fracture. This may be a small puncture wound caused by the sharp end of the fractured bone penetrating the skin or it may be gross destruction of the skin and muscle caused by a vehicle or ballistic weapon. In either case the presence of a skin wound increases the likelihood of osteomyelitis.

The clinical signs of a fracture are *local*, i.e., those related to the changes at the fracture site and *general* signs.

Local signs consist of pain, deformity, crepitus and abnormal mobility. Fractures are almost invariably painful, particularly when the injured part is moved. Deformity depends upon the displacement of the fractured bone end and the amount of soft tissue swelling and damage at the fracture site. Crepitus describes the grating sound produced when the two ends of a fractured bone rub together. Abnormal mobility is generally evident if the fracture is complete.

General signs include loss of function, haemorrhage and shock. Dogs generally carry the leg if the fracture involves a limb, but they may be unable to stand if it involves the spine, pelvis or more than one leg.

Fractures of the head and face often appear dramatic due to the associated blood loss. A dog with a fractured lower jaw is unable to close its mouth and drools blood-stained saliva. Fractures involving the nose usually bleed even more profusely. In both instances the haemorrhage can be seen, that is if it is external haemorrhage. Internal haemorrhage is not immediately apparent since it is not visible, yet it is often serious and may be life threatening. There is usually considerable haemorrhage around a fracture site, particularly if the bone is surrounded by a large muscle mass. Bleeding into the chest or abdomen is potentially even more serious and is a common cause of shock.

Profuse haemorrhage and shock are complications of fractures that demand immediate treatment. This often requires intensive nursing, is time-consuming and can be expensive. Equally, it can be most rewarding if the patient survives.

Fractures involving the skull and spine are serious fractures, since they may cause severe neurological disturbances. A depressed fracture of the skull will cause increased pressure on the underlying brain, which requires emergency surgery to relieve it. Fractures of the spine may cause pressure on the spinal cord, resulting in paralysis of the limbs. These too are serious fractures that require emergency treatment. Unfortunately, not all dogs recover from such fractures and for some euthanasia is the only humane solution.

FIRST AID FOR FRACTURES

(see Chapter 26 First Aid)

The aim of first-aid treatment of fractures should be to minimise further damage to the injured part, to make the dog as comfortable as possible and to control any associated haemorrhage. If the fracture involves the head or face it is essential that the dog's airway is kept unobstructed by removing any blood, mucus or other foreign material from the mouth and throat. Wounds may be covered with a clean dressing or cotton material. Immobilisation of the injured limb will do much to prevent further damage and reduce pain. If skilled help is unavailable it is best to support the fractured limb, holding it in as comfortable a position as possible. Careless handling, or unskilled attempts at bandaging fractures which have little overlying muscle, may convert a closed fracture into an open one. However, a temporary splint, using a rolled-up newspaper, a piece of wood, or something similar, will provide good support, particularly when the fracture is below the elbow or hock. Dogs that are unable to stand may have neurological injuries and should be lifted on to a flat board or tray and moved very carefully.

TREATMENT OF FRACTURES

Unless there are life-threatening problems most veterinarians will defer treatment of fractures for two to three days. This is to provide time to treat the dog for its other injuries, to treat blood loss and damage to internal organs and to ensure that the dog has no other life-threatening problems.

The treatment of a fracture will vary depending upon its type, the amount of soft tissue damage, the age of the dog and the future activity expected of it. In all cases, however, the fracture must be reduced, aligned and immobilised. Reduction and alignment ensure that the fractured bone ends are fitted together accurately and the previous shape and contour of the bone is restored. The fracture is then immobilised by external or internal fixation.

External immobilisation includes the use of casts, splints and devices such as Kirschner splints. Casts have traditionally been made of plaster of Paris, but several fibre-glass based materials are now available. These are much stronger, lighter and more durable. Casts are really only suitable for immobilising fractures of the lower limbs since, to counteract the rotational forces at the fracture site, the cast must immobilise the joint above and below the fracture. Casts must be checked regularly to ensure that they are not rubbing or causing pressure sores. They are normally applied for four to six weeks, but it may be necessary to replace them more frequently, particularly when they become wet or soiled. They may also require replacing more frequently in rapidly growing puppies.

Kirschner splints and their variations employ pins that are driven through the skin into the underlying bone (Fig. 143 on following page). The pins are then connected together by clamps and further pins, or by acrylic cement, so that the fracture is supported by an external frame. These splints are extremely useful in the treatment of infected fractures or where the fracture is accompanied by gross soft tissue damage.

Internal fixation of fractures include the use of intramedullary pins, bone plates, screws and orthopaedic wire. This type of fixation is generally reserved for those fractures that are not amenable to external fixation or where a return to athletic function is desired.

Intramedullary pins are generally used to immobilise fractures of long, straight bones such as the femur. The fracture must be relatively transverse, so that the bone ends do not override when the dog puts weight on the limb. Intramedullary pins do not provide good rotational stability since they are round in cross-section. If the fracture is oblique, this disadvantage can be overcome by the addition of encircling wires (Fig. 144). Alternatively, additional stability can be achieved by using several small intramedullary pins, rather than one large pin, using a technique called stack pinning.

Internal immobilisation of fractures using bone plates and screws provides a very stable form of fixation. A wide variety of plates is available, but they fall basically into two types. The first type of plate, of which Venable and Sherman plates are examples, is attached to the bone by self-tapping screws. Both the plates and screws must be of the same metal, which is generally a surgical grade of stainless steel. Plates enable the surgeon to repair more complicated fractures and to bridge defects in the bone when an area is so comminuted that it is impossible to include the fragments in the repair.

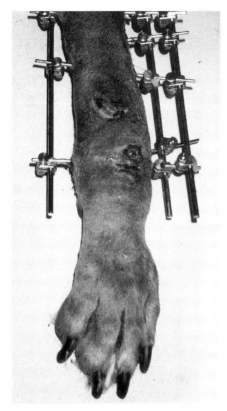

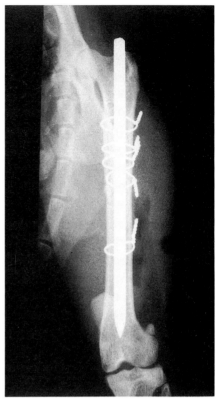

Figure 143 Kirschner splint applied to an infected fracture of the radius

Figure 144 Intramedullary pin and five cerclage wires immobilising a comminuted femoral fracture

The second type of bone plate has been developed by a Swiss company and these plates are often referred to as AO plates. They have been designed to create compression across the fracture site so that the fracture heals by a process called primary bone union. This means that the fracture heals by bone growing from one fractured bone end to the other without the formation of callus (Fig. 145). Callus is only produced when there is movement at the fracture site and the aim of AO plates is to create such high interfragmentary forces at the fracture site that all movement is eliminated and no callus is formed.

In some instances the formation of callus may be unimportant, but if it becomes adherent to adjacent muscles or tendons it will impede the function of these structures and the dog may remain permanently lame. It is especially important that fractures involving joints heal without the formation of callus, since the presence of any new bone in the joint will lead to the development of osteoarthritis.

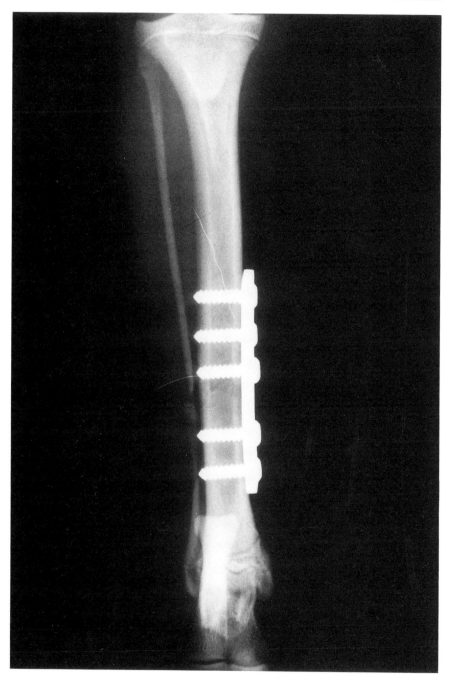

Figure 145   Primary bone union. The fractured tibia has healed without the formation of callus

The most commonly used AO plate is called a dynamic compression plate. This has elliptical screw holes rather than the round holes of a Venable or Sherman plate. The design of the holes is such that, when the screws are placed and tightened in an eccentric position within the hole, the bone moves relative to the plate and compression is created across the fracture. The screws used with AO plates are not self-tapping, so that a thread has to be cut in the bone with a special bone tap. This, combined with the design of the screw itself, means that the screw is less likely to pull out of the bone.

AO plates are stronger than conventional plates and are produced in a much greater variety of shapes and sizes. Thus it is possible to repair a greater range of fractures with this system of plating. The biggest advantage of AO plates, however, is that greater stability is created at the fracture site. This enables the dog to begin weight-bearing on the operated limb very soon after surgery and encourages the fracture to heal. Early weight-bearing also reduces joint stiffness and muscle atrophy due to inactivity. It is important to limit the dog's exercise to lead walking for approximately six weeks after the surgery so that the forces generated by weight-bearing do not stress the plate excessively.

Fractures of long bone are rarely repaired using screws or wire alone, since these implants are insufficiently strong to be used on their own. Screws are often used, however, to join a small piece of bone to a larger piece (Fig. 146). In these instances, since callus is undesirable, compression is created at the fracture site using the lag screw principle. This means that the smaller part of the fractured bone is free to slide along the screw while the screw threads grip the larger part of the bone. Thus, interfragmentary compression is created as the screw is tightened.

Compression using orthopaedic wire can be achieved by using a figure-of-eight tension band wire. This is particularly useful when treating fractures that are distracted by the pull of a muscle or tendon (Fig. 147). The 'figure-of-eight' wire converts the distractive forces into compressive forces at the fracture site, encouraging repair by primary bone healing.

Fractures involving growth plates are important, since if the growth plate is damaged sufficiently to cause it to close, i.e., to become inactive, it may result in shortening or deformity of the limb. Growth plate fractures must be aligned accurately and immobilised for as short a period as possible. Any implant placed across a growth plate should be removed as soon as the fracture has healed so that it does not encourage premature closure of the plate.

Fractures are a common cause of lameness and are important, not only because of their frequency but also because many of the dogs involved are young and otherwise healthy. Fortunately with careful management many can be treated successfully and the patient can regain its former role, whether it be a pet or a working dog. If a return to previous athletic

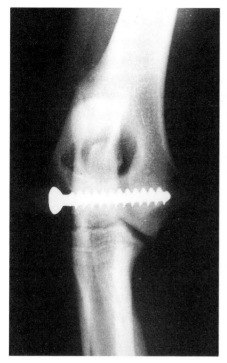 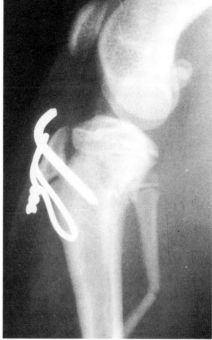

Figure 146 A fracture of the lower end of the humerus repaired with a lag screw

Figure 147 A fractured tibial crest repaired with a figure of eight tension band wire

performance is impossible, at least with modern orthopaedic techniques it is possible to restore pain-free movement so that the dog can enjoy life as a pet or be used for breeding.

Diseases of joints

HIP DYSPLASIA

The term dysplasia means abnormal growth; thus hip dysplasia is a developmental condition that results in abnormal looseness or laxity of the hip joints. It is currently accepted to be a multifactorial disease with heredity, nutrition, trauma, exercise, etc., all influencing the outcome of the condition. The inherited component is caused by the interaction of many genes – hence it is a polygenic condition. However, the expression of these genes may be modified by the environmental factors listed above. These environmental factors do not cause hip dysplasia but they may influence how unstable the hip joint becomes and how much osteoarthritis ultimately develops as a result of that instability.

The hip joints of all puppies are reported to be normal at birth, but some time after two weeks of age the femoral head of a dysplastic puppy fails to sit firmly within its acetabulum, or socket, and the joint becomes unstable. As a result the joint capsule becomes stretched, the ligament that holds the head of the femur into the acetabulum (the teres ligament) becomes stretched and the articular cartilage becomes eroded. In an attempt to re-establish stability the joint undergoes remodelling changes and new bone develops around the margins of the femoral head, neck and acetabulum (Fig. 148). The rate of development of this osteoarthritic new bone depends upon the individual puppy and upon the environmental factors cited above.

The clinical signs of hip dysplasia may become apparent as early as four to five months of age or lameness may not develop until the osteoarthritis becomes significant. This may be as early as 15 months or may not occur until middle or old age. The usual signs in the young puppy range from reduced exercise tolerance to a crippling lameness. The dog may be reluctant to sit or to rise from a lying position, it may have a 'bunny hopping' gait that gets worse with exercise or it may be stiff after rest, especially following exercise. A clicking sound can sometimes be heard as the femoral heads subluxate. In severe cases, puppies will shift more of their weight forwards to relieve the weight on their hips, and in consequence develop well-muscled forequarters and poorly developed hindquarters (Fig. 149).

Figure 148 Osteoarthritis as a result of hip dysplasia. Note the extensive new bone formed around the joints

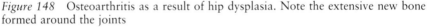

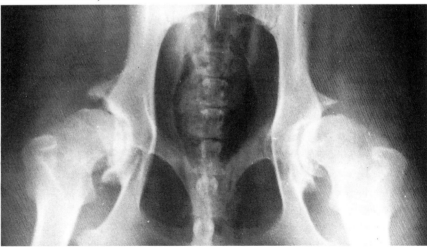

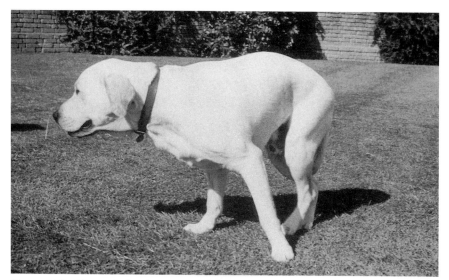

Figure 149 Young Labrador Retriever with severe hip dysplasia. Much of the weight is taken on the forelimbs

Figure 150 Ventro-dorsal radiograph of a dog with good hips

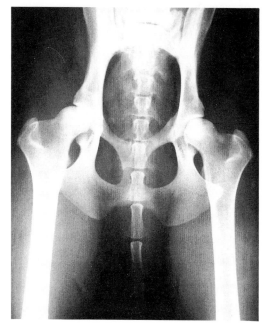

The diagnosis of hip dysplasia is made on a physical examination supported by radiographic evidence. The radiograph is taken with the dog placed on its back with its pelvis symmetrical and both hindlegs extended and parallel (Fig. 150). It is generally necessary to anaesthetise the dog to position it correctly, although on occasions sedation alone may be adequate.

The radiograph is assessed in a standard fashion allowing for variations between breeds and age. The parameters assessed are:

the degree of subluxation of the femoral heads;
the condition of the dorsal, cranial and caudal acetabular rims;
the shape of the femoral heads and necks;
new bone formation and other evidence of osteoarthritis.

The control of hip dysplasia depends upon selectively breeding for normal progeny. Potential breeding stock should be radiographed when they are 12 months or older and the radiographs submitted to the British Veterinary Association/Kennel Club (BVA/KC) hip dysplasia scheme. Each radiograph must bear the dog's Kennel Club registration number photographed on to it for identification. Each hip is given a score, based upon the above parameters, from 0 to 54, making a total of 108 for both hips. The lower the score the better the radiographic appearance of the hips, and a dog is acceptable for breeding if it scores eight or less, with neither hip scoring more than six. Dogs with greater scores should only be bred from as part of a carefully controlled programe. This may be necessary in breeds that have a high average score or the gene pool would be unduly restricted. However, it should always be the aim to select breeding stock with a score less than that of the breed average.

Treatment will depend upon the individual dog and the stage and severity of the condition. Young puppies with unstable hips often respond to limited exercise and strict maintenance of their correct body weight. This conservative management is often sufficient to allow the hip joints to stabilise by the time the dog is 15 to 18 months old. It is sometimes necessary to provide analgesia with non-steroidal anti-inflammatory drugs (NSAIDs) during this time. Alternatively, surgery may be advised. The simplest surgical relief is usually offered by pectineal myectomy. This involves removing part or all of the pectineus situated on the inside of the thigh. It is a simple procedure which can relieve pain for several months, but it does not reduce the amount of osteoarthritis that develops as the hip joints stabilise.

Puppies with severe dysplasia are best treated surgically. This involves cutting either the pelvis or femur to improve the congruency of the hip joint. By improving the way the joint surfaces fit in the puppy, it is possible to reduce the severity of the osteoarthritis that will eventually develop. Post-operatively, it is important that these puppies start to walk on the operated limbs as soon as possible, for this will encourage the hip joint to remodel and fit together.

Older dogs with established osteoarthritis can be treated with pain-killers (NSAIDs). Alternatively, surgical removal of the femoral head by an excision arthroplasty will encourage the formation of a non-painful

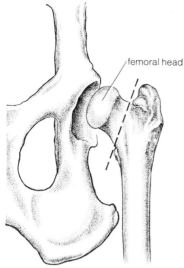

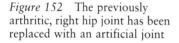
femoral head

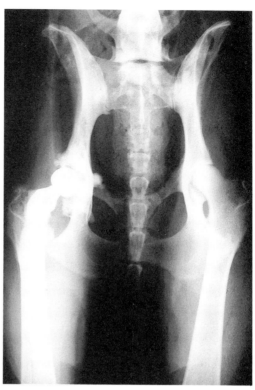

Figure 151 An excision arthroplasty involves removal of the femoral head and neck to promote a fibrous joint

Figure 152 The previously arthritic, right hip joint has been replaced with an artificial joint

fibrous joint (Fig. 151). This is satisfactory for medium-sized dogs but inadequate for large dogs.

Total hip replacement is available at specialist centres. This entails replacement of the femoral head with a stainless steel prosthesis and the acetabulum with a high-density polypropylene socket. The surgery is difficult and expensive, but creates a fully functional joint from an arthritic one (Fig. 152).

NECROSIS OF THE FEMORAL HEAD

This is also called Legg Calvé Perthes disease or sometimes just Perthes disease. It affects the femoral head or heads of the smaller breeds, particularly the terrier breeds. Lameness is generally insidious in onset, but slowly becomes worse, so that eventually the affected limb is carried. The muscles of the thigh and upper leg disappear due to disuse and the femoral head becomes distorted (Fig. 153). This encourages the formation of osteoathritis and further joint pain. The condition is thought to be inherited.

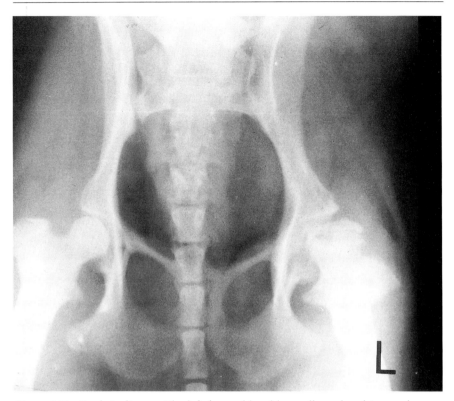

Figure 153 Perthe's disease. The left femoral head has collapsed and is grossly misshapen

In advanced cases the treatment of choice is removal of the femoral head by an excision arthroplasty (see Fig. 151). This encourages the formation of a false fibrous joint which is non-painful.

OSTEOCHONDROSIS

Osteochondrosis is a generalised condition due to a failure of normal endochondral ossification. It might involve the growth plates, but more frequently it involves the articular cartilage of the joints. The cartilage becomes thickened and less able to withstand the normal weight-bearing forces imposed upon it. As a result the thickened cartilage becomes necrotic and breaks away from the underlying subchrondral bone, either as a flap of cartilage or as an osteochondral fragment – which contains bone as well as cartilage. The cause of osteochondrosis is discussed on page 307. The lesion occurs in the shoulder, elbow, stifle and hock joints of large and giant breed dogs. It is frequently bilateral, although, on occasions, lameness is only evident in one joint. Lameness generally occurs when the

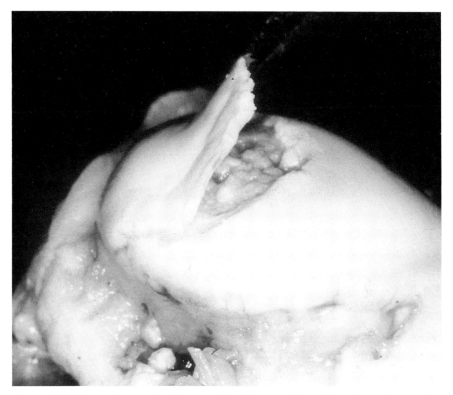

Figure 154 Osteochondrosis of the shoulder. There is a large flap of articular cartilage on the head of the humerus

dog is between five and nine months of age and it usually fails to respond to medical treatment. In general, treatment involves the surgical removal of the offending flap.

Shoulder

Osteochondrosis of the shoulder occurs in giant breeds such as the Irish Wolfhound and Great Dane. It is also seen in narrow-chested breeds such as the Collie and the Setter. The lesion classically involves the caudal aspect of the humeral head (Fig. 154). The most obvious clinical signs are pain on extension of the joint and, in long-standing cases, loss of muscle over the shoulder.

Elbow

There are four manifestations of osteochondrosis in the elbow. The two frequently seen in Labradors, Retrievers and Rottweilers are an articular flap in the cartilage of the medial condyle of the humerus or an ununited medial coronoid process (Fig. 155). Both present as pain on flexion of the joint, especially when combined with inward rotation of the carpus. Neither are easy to diagnose radiographically and it is usual to look for the earliest signs of degenerative joint disease to establish the diagnosis (Fig. 156).

The third form of elbow osteochondrosis involves the growth plate of the anconeal process (Fig. 157). This is seen most frequently in young, male German Shepherd Dogs, although many other breeds are involved. The elbow is painful on extension. The growth plate should close at four months of age and lameness usually begins around five to eight months.

The final form of elbow osteochondrosis occurs much less frequently. It is an ununited medial epicondyle of the humerus (Fig. 158). Treatment either involves removal of the fragment or, if it is large enough, lag screwing it back into position.

Stifle

Osteochondrosis of the stifle occurs as an articular flap on either femoral condyle. The joint is swollen, painful to manipulate and the dog walks by keeping the joint held stiffly.

Figure 155 Osteochondrosis of the elbow. The triangular shaped piece of bone is an unwanted coronoid process

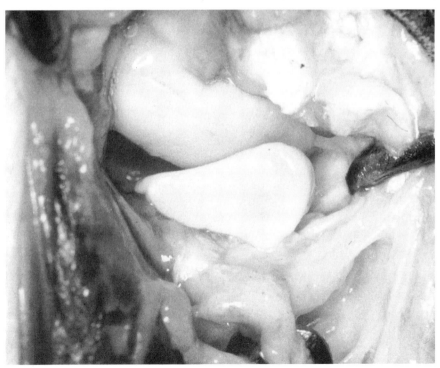

Figure 156
Osteoarthritis of
the elbow as a
result of
osteochondrosis.
There is new bone
(arrowed) on the
anconeal process
and on the head of
the radius

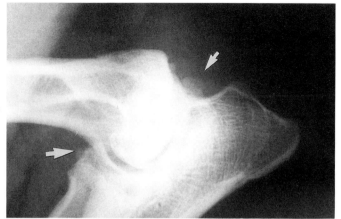

Figure 157 An
ununited anconeal
process

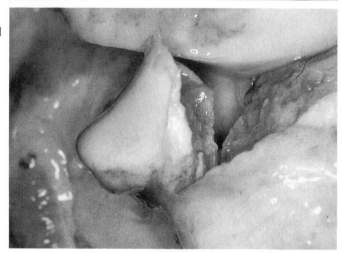

Figure 158
Radiograph
demonstrating an
ununited medial
epicondyle

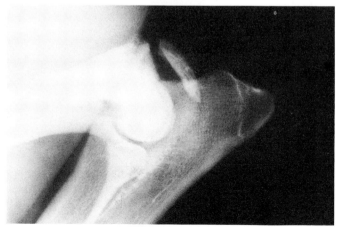

Hock

The lesion is usually an osteochondral fragment that occurs on the medial side of the tibial tarsal bone. The joint is painful on flexion and there is generally a moderate joint effusion.

There is some diversity of opinion as to the best form of treatment for osteochondrosis. Conservative treatment in the early stages of the disease, before the thickened articular cartilage pulls away as a flap, may be successful. The diet should be examined for evidence of over-supplementation and the dog's exercise restricted to prevent unnecessary trauma to the damaged joint. The response to surgical removal of the flap is variable, depending upon which joint is involved. The shoulder and stifle carry good prognoses. The elbow has a somewhat mixed response, while the hock joint carries the poorest prognosis.

TRAUMATIC JOINT CONDITIONS

The two common traumatic conditions of joints are sprains and disloca-tions. The stifle joint especially is frequently damaged and has its own special injuries due to its additional ligaments and associated structures.

Sprains

A sprain occurs when the ligaments and joint capsule are stretched or torn. It is usually the result of the joint exceeding the normal range of movement due to an accident such as a slip or fall. The joint quickly swells and becomes painful, especially when moved. The dog is lame, but not as lame as if it had fractured or dislocated the joint. However, the veterinary surgeon will often radiograph a joint with a suspected sprain to eliminate the possibility of damage to the adjacent bones.

Uncomplicated sprains are treated by rest, cold applications and bandaging until the acute inflammation and swelling has subsided. Once the swelling and pain have been relieved, gentle exercise is introduced to prevent the development of a stiff joint.

The carpus is frequently sprained by all types of dog. Uncomplicated sprains are treated as described above, but on occasions the supporting ligaments at the back of the joint are so severely damaged that further measures are required. These injuries are generally associated with the dog jumping or falling from a height and rupturing the relevant ligaments as they land. Splinting or casting the joint for four to six weeks may provide sufficient stability to allow these ligaments to heal, but generally it is necessary to fuse the joint. This is termed an arthrodesis (Fig. 159). It involves removing all of the articular cartilage so that bare bone is exposed, packing the spaces between these bones with small pieces of bone (bone

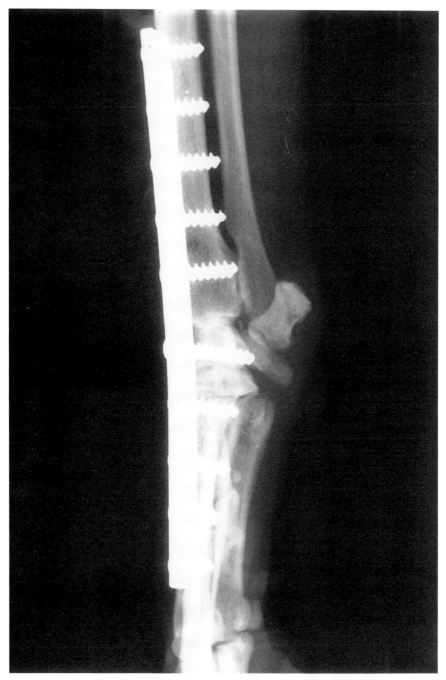

Figure 159   The carpal joints have been fused, creating an arthrodesis. The bones are immobilised with a plate and screws until they fuse

graft) taken from elswhere in the dog, and immobilising the joint with a bone plate. Fusion of all the bones should occur within six to ten weeks, after which time the dog is able to exercise without pain. The lack of movement in the carpal joint does not inconvenience the dog, although it has to alter its gait to accommodate this immobile joint.

Sprains of the toes are a common injury in racing greyhounds and other working dogs. Frequently, sprains of the toe joints are accompanied by rupture of one or both collateral ligaments. In these cases there is excessive movement of the joint and there may be an associated small skin wound. The torn ligament(s) are generally repaired surgically and the dog confined to lead exercise for at least a month. Amputation of the affected toe is sometimes indicated, but will have an adverse effect on the dog's subsequent performance. The middle two toes of any foot, the inside toe of the left forefoot and the outside toe of the right hindfoot are particularly important to the dog's ability to corner when running anti-clockwise.

Dislocations

The terms dislocation and luxation are synonomous, that is they refer to the displacement of the opposing surfaces of the bones that form a joint. A partial dislocation is sometimes called a subluxation.

Dislocations may be the result of congenital or developmental problems, but most are caused by trauma. The dog is unable to use the joint and the limb is often held in an unnatural position. The joint is painful and swollen. No attempt should be made to try to put the joint back in its correct position. It must be realigned (reduced) under general anaesthesia, since manipulating the joint is a painful procedure and the surrounding muscles must be relaxed. Following reduction, the joint is generally bandaged for 7 to 10 days. If it reluxates after this time it may be necessary to operate to prevent future dislocation.

Dislocation of the elbow

This is one of the more common forelimb dislocations. The dog is unable to use the limb and there is obvious deformity of the joint. The elbow and lower limb are rotated outwards and the leg is held semi-flexed.

Dislocation of the hip

The hip joint is the most commonly luxated joint in the dog. It may occur as a result of jumping or falling awkwardly, or it may be the result of a traffic accident. The leg is carried, often with the thigh rotated outward, but, because the hip joint is surrounded by a large amount of muscle, deformity may not be readily apparent.

Following reduction of the joint under general anaesthesia, the leg is generally bandaged with a figure-of-eight bandage to encourage the head of the femur to stay within the acetabulum or socket. This bandage is generally maintained for a week or so while the damaged tissues around the joint have a chance to heal. If the dislocation recurs there are a number of surgical options that are available. The torn ligament between the femoral and head and acetabulum may be replaced with an artificial one in an operation called a 'hip toggle' procedure. Alternatively, the joint may be stabilised by the strategic placement of a steel pin – the Tranacetabular pinning technique. If the recurrent dislocation is due to a previously dysplastic joint the femoral head can be removed (see Fig. 151). This permits the formation of a fibrous union between the femoral neck and the acetabulum and is very successful, particularly in small dogs. This surgery may be termed an excision arthroplasty or a femoral head osteotomy. A further option, especially in large dogs, is to perform a total hip replacement.

Dislocation of the stifle

Dislocations of the patella or knee-cap are common, particularly in small breeds of dog. Most are due to congenital causes, but occasionally a patellar luxation is caused by an indirect force, especially when the dog turns at high speed. Generally the patella dislocates medially, but lateral luxations are not uncommon in large and giant breed dogs. Surgical correction is almost invariably required. The type of surgery depends upon the underlying cause. Some of the more common procedures include transplantation of the tibial crest (Fig. 160) and an operation called a

Figure 160   Transplantation of the tibial crest involves a) cutting the crest from its original position with a saw and b) wiring it in a position which allows the patella to run within the trochlea (groove) of the femur

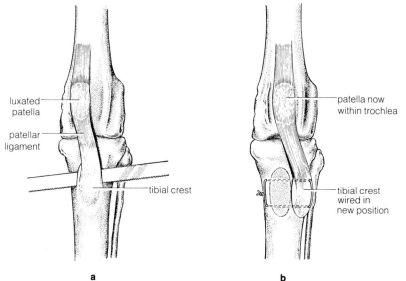

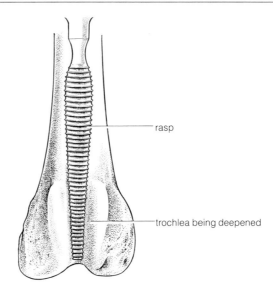

Figure 161 A trochleaplasty is performed by deepening the trochlea or groove of the femur with a rasp

rasp

trochlea being deepened

trochleaplasty (Fig. 161). The former involves the realignment of the direction of the patella by moving a small piece of bone, to which the patellar ligament is attached, to a more favourable position. A trochlea-plasty involves the deepening of the groove that the patella normally runs in.

Rupture of the cruciate ligaments in the stifle joint

The cranial and caudal cruciate ligaments cross each other within the stifle and are important structures in maintaining joint stability (see Fig. 138). Rupture of the cranial cruciate ligament is a common injury, especially in older, overweight, large breed dogs. Sometimes the onset of lameness is sudden, on other occasions the dog shows a mild intermittent lameness that gets slowly worse. The affected limb is held semi-flexed with possibly just the toes touching the ground. The stifle is swollen but not unduly painful. The diagnosis is confirmed by the demonstration of a cranial drawer movement, i.e., by showing it is possible to move the tibia forward on the femur.

Treatment depends upon the size of the dog and the exercise expected of it. Lameness in a small dog will improve with rest and these patients often resume an active life in a few months. Lameness in larger dogs, or working dogs, will improve initially, but these animals generally require surgery to stabilise the affected joint in order to prevent the development of osteoarthritis.

There are many different surgical techniques to stabilise the stifle. A commonly performed procedure is the replacement of the ruptured ligament by a new ligament constructed from adjacent tissue. This ligament

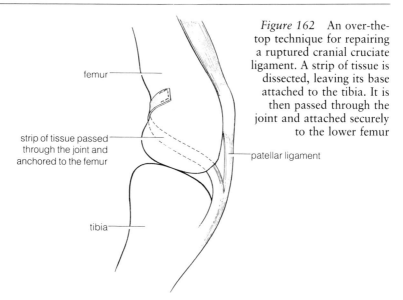

Figure 162 An over-the-top technique for repairing a ruptured cranial cruciate ligament. A strip of tissue is dissected, leaving its base attached to the tibia. It is then passed through the joint and attached securely to the lower femur

femur

strip of tissue passed through the joint and anchored to the femur

patellar ligament

tibia

is taken from the tibia, passed through the joint and over the lateral condyle of the femur before being anchored to this part of the lower femur. This is called the 'over-the-top' technique (Fig. 162). An alternative procedure is to pass a heavy suture from the lower femur to the tibia so that the two bones are held in the correct position. This suture is called a lateral retinacular suture.

Whatever the type of surgery, all the procedures rely on careful post-operative nursing to protect the joint until it has healed. A typical regime is two to three weeks of total rest, followed by four to six weeks of lead exercise and a further four to six weeks of limited exercise.

Large dogs such as the Rottweiler and Labrador may suffer a rupture of the cranial cruciate ligaments of both their stifles well before they are middle-aged. The reason for this is unclear, but it seems that their ligaments undergo a premature 'ageing' process and are weaker than normal. Usually these ligaments rupture a little at a time so that the dog experiences bouts of mild lameness – until the final fibres disintegrate and the dog becomes acutely lame. However, because of the pre-existing instability, which may have been present for months or even years, the joints will already be osteoarthritic when the dog suddenly goes lame. Such cases may require surgery, but if the degenerative changes are severe, the treatment may comprise controlled exercise, attention to the maintenance of correct body weight and the tactical use of analgesics.

Meniscal damage

The stifle joint contains two C-shaped fibrocartilaginous structures called the lateral and medial menisci. These roll back and forth as the joint flexes and extends and contribute to the congruency of the joint surfaces. In addition, they are part of the anti-concussion mechanism of the joint, acting rather like shock absorbers. The menisci have a poor blood supply, hence they are slow to heal when damaged.

Tearing of the medial meniscus is a common complication associated with rupture of the cranial cruciate ligament. Generally the torn portion is sufficiently extensive that the entire meniscus must be removed. This is done at the same time as the cruciate repair.

Dislocation of the hock

This is an infrequent injury caused, generally, by a small fracture at the origin of one or both collateral ligaments. This type of fracture can be repaired using a tension band technique (see Fig. 147). Dislocations of the hock are also caused by the dog being dragged along the highway by a car, during which time the side of the joint is ground away, rather like being removed with a plane. There is extensive loss of soft tissue and the wound must be left open until all the infection is controlled and granulation tissue begins to form. At this stage it is possible to reconstruct an artificial collateral ligament to stabilise the joint.

A second type of hock dislocation occurs at one of the joints called the proximal intertarsal joint (Fig. 163). This is usually a subluxation and commonly occurs in Collie breeds, especially the Shetland Sheepdog. It is generally occurs in middle-aged dogs who are overweight. The injury occurs spontaneously, often as a result of the dog merely running in the garden, and sometimes both hock joints are affected. The subluxation is due to rupture of the plantar ligament. Since the joint normally has very little movement, it can be fused (arthrodesed) with little effect on the dog's gait.

Diseases of muscle

Muscles have a rich blood supply and small defects in their tissue may regenerate. However, large defects become filled with non-elastic fibrous tissue and this may result in a muscle that is unable to stretch as much as previously. As a consequence, range of movement in adjacent joints is reduced and the dog may develop a mechanical lameness.

Although muscle injuries are seen in all breeds of dog they are most frequently seen in racing Greyhounds. Such injuries may be classified as contusions, lacerations, ruptures and contractures.

CONTUSIONS

Contusions generally result from falls, fight wounds or other penetrating injuries, and blows. The overlying skin is often discoloured and the affected

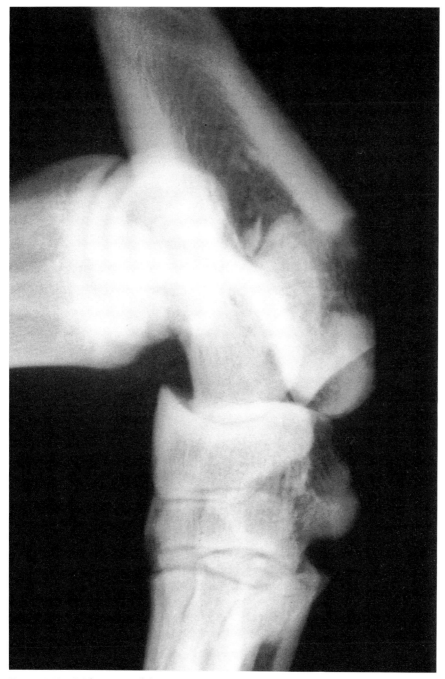

Figure 163 Dislocation of the proximal intertarsal joint. The back of the hock should be straight

muscle is hot and painful. A specific contusion known as 'track-leg' occurs in the Greyhound. This is a swelling of the muscles covering the inner aspect of the lower third of the tibia and it is due to the inside of the lower limb striking the outside of the elbow. The left leg is usually involved. The injury occurs as the hindlimb advances beyond the forelimb when the dog is at a full gallop. Most contusions do not require treatment other than rest. However, if a 'track-leg' occurs as a result of the Greyhound altering its gait due to some other injury the problem may recur. In these recurrent cases the inflammation may become more extensive and have greater consequences. If it extends to the underlying tibia, the periosteum of the bone will become damaged and new bone will be laid down at the site of this inflammation. This will then contribute to the problem and a vicious circle will be set up. In mild cases greasing the affected areas will help to reduce the problem.

LACERATIONS

Lacerations may either occur in the direction of the muscle fibres (when they will appear split) or across the fibres. Sometimes the gap may be felt; on other occasions it will become filled with a large blood clot (haematoma) formed as a result of damage to the local blood vessels. Small lacerations will heal with rest. Large defects will require veterinary attention.

RUPTURES

A muscle may rupture from a direct blow or, more commonly, by sudden forces imposed by an inco-ordinate movement or unusually violent exercise. The dog may carry its leg or it may change its gait. The affected area becomes swollen, warm and painful. Small ruptures will heal if the affected area is rested for two to three weeks. Complete ruptures require surgical repair, followed by immobilisation of the limb for several weeks.

Ultrasound therapy may encourage healing and reduce scar tissue formation during the healing phase. A typical regime would be to rest the area for the first four days and then follow this with ultrasound therapy twice daily for a further four to five days. Therapy might then be reduced to daily treatment over the next 10 days or so.

Muscle ruptures are an important cause of lameness in the racing Greyhound. They tend to occur at the same sites, since the dogs always race at speed around an oval or circular track in an anti-clockwise direction. The commoner muscle ruptures are listed below:

Infraspinatus and trapezium muscles

These shoulder muscles are frequently injured and result in loss of stride length. Dogs consequently become slower, particularly on cornering.

Triceps

This muscle has four heads which join to form a major muscle of the upper foreleg. The long head is the common site of injury. Either the muscle pulls away from its attachment to the scapula or the rupture occurs within the body of the muscle. The rupture is frequently accompanied by a haematoma, which is easily felt. Conservative management often allows a return to racing, although the dog's performance is reduced. Early surgical reattachment of the damaged muscle to the scapula is indicated, but the repair may break down especially if the shoulder is over-extended during the post-operative period.

Gracilis

The gracilis muscle lies on the inner aspect of the thigh. Although the rupture may occur anywhere along the length of the muscle it generally occurs in its caudal portion. It is a serious injury that frequently signals an early retirement from the track and always merits veterinary attention. Within 12 to 24 hours of the injury the overlying skin becomes discoloured and a painful swelling develops. The torn muscle 'drops' and a gap in the muscle tissue fills with a haematoma. The injury should be treated as soon as possible with ice packs and support bandaging. Surgical removal of the haematoma and repositioning of the torn muscle is indicated in all but the most minor of tears. The area should be bandaged post-operatively for approximately a month and the dog rested for three months. A gradually increasing exercise regime should be instituted to limit the formation of restrictive scar tissue, but this is not always successful.

Tensor fascia lata

This muscle lies superficially on the lateral aspect of the thigh and commonly ruptures where its muscular portion joins the tendinous part. The Greyhound will show pain on extension of its hip and a depression can be palpated at the site of the rupture. The rupture can be repaired successfully, although the dog may not always return to its former athletic performance.

CONTRACTURES

Permanent contracture or shortening of a muscle may follow an injury to the muscle itself or to the nerve that activates it. In either case the muscle is replaced by non-elastic fibrous tissue. These injuries are uncommon but result in a mechanical lameness. The following contractures have been seen:

Infraspinatus

This is most commonly seen in working dogs or in dogs that lead an active life. It is believed that trauma is responsible for at least some of the cases, although a single injury to the affected area often goes unnoticed by the owner. The elbow is pulled outwards by the shortened infraspinatus, which lies on the lateral aspect of the shoulder. Thus the dog's gait becomes altered. Treatment involves surgical excision of the fibrous tissue that has replaced the damage muscle. Exercise is commenced immediately after surgery to discourage further scar tissue from restricting shoulder movement. The response to treatment is good.

Gracilis

Contracture of the gracilis muscle is seen occasionally in the larger breed dogs. A taut fibrous band can be palpated on the caudomedial aspect of the thigh, instead of the usual fleshy muscle belly. A mechanical lameness is seen; the hock is suddenly snatched up and rotated outwards as the limb is advanced. Surgical removal of the fibrous tissue provides temporary remission of the signs, but the lameness returns within a few months. Thus it is dubious whether surgery is indicated. However, since the lameness is of a mechanical origin, and is not painful, these dogs continue to lead happy active lives.

Semi-membranosus and semi-tendinosus

These two muscles are situated on the caudal aspect of the thigh. Contracture is uncommon, but results in the foot suddenly being snatched backwards just before it strikes the ground. Treatment is unnecessary.

MYOSITIS

Inflammation of muscle is called myositis. It may be due to a number of causes, including trauma and infection. A specific myositis is myositis of the jaw muscles. This is a painful condition whose cause is unknown. The muscles are swollen and the dog is unwilling to open its mouth due to the pain. Later, the muscles waste (atrophy) and the skull becomes prominent as the dog loses the muscles on either side of its head. It is still unable to open its mouth, but the cause is now mechanical, since the muscles are replaced with non-elastic fibrous tissue.

During the initial inflammatory phase the dog is treated with painkillers and anti-inflammatory drugs. When the muscle has been replaced with fibrous tissue, drug therapy is unsuccessful. In these cases, it is necessary for the veterinarian to break down this fibrous tissue by forcible opening the dog's mouth under general anaesthesia. Unfortunately, the scar tissue tends to re-form and the treatment has to be repeated on several occasions. Most dogs are left with permanently restricted jaw movement, but they are capable of opening their mouths sufficiently to eat soft food.

GREYHOUND CRAMP

There are many terms associated with this condition. 'Cramp', 'myoglobi-nuria', 'exertional myopathy' and 'azoturia' are frequently used to describe different degrees of this single condition. It affects the skeletal muscles, especially those of the hindlimb, back and forelimbs, and is associated with exercise.

Cramp is regarded as being the mild form of the condition, while the term exertional rhabdomyolysis is used for the severe form. Exertional rhabdomyolysis means disintegration of the skeletal muscles associated with exercise. There are several circumstances when this condition is likely to occur. It is commoner in hot, humid weather, especially following a long car trip. Excitable dogs that bark, whine or pant incessantly when kennelled prior to a race are prone to the condition. Dogs running for the first time over a longer distance, or those that return to the track after a prolonged rest period, may also be more prone to cramping.

The main signs of cramp are extreme muscle pain, with dragging of the nails. The dog is agitated and its breathing is laboured. Signs of severe rhabdomyolysis include swollen and excruciatingly painful back muscles and port-coloured urine. The dog assumes a hunched appearance, goes off its food, drinks excessively and is ill. It may lose weight and take several months to recover fully.

There are several factors implicated in this condition. A relative lack of oxygen towards the end of the race causes lactic acid to build-up in the muscles. This destroys muscle tissue and the breakdown products spill over into the blood and are excreted by the kidneys. This is the reason why the urine is discoloured in severe cases. The lack of oxygen also affects the outer membrane of the cells causing the inside of these cells to be more acidic than normal. A relative lack of potassium, due either to a diet deficient in potassium or the excessive loss because of excitement and panting before a race, causes a reduced blood flow to the muscles. Finally, some families of greyhounds appear to have a genetic predisposition to the problem.

Treatment of cramp should include rest, careful training of the dog and attention to its diet. However, some dogs appear to be prone to the condition and suffer recurrent attacks.

Diseases of tendons

RUPTURE OF TENDONS

Rupture of a tendon may follow a sharp blow, lacerations, falls or inco-ordinate movements. Any violent contraction of a muscle against a fixed joint or bone is likely to result in rupture of either the muscle or its tendon, particularly in older, overweight, unfit animals.

The healing of a ruptured tendon can be conveniently divided into two phases. During the first three to four weeks the gap between the ruptured tendon ends fills with newly formed, randomly orientated collagen fibres. This random orientation is much less strong than the original parallel arrangement of the fibres. During this stage of healing the tendon must be protected from weight-bearing forces by putting the limb in a cast. The second phase of tendon healing occurs over the next six to eight weeks and involves the re-orientation of the collagen fibres under the influence of limited weight-bearing forces.

Tendon adhesions are prevented by gentle handling of tissues during surgery and the elimination of any infection. Generally, when a ruptured tendon is accompanied by a grossly contaminated wound it is advisable to defer surgical repair of the tendon until after the infection has been controlled.

COMMON TENDON INJURIES

Rupture of the Achilles tendon

The Achilles tendon is the largest tendon in the dog and consequently it takes the longest time to heal. The rupture may be partial or complete and is frequently caused by a laceration above the point of the hock. The skin wound is usually small yet the damage to the underlying tendon can be devastating. The dog is unable to use its leg or will walk with its hock dropped flat to the ground.

The tendon must be repaired surgically if the dog is to regain satisfactory function. Post-operatively, the limb is immobilised with the hock in extension for several weeks, followed by a support bandage for another month to six weeks.

An alternative to casting the limb is to immobilise the hock joint with a bone screw (Fig. 164). This is removed once the tendon has healed. The advantage of this technique is that it avoids the use of a cast and is more comfortable for the dog.

Rupture of the digital flexor tendons

These tendons are frequently lacerated by dogs walking on pieces of glass or other sharp objects. They may also be stretched and torn in racing Greyhounds. Lacerations are generally accompanied by profuse haemorrhage, which tends to obscure the full extent of the damage to the underlying tendons. Severance of the superficial flexor tendons does not unduly affect the position of the toes. In contrast, lacerations of the deep digital flexor alter the posture of the toes when the dog puts weight on its

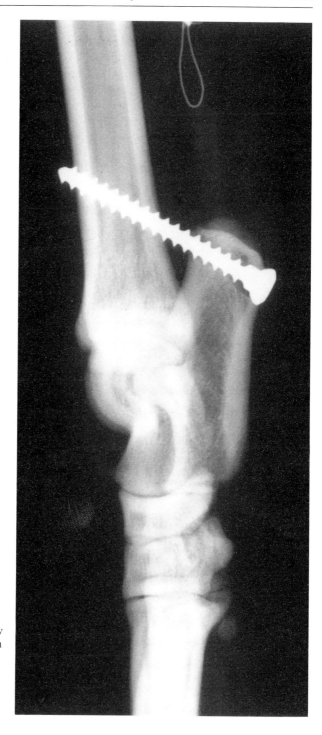

Figure 164 The hock has been immobilised temporarily with a screw to reduce the tension on the Achilles tendon. A wire suture used to repair the tendon is visible at the top of the radiograph

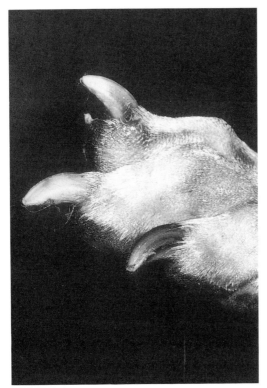

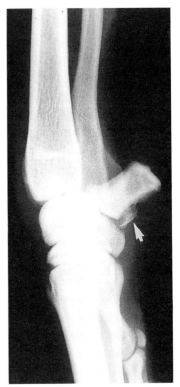

Figure 165   A 'knocked up' toe in a racing
Greyhound

Figure 166   A chip fracture of
the accessory carpal bone
(arrowed)

foot. If the laceration is above the second phalanx the affected toe(s) will
be dropped, i.e., lower than the other toes; if the tendon is severed close
to the end of the toe, the toe will be raised from the ground (a so-called
'knocked-up' toe) (Fig. 165).

Lacerations of both the superficial and deep digital flexor tendons
should be repaired surgically. Post-operatively the foot is immobilised in
a cast for three weeks, followed by three weeks in a padded bandage.
Limited exercise on a lead is mandatory until healing is complete.

Superficial digital flexor tendon injuries are a frequent cause of lameness
in the racing Greyhound. They generally involve the fifth toe of the left
forelimb or the second toe (the inside toe) of the right forelimb. The
tendons usually tear at the level of the metacarpal or metatarsal bones and
take at least three months to heal. Complete ruptures are repaired
surgically while partial tears are treated conservatively by resting the dog.
Numerous linaments, lotions, poultices and other local applications have
been advocated to encourage healing, but their value is equivocal.

Rupture of flexor carpi ulnaris

This muscle has two tendons which insert independently on to the accessory carpal bone. The tendon of the larger head may tear near its insertion, while excessive tension on the smaller head usually causes a chip fracture of the accessory carpal bone (Fig. 166). Chips should be removed, or re-attached if they are large enough, while tears in the tendon should be sutured. Post-operative management comprises a minimum of four to six weeks support bandaging before allowing a gradual return to work.

Displacement of the superficial flexor tendon

This injury is seen occasionally in the racing Greyhound and also in the Collie breeds, especially the Shetland Sheepdog. The dog is able to take weight on the limb, but the hock is flexed excessively ('dropped'). A swelling is palpable over the point of the hock and the tendon can be felt to slip on and off the end of the point of the hock. It can be sewn back into place and full function is usually restored.

20

THE CANINE IMMUNE SYSTEM

Dogs, like ourselves and other animals, have a series of defence mechanisms to protect them from disease caused by invasion by foreign organisms, tissues or other substances. The healthy skin acts as a barrier, preventing entry of microbes and other potentially harmful substances. Mucous membranes in the nose trap substances that are breathed in. Coughing prevents the ingress of invaders to the lungs, while the mucus lining the airways acts as a further barrier. Stomach acid and the mucus produced by the small bowel are further examples of defence mechanisms, as is the action of liver in destroying toxins produced by bacteria.

Should all these primary defence mechanisms fail and potentially harmful organisms or substances enter the body (antigens), then the body will mount a second line of defence via the immune system.

STRUCTURE

The immune system consists of the lymph nodes together with the spleen, thymus, lung, liver and a variety of cells formed in the bone marrow that circulate in the blood and are collectively known as leucoyctes or white blood cells. There are five types of white blood cells recognised by their appearance (see Chapter 9 Haematology). These are lymphocytes, polymorphonuclear leucocytes or neutrophils, monocytes (which are called macrophages when they are found in tissues), eosinophils and basophils. Lymphocytes, neutrophils and monocytes are the most important in defending the body against invasion by micro-organisms.

Neutrophils and macrophages (monocytes) are scavenger cells. They engulf particulate matter such as bacteria by a process called phagocytosis. Once engulfed, these bacteria are killed and broken down by enzymes released within the scavenger cells. As a general rule neutrophils are a highly mobile defence system arriving first at the site of inflammation or tissue injury, while monocytes (macrophages) arrive later in the inflammatory process. Macrophages are often found within tissues through which large numbers of potentially pathogenic organisms pass, hence there are large numbers of macrophages present in the lungs to remove airborne micro-organisms and in the liver to filter out harmful bacteria (pathogens) arriving in the blood from the gut.

NON-SPECIFIC IMMUNITY

A healthy dog is protected from potentially harmful micro-organisms in the environment by a number of effective mechanisms present at the time of birth. These primary defences do not depend on the dog having any previous experience of the particular infection and are generally effective against a wide range of potentially infective agents. Thus they are truly non-specific. Such defences may be physical, as previously described in the case of the tough, waterproof layer of skin on most of the body's surfaces. The layer of mucus coating the surface of the respiratory tract also acts as a physical trapping mechanism for small particles. In addition the action of the fine, hairlike cilia within the mucus moves it in the direction of the mouth, from where it may be swallowed or coughed out.

Other primary, non-specific defences may be chemical in nature. The previously mentioned acidic juices present in the stomach kill many micro-organisms in the gastrointestinal tract. Natural lubricants such as saliva, tears and nasal secretions contain substances capable of deactivating some viruses as well as lysosymes, which are enzymes capable of killing some types of bacteria. Antifungal agents can also be present in the secretions, as well as cells such as neutrophils and macrophages capable of engulfing bacteria and killing them.

Table 20 Mechanisms of resistance

Non specific resistance	*Specific Acquired Immunity*
is inborn	is acquired:
	(a) by exposure to antigen
	(b) by passive transfer of antibody in colostrum and across placenta
Includes:	Includes:
(a) the presence of intact barriers, e.g., skin and mucous membranes	(a) production of specific antibody from 'B' cells
(b) flushing action of milk, tears and urine	(b) production of sensitized or aggressive 'T' cells
(c) cough and blink reflexes	(c) production of lymphokines from 'T' cells
(d) acidic secretions, e.g., in vagina and stomach	
(e) enzymes in secretions and tissue fluid, e.g., lysosyme	

SPECIFIC IMMUNITY

The circulating white blood cell population of the dog consists of 12–30 per cent lymphocytes. These are present in particularly large numbers in those tissues engaged in the production of antibody, i.e., the lymph nodes, the spleen and bone marrow. At these sites pieces of the infective agent consisting of large molecules called antigens are presented to special small lymphocytes known as B cells. The antigens become bound to the B cells at special receptor sites on the cell surface and this stimulates the B cell to divide, producing a group of cells known as a clone of plasma cells, each of which is capable of producing a specific substance that can combine with the antigen and render it harmless. This substance is known as antibody, and antibody molecules are specific to a particular antigen. The analogy of the lock and key perhaps explains this more easily. If the antigen is thought of as a key then there is only one lock, antibody, that the key will fit (Fig. 167). In other words, antibody produced by a particular antigen combines with that antigen only. The number of antigens that can result in an antibody response is immense, running into many millions. Simply, antigens can be thought of as any form of foreign protein, i.e., not of the body, and may be parts of bacteria or viruses or other foreign proteins that have entered the body.

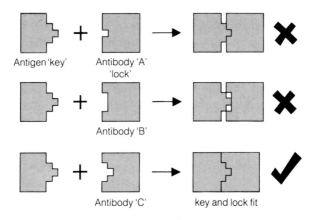

Figure 167   Lock and key analogy of antibody specificity

Antibody molecules produced may have one of a number of functions. They may (1) render inactive or neutralise the bacterial toxins, (2) promote breakdown (lysis) of bacteria, viruses or protozoa, (3) promote ingestion (phagocytosis) of particles by scavenger cells by coating the particles and making them more 'sticky', and (4) trigger other defensive enzyme systems, e.g., the complement system. This consists of complex protein enzymes occurring in normal serum which interact to combine with the antigen/

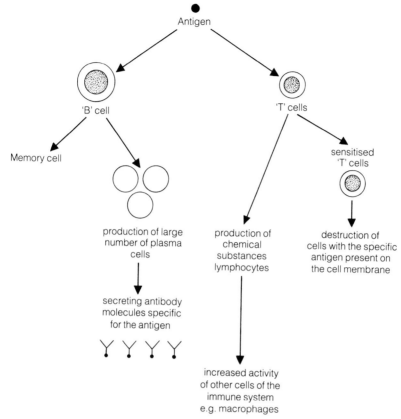

Antigen

'B' cell

'T' cells

Memory cell

sensitised
'T' cells

production of large
number of plasma
cells

production of
chemical
substances
lymphocytes

destruction of
cells with the specific
antigen present on
the cell membrane

secreting antibody
molecules specific
for the antigen

increased activity
of other cells of the
immune system
e.g. macrophages

Figure 168   Humoral and cell-mediated immunity

antibody complex to destroy the antigen when it happens to be a complete cell.

The production of antibody is known as the humoral response. At the same time there is also another response taking place. This is known as the cell-mediated response or cell-mediated immunity (Fig. 168). While the small lymphocytes (B-cells) are producing antibody, antigen is also presented to the large lymphocytes, which are known as T-cells. This triggers the production of sensitised (aggressive) T-cells specific for a given antigen. These sensitised T-cells are capable of recognising antigen on cell surfaces and can directly kill these target cells, e.g., virus-infected cells, tumour cells, etc.

The production of such specific immune responses is a slow process. Detectable amounts of antibody cannot normally by demonstrated in the circulation until at least five days after the antigen is first presented. Peak levels usually are not reached for approximately two weeks. However, when the same antigen or infection occurs on a second or subsequent occasion, the animal's immune system responds rapidly and peak response is usually present within two or three days and is usually very much higher than the initial response. It is upon this immune response that vaccination depends for its success.

Although, as previously mentioned, the physical defences are present in the young puppy from birth, immunologically the puppy is incompetent for some weeks, but protection is afforded by the bitch, who provides some of her circulating antibodies, which are either transferred across the placenta before the puppy is born or absorbed across the gut in early life from the first milk or colostrum. The presence of this antibody, which is called passive antibody since it has not been produced by the puppy itself, gives the puppy protection against those diseases that the bitch has herself encountered or been protected against by vaccination. This maternally acquired immunity is of only a temporary nature and starts to fade as the puppy's own immune system becomes competent. However, its presence can sometimes interfere with the development of immunity and production of antibodies by the puppy at the time of vaccination against one of the major diseases and thus necessitates the use of two or more doses of vaccines several weeks apart. This commonly occurs in the case of canine parvovirus, the maternally derived antibodies to which, in the puppy, may last as long as 20 weeks compared with an average of 12 weeks in the case of the other diseases commonly vaccinated against, e.g., distemper. Recently much research has been directed at the problem of ensuring early protection of the puppy in spite of high levels of circulating maternal antibody.

The presence of high circulating antibody levels does not necessarily guarantee protection from infectious disease. In certain circumstances the production of local antibody gives better protection. An example of this is kennel cough, due to *Bordetella bronchiseptica*. Local immunity produced by the administration of an intranasal vaccine gives much better protection than Bordetella vaccines introduced more conventionally.

Protection may also be a function of some aspect of cell-mediated immunity.

AUTO-IMMUNITY

The immune system is primarily concerned with the elimination of antigens from the system. These are usually foreign proteins and may be from bacteria, viruses, parasites or other pathogens. Similar proteins are present as part of the body's own tissues and therefore it is important that the immune system recognises 'itself' from 'non-self'. During development of the puppy at around the 42nd day of gestation an inventory of all the antigenic material present is taken and this is designated as 'self'. Any proteins (i.e., antigens) introduced in later life are then recognised as 'foreign' and an immune response is mounted against them. Utilising this method of recognition, disease-producing organisms (pathogens) that do invade the body are usually eliminated rapidly and it has long been recognised that individuals who recovered from attacks of disease were spared further attacks. An example of this was smallpox in man and we know today that the disease did not recur in the recovered individual due to the development of immunity against the foreign protein (antigen), in this case the smallpox virus.

When an immune response is mounted against self 'tissue' it represents a severe breakdown in the finely tuned immune system. Diseases caused by such a breakdown are termed *auto-immune*. They include such conditions as:

Auto-immune haemolytic anaemia (AIHA)
Immune mediated thrombocytopaenia (IMT)
Systemic lupus erythematosus (SLE)
Auto-immune thyroiditis

In all these diseases 'self' protein is mistaken for a foreign antigen. There are thought to be a number of reasons for the lack of recognition of the self tissues. These include:

1. Neoplastic conditions (cancers) of the lymphoid or immune system itself.

2. Formation of new antigens during the animal's development. Such potential antigenic substances as spermatozoa and lens protein from the eye are normally shielded from the body's immune system, but when such barriers break down auto-immunity can result.

3. It is known that the presence of viruses in association with some of the body cells may stimulate an immune response which not only damages the virus but can affect the cell with which it is associated.

4. Drug molecules, in themselves too small to stimulate an immune response, may become attached to protein molecules in cell walls or as free proteins in plasma and thus increase their overall molecular size, enabling them to stimulate an immune response. The resulting immune response can be directed against both the drug and the cell's wall, again causing damage to the cell, or the response can result in the production of circulating antigen/antibody complexes. These can become bound to circulating red blood cells or blood platelets and so result in their damage. It appears that examples of drug-induced auto-immunity are less frequent in the dog than in man.

Now let us look at some of the more important auto-immune diseases encountered in the dog.

Auto-immune haemolytic anaemia (AIHA)

AIHA is the production of antibodies against circulating red blood cells (erythrocytes), leading to the destruction of these cells in the liver and spleen. Less commonly the production of such antibodies can occur secondarily to a number of infective, neoplastic or other auto-immune diseases. The disease is more common in bitches than in dogs and is often seen in young adults. It can occur in any breed. Different forms of AIHA are recognised according to the characteristics of the antibody involved and the temperature at which the antibody is maximally destructive.

Thus there are so-called 'warm-antibody' and 'cold antibody' types.

Clinical signs   Clinical signs of AIHA include progressive exercise intolerance, lethargy and weakness, inappetence, increased thirst, raised heart and respiratory rates and vomiting. Frank bleeding is not commonly a sign of AIHA, although haemoglobin (red blood pigment) may be apparent in the urine. Diagnosis depends on laboratory testing.

Treatment   Treatment consists of large doses of corticosteroids, sometimes supplemented with other immunosuppressive drugs over a period of weeks to months and even years. Responses to treatment are often good, although some individuals have periodic relapses and a few fail to respond at all. There is some evidence that failure to respond to treatment is related to the characteristics of the antibody involved. Neutering may be useful in bitches, as relapses have been seen to occur with the onset of oestrus.

Immune mediated thrombocytopaenia (IMT)

IMT is more rarely encountered than AIHA, which is itself not all that common. Clinically it is associated with acute or chronic bleeding due to a reduction in the number of circulating blood platelets, which are the small blood cells whose function is to plug the gaps in any damaged blood vessels.

Clinical signs   Clinical signs include the presence of blood in urine and faeces, nose bleeds (epistaxis), excessive bruising from the slightest blow or knock and the presence of small haemorrhages on the gums. Excessive bleeding from any wound, surgical or traumatic, is also a feature. It should be borne in mind that similar clinical signs could be due to ingestion of Warfarin, a commonly used rat poison, in certain circumstances. Diagnosis again depends on sophisticated laboratory tests.

Treatment   Treatment, as with all the auto-immune diseases, depends upon administration of corticosteroids and other immunosuppressive drugs. Treatment is usually successful in those animals that do not have serious underlying disease or organ failure.

Systemic Lupus erythematosus (SLE)

This disease affects many systems of the body and is associated with the formation of antibodies to the nucleus of body cells (anti-nuclear antibody).

Clinical signs Arthritis affecting several joints of both forelegs or both hindlegs or all four legs is a common sign, together with anaemia, skin lesions, muscle stiffness, enlarged lymph nodes and recurrent fever. Central nervous system disorders, including encephalitis and meningitis, also occur. The respiratory tract may also become involved. Because of the varying clinical signs of SLE, diagnosis can be very difficult. It depends on the clinical signs and also the involvement of more than one organ system. Anti-nuclear antibody must be demonstrated in the blood by laboratory tests before a definite diagnosis can be given. Bitches are more often affected than dogs, and in one survey German Shepherds and Irish Setters appeared to predominate.

Rheumatoid arthritis

Rheumatoid arthritis (RA) is a chronic destructive inflammatory disease involving the synovial membrane (lining) of the joint. It involves the deposition of antibodies to the dog's own immunoglobin molecules in the synovial membrane.

Clinical signs Clinical signs include morning stiffness and swelling and pain in the joints. Different joints may be affected at different times or symmetrical joints may be affected. Fever, inappetence and lethargy may occur. Unlike the condition in man, the development of rheumatoid nodules in the skin or involvement of the heart and lungs have not been reported in the dog. The distension of the joint capsule, weakening of the ligaments and destruction of the cartilage and bone can lead ultimately to permanently deformed joints. Diagnosis depends on radiography of the affected joints and sampling of the joint fluid, together with the synovial membrane lining them for laboratory tests.

Treatment The condition in the dog is as difficult to treat as that in man. It can only aim to reduce inflammation and pain, enabling the animal to move more freely. A main object of treatment apart from prevention of pain and inflammation is to delay the destruction of the joint, since there is no cure for rheumatoid arthritis. The disease is always progressive with time.

In many cases treatment results only in slight relief from pain and the doses of drug used frequently have to be increased as the disease progresses. Management becomes a major commitment, both for the owner and the veterinary surgeon. Controlled exercise plays an important part in management. Swimming, regular lead exercise and joint manipulation all play a part in maintaining joint mobility. One should never lose sight of the dog's quality of life, and if this is considered unacceptable, euthanasia is often the only course of treatment left open. Drug therapy, including corticosteroids and immunosuppresants, feature prominently. Pain-killing and anti-inflammatory drugs such as aspirin are also very useful. Injections of gold salts have been helpful in some cases and surgery is at times resorted to, to repair damaged ligaments or stabilise affected joints.

Auto-immune skin diseases

Pemphigus This term covers a group of non-infectious blistering or ulcerative skin disorders due to auto-antibodies produced against various components of the skin. Lesions can occur anywhere on the body, although the mucocutaneous junctions (those areas where the mucous membrane meets the skin), such as around the muzzle, the ears, eyes and anal region, are most commonly affected.

Signs Lesions are sited primarily at the junctions of haired skin and mucous membrane (mucocutaneous junction). Nail beds may be affected and nails lost. There is hair loss, loss of pigment, crusting, variable irritation and the formation of blisters and ulcers. When antibodies are produced against the 'cement' which binds cells together in the epidermis, the condition is called *Pemphigus foliaceus*.

Other forms of Pemphigus more rarely encountered in the dog include *Pemphigus vulgaris*, *Pemphigus vegetans*, *Pemphigus erythematosus* and *Bullous pemphigoid*. Differentiation of the types of Pemphigus is made after microscopical examination of sections of the skin.

Treatment Treatment of Pemphigus, like the other auto-immune disorders, involves the use of corticosteroids and other immunosuppressive drugs, sometimes in conjunction with antibiotics to counter bacterial skin infections. Treatment is long and slow, first aiming to achieve remission of clinical signs and secondly to maintain that remission. Unfortunately treatment is not always successful, but where it is lifelong therapy is usually required. A minority of cases will go into spontaneous remission and therapy can be stopped.

Discoid lupus erythematosus (DLE)

This is an auto-immune disease of the skin of the dog, which, unlike systemic lupus erythematosus, affects many of the systems of the body.

Clinical signs   Clinical signs include loss of hair, crusting, loss of pigment, reddening of the skin and sometimes ulceration. Lesions are always symmetrical and occur on and spread up the bridge of the nose. Sometimes the face and lips are involved. This is one of the causes of 'collie nose' and is seen in Collies, Shetland Sheepdogs and German Shepherd Dogs. Laboratory tests may be used to demonstrate deposits of antibody at the dermal/epidermal junction within the skin.

Treatment   Corticosteroids are employed, either by mouth or locally in the form of creams. Use of high-factor sunblocks and avoidance of strong sunlight can also help. In some countries tattooing has been used to alleviate the condition.

Other immune mediated diseases

Myasthenia gravis   The form of *Myasthenia gravis* seen in adult dogs is like the late onset form of the disease in man. It involves the formation of auto-antibodies against acetylcholine receptors on skeletal muscle fibres. Acetylcholine is an important transmitter of nerve impulses to the muscles and antibodies formed sit on the acetylcholine receptors, blocking its action and therefore nerve transmission. Clinically this appears as weakness and greatly reduced exercise tolerance. Oesophageal dilation (Megaesophagus) may also be present and lead to regurgitation of food. Treatment is possible using the drug neostigmine, which enhances the effects of acetylcholine. Corticosteroids are also often used at the same time in an attempt to reduce auto-antibody formation.

Auto-immune thyroiditis   Many dogs with hypothyroidism, a deficiency of thyroid gland activity, have been found to have auto-antibodies to thyroglobulin, which is a stored form of thyroid hormone found within the gland. As a result of this auto-immune reaction the glandular tissue is gradually replaced with fibrous tissue. Hypothyroidism is more fully discussed in Chapter 14 on the endocrine system.

Glomerulonephritis   When antibody reacts with antigen (foreign protein) under conditions where the number of antigen molecules greatly exceeds those of antibody, large networks of so-called antigen/antibody complexes are formed. These circulate in the blood, finally accumulating in the capillary walls of the kidney glomeruli (filtration units). They then trigger a series of complex enzyme reactions known as the complement cascade, resulting in irreparable damage to the cells of the kidney filtration system. Such events have been reported to occur with a variety of disease conditions, including infections e.g., pyometra, auto-immune disease, e.g., systemic lupus erythematosus and neoplasia (cancer).

Successful treatment of the underlying disease will stop progression of the glomerular nephritis, but cannot reverse the damage which has already occurred. Attempts to identify the auto-antibody to components of the kidney glomerulus have not far been successful.

Considerations of treatment of auto-immune disease

It is important to remember that canine patients undergoing treatment for auto-immune disease are very often not going to be cured but rather have the clinical signs of the disease suppressed by the use of drugs. The aim of this palliation is to ensure a reasonable quality of life for the dog, but a great deal of owner dedication is required in the management. Some cases, e.g., rheumatoid arthritis, will not be suppressed for very long.

The drugs used are themselves not without side effects; many will reduce the dog's ability to heal after minor surgery, make the animal more susceptible to other infections or produce side effects which cannot be controlled and therefore make their use unsuitable in that particular patient. Regular monitoring is essential for the dog's well-being. Veterinarians will advise regarding suitable monitoring regimes. It is really important to observe these and to take your dog back to the vet when requested to do so.

Postscript: Without doubt our knowledge of the role of the immune system in the progression of many diseases is still in its infancy. As our knowledge increases so our attitudes to the prevention and treatment of disease is going to change rapidly. This chapter is out of date already, so fast is our knowledge in this field expanding.

Infectious Diseases

21

INTRODUCTION
TO INFECTIOUS DISEASES

Infectious diseases are illnesses caused by the growth or development of another living organism, 'the infectious agent', in or on an animal. Infectious diseases of dogs include some of the best-known canine diseases, such as distemper and parvovirus infections, and are important causes of illness and death. Some infectious diseases of the dog can also be transmitted to humans and are therefore also important from a public health point of view.

It is often thought that all infectious diseases are caused by viruses or bacteria, the two best-known types of infectious agents, but, in fact, a large number of different types of living organisms can give rise to infectious disease. These are viruses, bacteria, mycoplasma, rickettsia, chlamydia, fungi, algae, protozoa, helminths and arthropods. The last three types of organisms, i.e., protozoa, helminths and arthropods, are also commonly known as parasites.

Resistance to infection

Infectious disease requires not only an infectious agent but also a susceptible 'host' or animal in which that agent may grow. Animals may be resistant to particular infectious diseases for a variety of reasons. Many infections, especially viral and parasitic ones, are relatively 'species specific' which means they will cause disease in only one type of animal. For example, *Demodex canis*, which causes mange, a skin disease, does so only in dogs, not in cats or other species. This limitation of infection to one species of animal is a type of natural or genetic resistance. Age resistance is important in some infections; canine herpesvirus infection kills pups less than 2 weeks old, but is very unlikely to cause severe disease in older animals.

However, the most important factor determining whether an animal is susceptible to an infection is undoubtedly whether that animal has an acquired resistance or immunity. As everyone knows, it is uncommon to suffer more than once from major infections, such as measles in man or distemper in dogs. This is because the body's specific defence mechanisms, its immune system, can remember or recognise infections which it has met before and is able to prevent them developing again – the animal is then said to be immune to that particular disease. The immune system is also responsible for fighting and eliminating diseases when they are encountered for the first time.

In pups, the immune system develops in the womb in the second half of pregnancy and in the first few weeks after birth. By four weeks of age the pup is immunocompetent, i.e., it has a fully developed immune system capable of responding to infections. Animals may become immune to a particular infection by being naturally exposed to it or by being immunised or vaccinated against it. Immunity to serious infections like distemper usually lasts for many years, even for life, but for minor infections, such as kennel cough, immunity is often relatively short-lived, so the animal may suffer repeatedly from the same infection.

In animals which are in poor condition, whether because of serious illness, starvation or some other reason, the immune system may not work as well as it should. Such animals are said to have an acquired immunodeficiency or to be immunosuppressed, and are more likely to contract infectious diseases or to be seriously affected by them. Some drugs, especially those used to treat cancer or to control allergies and inflammation, can also cause immunosuppression and extra care may need to be taken to prevent infections in animals receiving these substances. Very occasionally, animals are born with an immune system that is not properly developed or is even absent. These animals, which are said to be congenitally immunodeficient, cannot defend themselves against even minor infections and usually die early in life as a result of severe or repeated infections.

Patterns of infectious disease

Strictly speaking, 'infectious' means only that a disease is caused by one of the types of infectious agents mentioned earlier. However, 'infectious' is often loosely used when what is meant is 'contagious'. A contagious disease is one which is transmitted between one animal and another by direct or indirect contact. Common examples of contagious disease in dogs are kennel cough and distemper.

Obviously, all contagious diseases are infectious, but not all infectious diseases are contagious. For example, an abscess that develops in the neck following a bite is infectious in that it is caused by bacteria introduced under the skin when the dog was bitten; but it is not contagious, in that the abscess cannot be transmitted to another animal by either simple direct contact, such as sleeping in the same basket, or by indirect contact, such as being groomed with the same brush.

Infectious diseases occur in a number of patterns, depending on the degree of contagiousness of the infection and the immunity of animals in the population.

1. *Sporadic disease* is where a few cases occur randomly – sporadic diseases, such as abscesses, are usually non-contagious.
2. *Endemic disease* is where cases occur regularly in a population – endemic diseases, such as distemper in large urban areas, are usually contagious, but adult animals are usually immune and disease is most likely in young or newly introduced animals.
3. *Epidemic disease* is where many cases develop within a short space of time in one area; for an epidemic to occur, the infection must be contagious and the population must have little immunity to it. Local epidemics, such as an outbreak of kennel cough, are usually the result of introduction of a disease which has not been present for some time into a group of animals. The introduction of a totally new disease, or a new type of disease, can result in very widespread epidemics or even pandemics, in which disease spreads from country to country. New types of influenza, such as Hong Kong flu, are the commonest cause of pandemics in man. In the dog, the best-known pandemic was canine parvovirus infection, which spread worldwide in 1978–80.

As mentioned above, some infections are found in only one animal species, but others can be transmitted to different types of animals, including man. An infection that is transmitted to man from any animal is known as a zoonosis. In fact, a better definition of zoonosis is an infection which is *shared* by man and animals, since zoonoses work both ways – animals can catch diseases from man as well as man from animals – and infection of both man and animal may result from exposure to a common source as well as infection of one by another. A number of infections of the dog are zoonotic (see Table 21, overleaf) and can cause diseases ranging from mild skin rashes (with the skin parasite *Cheyletiella*) to very serious illness or even death (with rabies). All responsible dog owners must take special care to control potential zoonotic infections in their animals.

Sources of infection

The many organisms which cause infectious diseases can be acquired from a number of different sources (Fig. 169, overleaf).

1. *Other animals.* The most common source of an infectious disease is another animal. Dogs showing clinical signs of a contagious disease are obvious sources of infection. A less obvious, and therefore more potentially

Table 21 Important zoonotic infections of the dog

Type of infection	Cause of infection	Name of disease
Virus	Rabies virus	Rabies (hydrophobia)
Bacterium	Salmonella	Salmonellosis
	Campylobacter	Campylobacterosis
	Leptospira	Leptospirosis (Weil's disease in man)
Fungus	Microsporum	Ringworm
Helminths	*Toxocara canis*	Toxocariasis (Visceral larval migrants in man)
	Echinococcus granulosus	Echinococcosis (Hydatid disease in man)
Arthropods	*Cheyletiella parasitovorax*	Cheyletiellosis
	Sarcoptes scabei	Sarcoptic mange (Scabies in man)

serious, source is the carrier animal. This may be an animal that is recovering from disease but which is still excreting the organism responsible, or it may be an animal which has contracted infection without showing any signs of illness – this is termed subclinical or asymptomatic infection. The length of time for which an animal will excrete an infectious agent varies widely depending on the agent involved. It may be only a few days (with some viruses) or many months (for some parasites). Other animal species can also act as sources of infection or reservoirs for some diseases of the dog; probably the best-known example is rabies, which exists in wildlife such as the fox in Europe and is occasionally transmitted to dogs.

Figure 169 Sources of infection and routes of transmission

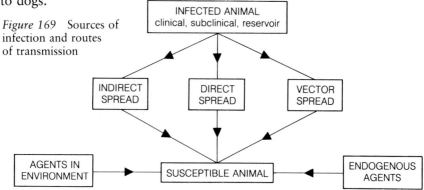

Method of spread to man	Disease in dog	Disease in man
Bite wound or licking of cut	Nervous disease and death	Nervous disease and death
Faecal contamination	Gastroenteritis	Gastroenteritis
Faecal contamination	Gastroenteritis	Gastroenteritis
Urine contamination	Liver and kidney disease	Liver and kidney disease and meningitis
Direct contact	Skin disease	Skin disease
Faecal contamination	Roundworms in intestine	Liver and eye disease
Faecal contamination	Tapeworms in intestine	Large cysts in liver, lungs and brain
Direct contact	Scurfy skin	Marked itching and rash
Direct contact	Skin disease	Skin disease

2. *The environment.* A few infectious agents exist naturally in the environment and are picked up directly from it. Examples are some bacterial infections such as tetanus and many fungal and algal diseases.

3. *Endogenous infection.* A number of organisms which have the potential to cause disease are also found as normal inhabitants of some parts of the body, especially the skin, the nose and the gut. These organisms, collectively called the commensal flora, will usually cause disease only in special circumstances. They may, for example, invade wounds and complicate diseases due to some other cause, when they are known as secondary invaders. They may also take advantage of immuno-suppression due to stress, some other infection or drug treatment to multiply and cause disease. Consequently, such endogenous infections are often known as opportunists.

Transmission of infection

For the various contagious diseases, transmission of infection between one animal and another can also be achieved in a variety of ways (see Fig. 169).

1. *Direct contact.* This is the simplest method of spread of infection between animals. It is also one of the commonest routes of transmission

in canine infections because of the way in which dogs normally lick, sniff and rub against each other when they meet. Special forms of direct contact transmission include venereal spread, i.e., spread during sexual contact (important in canine brucellosis), and prenatal or transplacental spread, i.e., where an infection is spread from the dam to her pups while they are still in the womb.

2. *Indirect contact.* This is also a common method of spread of contagious disease and is much more difficult to control than direct contact. Indirect contact can occur by environmental contamination, where, for example, faeces containing an infectious agent are passed on to the ground. Contamination of common exercise areas may result in transmission of infection to many dogs.

Food and water contamination are other forms of indirect contact that can spread infection to large numbers of animals. Another major type of indirect contact is contact via fomites. Fomites are inanimate objects that can carry infection between animals and include such obvious things as food and water dishes, grooming equipment and wellington boots as well as less apparent objects such as surgical instruments and other technical equipment.

The other major form of indirect contact is airborne or aerosol spread. This is especially important in respiratory infections such as kennel cough, when infectious particles coughed or sneezed out by an animal can travel over some distance. Because there is no physical agent (other than air) between the animals involved in airborne transmission, it is sometimes considered as a form of direct contact.

3. *Vectors.* These are living animals that transport infectious agents between animals. Many vectors, such as flies, birds or rodents, act purely mechanically, i.e., they are the living equivalent of fomites. However, with some diseases, the infectious agent actually multiplies within the vector. The most spectacular example of this (fortunately not present in Britain) is bubonic plague, where the bacterium responsible, *Yersinia pseudotuberculosis pestis*, multiplies within the fleas which transmit the infection. In still other diseases, especially parasitic ones, part of the life cycle of the infectious agent must take place within the vector before the infection can be transmitted further; the vector is then known as an intermediate host.

The importance of different routes of transmission varies with the agent involved and its ability to survive outside the body of an infected animal. Direct contact is particularly important for sensitive organisms, such as canine distemper virus, which are rapidly destroyed by environmental conditions. Indirect contact is much more important with highly resistant organisms, such as canine parvovirus or the eggs of nematode parasites (worms), which can survive on the ground or elsewhere in the environment for many weeks or months. In general, it is more difficult to control infections that are spread by indirect rather than by simple direct contact.

The different types of infectious agents

VIRUSES

Viruses are, in some ways, the simplest of the agents that cause infectious disease – they are certainly the smallest. Viruses are so small they cannot be seen even using an ordinary microscope. In scientific terms, they range in size from 10–400 nanometers in diameter (a metre contains one thousand million nanometers!). In more simple terms, one million parvoviruses (the smallest dog virus) laid end-to-end would measure less than one inch.

Viruses also have a relatively simple structure: a central core containing one of two types of nucleic acid – DNA or RNA; a surrounding shell of protein; and, in some viruses, an outer delicate membrane or envelope of lipoprotein. Viruses, unlike many other infectious agents, can only grow within the living cells of an animal. The outer protein shell or the envelope (when present) is responsible for allowing the virus to invade animal cells, while the central nucleic acid core holds the genetic information required for virus multiplication once inside the cell. Different viruses prefer to grow in cells from different parts of the body and this explains why viruses cause such different diseases – canine adenovirus, for example, grows well in liver cells and causes hepatitis, while rabies virus prefers nervous tissue cells, resulting in nervous disease.

Most viruses (such as canine parvovirus) cause disease because they take over the normal processes of the host cells in order to multiply and, in doing so, kill the cell they have invaded. Some viruses, such as herpesvirus, do not kill all the cells which they infect but 'hide' within a few cells only to flare up and cause further problems months or even years later; these are called latent infections. Another way in which viruses produce disease is by causing cell proliferation rather than cell death. A common example in the dog is papilloma virus, which causes warts. A very few viruses can cause more serious tumours or 'cancers'. The best-known virus of this type is the leukaemia virus of cats. It is possible that similar leukaemia viruses exist in the dog, but this is not yet known.

Because viruses grow in living cells, using the cells' own processes to multiply, it is difficult to treat virus infections. Drugs that interfere with virus growth also interfere with normal cell function, with serious effects on the animal. Treatment of virus infections is therefore aimed at combating the effects of disease until the animal's immune system can eliminate the infection. The fact that viruses grow only in living cells also explains why it can be difficult, and sometimes expensive, to confirm that a disease is caused by a particular virus; if the virus has to be isolated then this requires a specialist laboratory and quite expensive and sophisticated techniques.

Viruses vary widely in their ability to survive in the environment outside the body of an animal. Some, especially large enveloped viruses such as distemper, are readily destroyed by light or drying as well as by chemicals such as disinfectants. Others, especially small unenveloped viruses such as parvovirus, are extremely resistant, even to disinfectants, and can survive in the environment for many weeks or even months.

BACTERIA

Bacteria are much larger and more complex organisms than viruses. They are single-celled organisms, 0.1–1.0 microns (one million microns to the metre) in diameter and 1–10 microns long. They can be seen with ordinary microscopes and are usually spherical (cocci) or rod-shaped (bacilli) structures, though some are spiral. Bacteria usually have a rigid outer wall, which encloses not only the nucleic acids (bacteria have both DNA and RNA) that allow the bacteria to replicate but also other structures which permit the bacteria to produce energy and make new cell constituents from simple substances. This means that bacteria, unlike viruses, can grow and multiply outside other living cells provided they have a suitable source of energy. Most bacteria can be fairly easily grown in non-specialist laboratories.

Most bacteria are, in fact, free-living organisms, widely distributed in the environment. They are responsible for the decomposition and recycling of living tissues and are essential to the continuance of life as we know it. Most bacteria are totally harmless and, indeed, all normal animals have large populations of bacteria living on their skin and on internal surfaces such as the nose, mouth and intestines. These bacteria, the normal flora, live in harmony with their host and are often termed commensals. In animals such as the cow, the normal flora is actually essential to normal function of the intestines and in all animals the normal flora tends to resist the growth of more harmful, or pathogenic, bacteria.

Pathogenic bacteria are generally those which have developed the ability to survive and multiply within living tissues. Most gain entry to an animal's body by the mouth or nose, or through scratches or wounds on the skin, but a few use other routes such as the urinary or genital tract. Once within the animal, pathogenic bacteria may stay in one part of the body, causing a localised pneumonia in the lungs, for example. Some can spread to nearby tissues or even, via the blood, throughout the body, causing septicaemia.

Most bacteria cause disease by multiplying within and destroying the host's cells or by producing substances, known as toxins, which either kill host cells or interfere with their normal functions. Toxins may act locally at the site of bacterial growth but may also spread in the blood and have effects elsewhere in the animal. In tetanus, for example, the bacterium responsible, *Clostridium tetani*, grows locally at a wound, but the toxin which it produces spreads through the body causing widespread paralysis. A few bacteria cause disease by inducing very severe reactions by the animal's own immune system; probably the best example of this is tuberculosis. In rare instances, bacteria cause disease by growing and producing toxins outside an animal, which only becomes ill if it eats the preformed toxin – some forms of food poisoning act in this way, e.g., botulism caused by *Clostridium botulinum*.

It must also be remembered that normal bacterial flora can cause disease in animals which are immunosuppressed or if these bacteria are introduced into an area where they are not usually present, e.g., perforation of the intestine by a bone will cause severe peritonitis due to introduction of normal gut flora into the abdominal cavity. Normal bacterial flora may also invade tissues damaged by other infectious agents such as viruses or by other disease processes such as tumours.

Since the structure and, to some extent, the function of bacteria differs from that of animal cells, it is possible to treat almost all bacterial infections with chemicals, such as antibiotics, which kill or prevent the growth of bacteria. Antibiotics must not, however, be used indiscriminately. Some antibiotics, especially in high doses, have adverse effects on organs such as the kidney. Antibiotics are also likely to damage or disrupt the normal bacterial flora, which, especially in the intestine, can in itself cause illness. Bacteria can also become resistant to the effects of antibiotics, especially if they are improperly used.

Bacteria, like viruses, vary in their sensitivity to environmental conditions such as heat, light and drying. Many are relatively easily destroyed, but some, such as the mycobacteria, which cause tuberculosis, can survive in the environment for weeks or months. A number of bacteria, such as the Clostridia – including the cause of tetanus – form special structures called spores when conditions become difficult. The spores are very resistant and can survive for months or years until conditions improve. Most bacteria are sensitive to common disinfectants, but mycobacteria and spores are more resistant.

MYCOPLASMAS

Mycoplasmas are similar to bacteria but lack their outer rigid cell wall. They are very variable in shape, are very small (only up to 1 micron in diameter) and are difficult to identify under the microscope. Mycoplasmas are commonly found as part of the normal flora of respiratory and genital tracts. Pathogenic mycoplasmas have been described in a number of animals, but in the dog they appear to cause problems mainly as secondary invaders complicating other infections. Mycoplasmas are very sensitive to environmental conditions and to disinfectants. They are also sensitive to some antibiotics.

RICKETTSIAE AND CHLAMYDIA

Both rickettsiae and chlamydia are like very small (0.5 micron diameter) bacteria. They have a cell wall, but unlike bacteria can grow only inside animal cells, which makes them difficult to isolate. Almost all rickettsial diseases are transmitted by biting arthropod (insect) vectors such as ticks and lice. Reservoirs of infection may exist in wild animals such as small rodents. Rickettsial diseases in dogs are very uncommon in the British Isles, but do cause problems in America and parts of Europe.

Chlamydia cause important diseases in man and a number of animals (including birds – chlamydia are the cause of psittacosis, 'parrot disease', in both parrots and man) but have not been recognised as producing illness in dogs. Both rickettsiae and chlamydia are surprisingly resistant organisms, but infection with them will usually respond to treatment with appropriate antibiotics.

FUNGI AND ALGAE

These primitive plant-like organisms are found throughout the environment. Algae are free-living single-celled organisms often found in water. Only one type, Prototheca, is commonly associated with disease, and animals affected are often immunosuppressed by other disease problems. Most fungi are also totally harmless organisms which are essential parts of the normal recycling process of living tissues, especially of plants.

Fungi exist in two main forms, microscopic, oval or round, single-celled forms called yeasts and long branching tubes or hyphae, which form a tangled and usually visible mass known as a mycelium. The blue, green and white 'moulds' found on bread and cheese are common examples of mycelial fungi. Most fungi reproduce by forming large numbers of very small but highly resistant spores. These are carried in the air for long distances and are common surface contaminants.

The main way in which both yeasts and mycelial fungi cause disease is by actively invading and growing in animal tissues – such infections are called mycoses. The commonest and most important of these are the superficial skin infections commonly known as ringworm. Superficial infections of other body surfaces, such as the respiratory and genital tracts, also occur, but are less common. Subcutaneous mycoses, where fungi invade tissues under the skin, are infrequent, while systemic mycoses, where fungi spread throughout the body are rarer still.

Superficial mycoses do occur in otherwise healthy animals, but subcutaneous and systemic mycoses are much commoner in immunosuppressed individuals. Over-enthusiastic or inappropriate antibiotic treatment may predispose to fungal, and especially yeast, infections by killing off normal bacterial flora and allowing unchecked growth of otherwise harmless fungi. Most fungi are unaffected by common antibiotics and special antifungal drugs must be used to treat infections with these agents.

A few fungi cause disease by growing on food and producing poisonous substances called mycotoxins, which are then eaten by the animal. Animals can also develop allergies to fungi, especially to the small spores which are easily inhaled. Neither mycotoxins nor fungal allergies are common causes of disease in dogs.

THE PARASITES

Protozoa

Protozoa are single-celled members of the animal kingdom. Most are free-living and some are harmless commensals which live in the alimentary tract. Some of the few pathogenic (harmful) protozoa, e.g., the Coccidia, are also confined to the alimentary tract, where they grow in the intestinal lining and cause enteritis. Coccidia are simply transmitted between dogs by oocysts (eggs) shed in faeces.

Other pathogenic alimentary protozoa, e.g., the Sarcocysts, have a more complex life cycle. Oocysts passed by infected dogs are picked up by, and develop in, other animals such as sheep (the intermediate host). Other dogs then become infected by eating poorly cooked or raw meat from an intermediate host. Dogs actually act as an intermediate host for one alimentary protozoan parasite of cats, *Toxoplasma gondii*, and may become ill due to multiplication of intermediate forms of this parasite in body tissues.

The other important types of pathogenic protozoa, such as the Trypanosomes and Leishmanias, affect cells of the blood and lymphatic systems rather than the intestine and are transmitted by biting arthropods (insects). The arthropods can be either simple mechanical vectors or true intermediate hosts, with part of the protozoan life cycle taking place inside the vector. Luckily, these serious infections, some of which can affect man, are almost unknown in Britain except in imported dogs.

Alimentary protozoal infections can be treated with appropriate drugs, but control can be difficult as oocysts are very resistant. Control of insect-borne protozoa is also difficult, firstly, because it is almost impossible to control insect vectors and, secondly, because reservoirs of infection exist in wild animal populations. Treatment is possible, but is often difficult, and may not be undertaken because of potential risks to human health.

Helminths

Helminths or worms are well known to all dog owners. Two main groups infect dogs: nematodes or roundworms, which are long and cylindrical in shape, and cestodes or tapeworms, which have a small head and a long ribbon-like body made up of flattened packets or segments. A third type, trematodes or flukes, occasionally infect dogs in the tropics.

The best-known roundworms are those affecting the intestine, such as ascarids (the large white worms found in pups) and hookworms (found mainly in kennelled dogs). In small numbers these may have no effect on an infected dog, but in larger numbers they can cause disease by interfering with absorption of food, blocking the intestines or causing loss of blood. Other types of roundworms can infect other sites in the body, such as the lungs and the heart and blood vessels, but luckily many of these do not occur in Britain or are very rare.

Most roundworms (with the exception of the heartworms) have a direct life cycle, i.e., they are transmitted from dog to dog usually by eggs passed in faeces. Many nematode eggs are very resistant and can survive in the environment for many months or even years. Humans, especially children, who ingest dog ascarid eggs can contract a disease called visceral larval migrans.

Adult tapeworms are found in the intestines of infected dogs, where they cause little disease. Tapeworms, however, have an indirect life cycle in which eggs passed in dog faeces are picked up by and develop in other animals. The importance of the tapeworms comes from the fact that the developing intermediate forms of the tapeworms can cause serious disease, and even death, in the intermediate hosts, which can include man as well as cattle and sheep.

The common roundworm and tapeworm infections of the dog are easily eliminated by appropriate drugs. Although human disease due to these dog parasites is uncommon, it cannot be emphasised too strongly or too often that all responsible dog owners should ensure their animals are treated regularly for these infections to remove any possible risk to human health.

Arthropods

There are two main groups of arthropod parasites, the six-legged insects, which include fleas and lice as well as flies and mosquitoes, and the eight-legged arachnids, which include mites and ticks. The arthropods are almost all ectoparasites, that is they live on the outside of the affected animal, on the skin. Most are visible to the naked eye, except for mites, which are usually microscopic.

Most of the arthropod parasites cause direct skin irritation by biting the host or burrowing in the skin. Dogs can become allergic as a result of repeated bites and will then develop intense irritation following even a single bite. Many of the arthropods, such as fleas or ticks, remove small amounts of blood from their host, but only the sucking lice remove enough to cause anaemia. The other main way in which arthropods are responsible for disease is by acting as vectors or intermediate hosts for other infectious agents such as viruses, bacteria, rickettsia, protozoa and helminths.

Some of the arthropod parasites, such as the lice and some mites, are host specific, but others will bite any mammal that happens to be convenient, as anyone who has picked up a flea will know.

Control of infectious diseases

Control of infectious diseases in dogs is important for a variety of reasons. Firstly, the illnesses that they cause result in physical distress to affected animals (and emotional distress to their owners). Secondly, some diseases are a potential hazard to human health and their control is therefore essential. Thirdly, many of the diseases result in serious economic loss to dog breeders and kennel owners.

Details on control of specific diseases are dealt with in the chapters dealing with these conditions. However, there are a few general principles that apply to the control of any infectious disease and a grasp of these is invaluable irrespective of the disease and the number of animals at risk.

The keys to infectious disease control lie in the factors illustrated in Fig. 169, i.e., sources of infection and routes of transmission. Briefly, there must be, first, a source of infection, second, a susceptible animal and third, spread from one to the other by direct contact, by indirect contact or by vectors. Measures to modify all three of these factors can be used in disease control.

1. Control of sources of infection

It is impossible to control the presence of the sporadic infectious agents that are normally found in the environment or which are part of an animal's normal commensal flora. However, simple measures such as cleaning bites or cuts and scratches will considerably reduce the chances of problems from these organisms.

Control of contagious infections carried by other animals should be easier. Obviously, one should not buy a pup or dog that is showing signs of disease, but remember that asymptomatic carriers do occur. Asking, or seeing, whether other dogs on the premises are healthy is therefore another sensible precaution. If you have a large number of dogs, it is wise to quarantine new animals for 2–3 weeks to ensure they are not incubating any infectious diseases. Quarantine facilities are also useful for isolating animals that suddenly become ill. Precautions like these are clearly more difficult in kennels with a constant throughput of dogs, such as boarding kennels or in rescue kennels, where dogs from any source must be kept.

Remember that some infections, especially bacterial ones, such as Salmonella, can be introduced by contaminated food or water. Scrupulous hygiene in food preparation is as important when catering for our dogs as for ourselves, and a good supply of clean water is essential.

2. Control of susceptible animals – vaccination

For major infectious diseases, the most reliable and easiest method of control is to ensure, by vaccination, that dogs are resistant or immune to infection. It is important that all dogs are vaccinated against the life-threatening infections of distemper, parvovirus, infectious hepatitis and leptospirosis.

In theory, vaccination is very simple: a harmless form of the infection is inoculated into the animal, which mounts an immune response to it. That immune response protects the animal if it meets the real infection. The infectious agent can be made harmless by killing it (killed vaccines) or by growing it in unusual conditions so that it loses the ability to cause disease (live attenuated vaccines).

Live vaccines actually grow in vaccinated animals and may be excreted from them; they usually give a good immune response. Killed vaccines may need to be given more than once, or with a special enhancer called an adjuvant, to give a good response, since they cannot grow in the animal. The duration of immunity following vaccination may not be lifelong and regular boosters are usually needed.

Great care must be taken to ensure that live vaccines cannot grow sufficiently to cause disease and that any vaccine excreted is harmless. It is also important that only healthy animals are vaccinated, since ill animals will not respond properly. Live vaccines are not usually given to pregnant bitches; growing vaccine could cause problems in pups in the womb even if it were harmless in adults or pups after birth. Adverse reactions to both live and killed vaccines do happen in healthy animals, but are very rare;

they range from a lump at the site of injection to more serious allergic reactions with collapse.

Effective vaccines regularly produce immunity in adult animals (other than the very rare dog which cannot respond because of some form of immunosuppression), but vaccination of pups is rather more complicated. This is because of maternal antibody. The first milk or colostrum that pups get from their dams in the first few hours after birth is a very special substance. In addition to the normal constituents of milk, it contains substances called antibodies produced by the dam's immune system. These antibodies are absorbed by the pup in the first 24 hours of life and give it temporary protection against all the infectious agents to which the dam is immune. The level of protection which the pups receive mirrors the bitch's immunity – pups from a bitch with high immunity to parvovirus but low immunity to distemper will develop a higher level of maternal antibody against parvovirus than against distemper. Maternal antibody in the pups breaks down or decays at a steady rate – roughly, the amount halves every 8–9 days.

This passive protection is very important and pups which do not receive colostrum are much more likely to die from infections in the first few weeks of life. However, the passive protection provided by maternal antibody also interferes with response to vaccines and pups cannot be successfully vaccinated until maternal antibody has worn off. Obviously, the time it takes for this to happen depends on the amount of antibody which the pup absorbed and how much immunity the dam had. Some pups will have lost maternal antibody and be able to respond at 6 weeks, while in others vaccines will be blocked to twelve weeks or even later.

Vaccination is therefore rather more complicated in practice than in theory and should be under strict veterinary control. Suitable vaccination programmes, especially for pups, may vary widely depending on the vaccines being used, the age of animal and the risks of infection in a particular neighbourhood.

Passive protection can also be provided for adult animals by giving them antibodies in the form of injections of antisera produced from the blood of immune animals. Like maternal antibody, this passive protection is only temporary and wears off in a matter of weeks. It is useful in only a few circumstances – if, for example, a dog is going into an environment known to be infected with a particular organism but there is insufficient time for it to be vaccinated. Antisera can also be given to newborn pups to replace colostrum if the bitch is ill and has no milk.

3. Control of transmission of infection

Control of direct transmission is self-evident: animals with contagious diseases should be isolated from healthy non-immune dogs until they have recovered and stopped excreting the organism responsible or until the organism has been eliminated by treatment. Control of disease vectors is also relatively straightforward: mice, rats, flies and cockroaches are all obvious potential carriers of disease, but remember that arthropod parasites such as fleas and ticks can be vectors for other infections as well as causing their own problems. Indirect transmission, whether by aerosol, fomites or general environmental contamination, is more difficult to control.

Aerosol spread, so important in respiratory disease such as kennel cough, depends on the excretion of infectious particles into the air to be inhaled by other animals. Obviously, the more animals there are in a single airspace, the smaller that airspace is, and the more poorly ventilated it is, the more likely it will be that infectious particles coughed or sneezed out by one animal will be inhaled by another. Several small kennel units with separate airspaces and good ventilation are much less likely to have severe kennel cough than a single large kennel area with a common airspace and limited ventilation. Providing such suitable accommodation can be expensive.

Spread by fomites, i.e., inanimate objects, can be controlled by a combination of good management and elementary hygiene. The main difficulty lies in recognising the risks. The range of inanimate objects, particularly in a kennel, which can carry infection is enormous: food and water bowls, grooming equipment, wellington boots and overalls, brushes and shovels are among the obvious. Where possible, such objects should be kept to their own kennel or group of kennels, and they should be regularly cleaned and disinfected.

Good management and hygiene will also help reduce general environmental contamination. Kennels and concrete exercise runs can certainly be cleaned and disinfected, but this is not feasible for grassy areas. Environmental contamination is a particular problem of highly resistant organisms such as canine parvovirus and it would be a very brave person who would guarantee to eliminate such an infection from a house or a kennel by cleaning and disinfection.

It cannot be over-stressed that thorough cleaning with lots of soap, water and elbow grease is the most essential part of good hygiene. Also a good drainage system is needed to carry away contaminated water. Disinfectants should be used after, not instead of, thorough washing. If you have a particular infectious disease problem, check that the disinfectant you use is active against the agent responsible. Most disinfectants will kill a wide range of bacteria, but bacterial and fungal spores and some viruses are resistant to several – if in doubt, ask your vet. Whichever disinfectant you use must be used at the correct concentration – if is too dilute, it will not work!

As already mentioned, details on specific diseases and their control will be found elsewhere. However, the basics of contagious disease control can be summarised very simply: ensure your dogs are vaccinated against the major infectious diseases, be scrupulous about kennel hygiene, and be responsible – if your dogs have a contagious disease problem, do something about it and do not knowingly allow it to be passed on to other people's animals.

22
VIRAL AND BACTERIAL DISEASES

Diseases caused by viruses and bacteria cause illness and death in thousands of dogs every year. Although viral and bacterial diseases often occur independently, mixed infections are common, especially in the lungs and intestines. It is therefore useful to consider bacterial and viral diseases together and this chapter deals with them mainly from the point of view of the types of problems that they cause.

The killers – the major canine infectious diseases

Several infections (distemper, parvovirus, infectious hepatitis, and leptospirosis) regularly cause severe illness and death. Nowadays, effective vaccines should ensure they do not occur in individual animals, although their control in kennels is more difficult. Unfortunately, unvaccinated and stray dogs, especially in urban areas, are a constant reservoir for these infections. Rabies is the other major infectious disease of the dog. Vaccines against rabies are widely used in America and Europe, but, thankfully, this horrific disease does not occur in Britain or Ireland at this time. Vaccination against rabies is therefore not required in the British Isles, although strict quarantine of imported animals is necessary to prevent its introduction.

CANINE DISTEMPER

Distemper is one of the oldest and best-known dog diseases. Most cases occur in unvaccinated dogs in urban areas between 3 and 18 months of age (Fig. 171). Stray animals carry infection into surrounding suburban or rural areas and are a constant hazard for unvaccinated dogs or dogs whose immunity has waned. Local epidemics of distemper often occur in dogs in

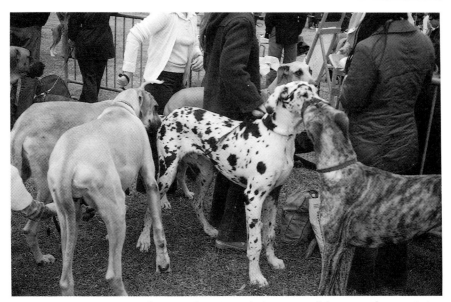

Figure 170 Direct contact between dogs is an obvious potential source of transmission of contagious diseases

rural areas if vaccination of local animals is allowed to lapse and an infected animal is brought in with holidaymakers. Distemper is also very common in rescue shelters because of the likely mix of unvaccinated animals and infected dogs.

Distemper is caused by a large RNA virus related to the human measles virus. The virus has a delicate outer envelope which is destroyed by heat and light. It cannot survive for long in the environment and infection is transmitted mainly by direct contact between animals or by aerosol spread over a short distance.

Development of disease

Dogs become infected by inhaling a virus which enters the bloodstream in the nose and throat and is carried to lymph nodes and other parts of the dog's immune system. Here, the virus starts to grow and a contest develops between the virus, which multiplies in and destroys the cells of the immune system, and the immune system, which tries to destroy and eliminate the virus. In many instances, the dog's immune system wins and the dog never shows signs of illness.

However, if the immune system loses, large amounts of virus are produced and spread to other parts of the body, including the lungs and nose, the stomach and intestines, the skin, and the brain and spinal cord. Further viral growth and cell destruction at these sites results in illness. Generally, it takes at least 2 weeks from initial infection for signs of respiratory and alimentary disease to become obvious, while nervous disease and skin problems are not usually seen until 3–4 weeks after infection.

In some dogs, the immune system stages a late recovery and only respiratory and alimentary tract signs occur. Dogs that develop nervous disease often die or have to be destroyed. Because the immune system is seriously damaged in distemper, secondary bacterial infections are very common and often make respiratory and alimentary disease worse. A small proportion of dogs which apparently recover from distemper, or are infected but show no obvious evidence of disease at the time, develop nervous signs many months or years later.

Clinical signs

The clinical signs of distemper are very variable. Probably over 50 per cent of infections are inapparent, while many others show only mild illness with decreased appetite, fever, slight discharge from the eyes or nose and a slight cough or mild diarrhoea. It is not usually possible to make a definite diagnosis in such cases.

More severe cases develop a more characteristic illness. At first, signs are similar to mild cases: a watery discharge from eyes and nose, slight fever, a mild cough and occasional vomiting. However, the oculo-nasal

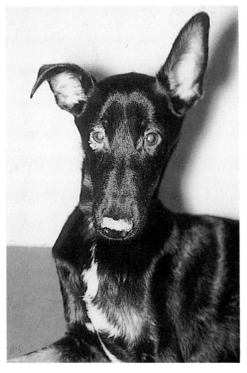

Figure 171 Canine distemper – this dog has a thick mucopurulent discharge encrusted round its eyes and nose

discharge becomes thick and purulent and the lining of the eye becomes reddened (Fig. 171). Fever persists, the cough becomes more severe and pneumonia may develop. Tonsils and lymph nodes are enlarged and the dog becomes depressed and unwilling to eat. Vomiting is very common and there is usually a light-coloured diarrhoea, occasionally with a few specks of blood. The dog often becomes dehydrated. These signs either worsen or start to improve over a period of 1–2 weeks and nervous signs and hyperkeratosis (hardpad) may then develop.

Many dogs with nervous signs due to distemper are restless and whine or whimper. The most serious sign is the development of 'fits'. In a mild fit, the dog twitches its eyes, champs its jaws and salivates slightly. In the most severe type of fit, a full epileptiform convulsion, the dog falls over, makes wild running movements with its legs, champs its jaws and salivates profusely; it may urinate and pass faeces. Recovery from such a fit takes some time and the most severely affected dogs will have repeated convulsions.

Dogs with 'nervous' distemper may also become paralysed – the hind limbs are usually affected and there may be loss of bladder and bowel control. Another nervous effect is the development of 'chorea' – a rhythmic twitch or spasm of a group of muscles (often on the head or legs). Chorea is usually permanent and animals which otherwise recover fully may be left with a lifelong twitch.

The classical skin lesion seen in distemper is hyperkeratosis or hardpad – the skin of the foot pads and nose becomes very thick and dry and may be cracked and painful (Fig. 172, overleaf). In addition, the skin is often generally scurfy and, especially in pups, flat, round pus-filled spots or pustules may develop on the skin of the groin or abdomen. Pups infected while their permanent teeth are developing will have brown pits visible in the white outer enamel of their adult teeth; this may be the only evidence they ever show of distemper infection. (See Chapter 29 Dentistry.)

Of dogs with enough clinical signs to make a definite diagnosis of distemper, about half will die or have to be destroyed, usually because of nervous disease. Recovery of those which survive may take two months or more. Infected animals may excrete virus for two months or more after infection, but fully recovered animals do not transmit the virus.

Treatment

No treatment will kill the virus in the body. Antibiotics are usually given to prevent or treat the bacterial infections that so often accompany distemper and other drugs may be needed to control vomiting, diarrhoea and fits. The most important part of treatment is good nursing to assist recovery. An affected dog should be kept clean, dry and comfortable. Many prefer dim lighting. The dog should be encouraged to drink small amounts of fluid frequently to prevent dehydration (intravenous fluids are

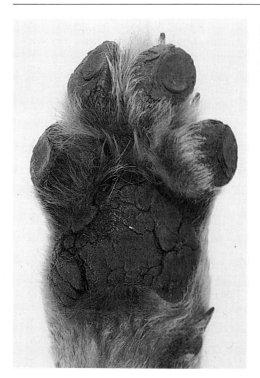

Figure 172 Canine distemper – the pads are very thickened and hard with deep cracks or fissures extending into the sensitive tissues

seldom necessary) and small amounts of light nourishing food should be offered. The eyes and nose should be cleaned regularly and a smear of Vaseline round these will help stop exudates drying into the skin. Creams may help to soften a dry, cracked nose or footpads.

Control

Safe, effective distemper vaccines have been available since the 1950s and all dogs should be vaccinated. In pups, vaccine may be given as early as 6 weeks of age, but, because of maternal antibody, a final vaccine must be given at 12 weeks or more to ensure that the pup responds. Pups should be isolated from possible infection until after this later vaccine has been given. The vaccination programmes used by different veterinary surgeons will vary depending on the age of a particular pup, its background and its chances of exposure to disease in a particular area. Booster vaccination may be required at intervals through life to ensure good immunity and no reputable boarding kennel or dog training club will admit animals which do not have a current vaccination certificate.

If distemper occurs in a kennel, sick dogs should be strictly quarantined – remember distemper is spread by direct and close aerosol contact. In-contact animals should be revaccinated. Ideally, when infected dogs are kept in the kennel, no new dogs should be admitted until a month after recovery of the last case. Kennels or kennel blocks which have housed infected dogs should be thoroughly cleaned, disinfected (all disinfectants will kill distemper virus) and left empty for a week. When infection occurs in a house, normal cleaning and heating at room temperature will kill distemper virus in a week, so a new dog can be acquired after 1–2 weeks.

PARVOVIRUS INFECTION

Canine parvovirus infection first appeared in 1978 and since then has been rivalled only by distemper as a cause of disease and death in dogs. Parvovirus arose from a mutation or change in a similar virus of cats, which allowed the new virus to grow and cause disease in dogs. Initially, all dogs were susceptible to parvovirus and the disease spread worldwide, causing massive epidemics between 1978 and 1980. Now the infection is endemic and disease is seen mainly in pups and young dogs that have lost their protective maternal antibody but have not yet been vaccinated. Disease occurs occasionally in isolated unvaccinated adults.

Parvovirus is a small DNA virus which is *extremely* resistant to environmental conditions and many disinfectants. It survives in faeces or faecally contaminated ground for many months and it is almost impossible to eliminate infection completely from a contaminated area. Indirect contact, by fomites – such as feeding bowls, brushes, etc., – or a contaminated environment, is the most important route of transmission, although direct spread also occurs.

Development of disease

Infection occurs by ingestion of the virus, which is taken up in the throat or intestine and carried in the blood to the lymphoid tissues of the animal. Parvovirus is such a small virus that it can *only* grow in those body cells which are themselves growing and multiplying. The lymphoid tissues contain such cells and large amounts of virus are produced in these organs. This virus is released into the blood about four days after infection and travels round the body looking for other suitable cells in which to grow.

In weaned pups and adult dogs, the most suitable cells are those at the bottom of the intestinal lining, which continually multiply to replace upper layers of the lining worn off in normal digestion. Growth of parvovirus in the multiplying cells destroys them and although the intestine can cope with the loss of some cells, a point is eventually reached where normal absorption of food and fluid can no longer occur and the animal develops enteritis and diarrhoea. Severe cases may have such severe intestinal destruction that bloody diarrhoea (dysentery) occurs. A good analogy is a pyramid of tins in a supermarket – a few tins may be removed without effect, but take out one too many and the whole pyramid collapses! Diarrhoea, which contains large amounts of virus, usually develops from

5–7 days after infection. By this time the dog's immune system is responding to infection and will eliminate virus from the body. If the damage to the intestinal lining is not too severe, or if the dog can be kept alive, the intestinal lining will eventually regenerate and the dog will make a full recovery.

A special situation occurs in pups that are infected in the first few days after birth. At this time, the intestinal lining cells are not multiplying fast enough to allow parvovirus to grow well in the intestine. However, cells in the heart are in their last phase of multiplication and infection in the few days around birth results in inflammation of the heart (myocarditis). Signs of heart damage do not usually become apparent until the pups become active at about 3–4 weeks of age.

Clinical signs

A typical case of parvovirus enteritis is a pup which is dull on the first day, vomiting on the second, has diarrhoea and becomes dehydrated on the third and is collapsed and dying with bloody diarrhoea or getting better by the fourth. However, there is wide variation in the severity and course of the disease. Many pups are only off colour for a few days, while others vomit occasionally or not at all or have only mild diarrhoea – foul-smelling bloody diarrhoea occurs only in severe cases. The course of the disease, especially in pups less than 10 weeks old, may be very short with pups going from being merely off colour to the point of death within 24 hours.

Figure 173 Canine parvovirus infection – both pups are very depressed and the small pup on the left is severely dehydrated. The skin of its back has stayed in a fold after being pulled up

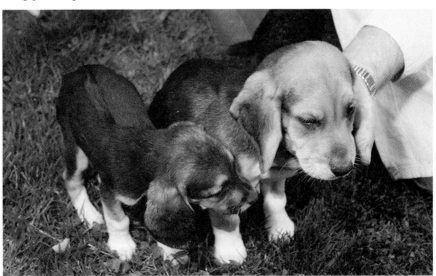

Pups of small breeds often become dehydrated and die rapidly with few other signs of illness. Dehydration is best seen as loss of elasticity of the skin – if the skin is pulled into a peak over the shoulders, it will take 1–2 seconds or more to flatten out (see Fig. 173). Signs in adult animals are similar.

The majority of animals infected with parvovirus show no evidence of disease. Only about 30 per cent of infected pups show any signs of illness and the *average* mortality in 8–10 week pups is about 10 per cent, although mortality in any particular litter may be 100 per cent. This means that infection (which can be carried into a kennel on boots or shoes) can be present in a kennel for some time without the owner being aware of the problem. The reason for this is that the severity of damage to the intestine, and therefore the severity of clinical disease, is directly related to the number of cells which are actively multiplying (and therefore able to be destroyed by virus) in the bottom layer of the intestinal lining.

In 'normal' pups, cell multiplication in the intestine is relatively low and so only a few cells are destroyed by virus – clinical disease is unlikely. However, several factors – other intestinal infections (e.g. worms), recent weaning, alterations in diet, and other forms of stress – increase the number of cells multiplying in the intestine and therefore the number of cells destroyed if the animal is infected by parvovirus. Pups in which such factors are present are much more likely to develop severe clinical signs (remember the tin can pyramid). It is not unusual, for example, for a pup to die of parvovirus enteritis within 7–10 days of sale, while pups still at the breeder's kennels, which have not been subjected to the stress of leaving home, are apparently normal. However, if blood samples from the 'normal' pups are checked they will have high antibody levels, showing that they have also been *infected*, though not *affected*.

The first indication of parvovirus myocarditis is the sudden death of previously fit healthy pups at about 3–4 weeks of age; pups may, quite literally, drop dead while playing or feeding. Pups which survive to 6–8 weeks may show more obvious signs of heart problems, such as failure to grow, difficulty in breathing or swelling of the abdomen. If myocarditis is confirmed in a pup then all the litter-mates are likely to be affected. Some may survive for many years, but others die of heart failure at several months of age and therefore none can be sold as normal animals. Weaned pups and adults with parvovirus *enteritis* do *not* develop heart problems.

Treatment

In mild cases of parvovirus enteritis, withholding solid food and giving frequent small amounts of fluid may be the only treatment needed. Remember that dogs, especially pups, can deteriorate very rapidly – it is much better to seek veterinary attention as early as possible. More severe cases may need special oral rehydration mixtures to counter the dehydrating effects of diarrhoea, while the most serious cases (those with continual vomiting, dogs with dysentery or those which are becoming severely dehydrated) will need intensive care with intravenous fluid drips. Antiemetics are often used to control vomiting and antibiotics are often given to prevent invasion of the damaged intestine by secondary bacterial infections or even normal bowel flora. Most animals recover quickly, but severe cases may be on a drip for several days while the intestinal lining regrows, and complete recovery may take a few weeks. A proportion of animals die despite the best intensive care. There is no effective treatment for parvovirus myocarditis.

Control

Effective vaccines based on the canine virus are available and all dogs should be vaccinated. As with distemper, vaccination may be begun at six weeks, but further vaccines will be needed because of the probability of interference by maternal antibody. Many bitches have high parvovirus antibody levels and maternal antibody can interfere with vaccination until 14–16 weeks or more. Once again, the vaccination programme recommended by a vet will vary, depending on the vaccine used and the chances of exposure to infection. Booster vaccinations for adults are recommended.

A particular problem exists in vaccinating pups on kennels where there is active parvovirus infection. Unfortunately, large amounts of 'wild' or virulent virus can 'break through' maternal antibody and cause disease several weeks before vaccine virus can protect pups. In such infected kennels, the obvious answer is to prevent, or reduce, the exposure of pups to virulent virus. However, since very large amounts of virus are produced by infected dogs (whether or not they show signs of disease), and the virus is very resistant, this can be very difficult to achieve.

First, scrupulous hygiene is essential to reduce the amount of environmental virus. Kennels must be thoroughly cleaned between use by each group of pups. Remember that parvovirus is resistant to many disinfectants (it is killed by 1:40–1:60 solutions of commercial – 11 per cent hypochlorite – bleach, by formalin fumigation and by a few commercial products which carry *specific* recommendations). Second, a vaccination programme should be formulated with your vet, using vaccines which have the best chance of breaking through maternal antibody, and, if necessary, taking blood samples for antibody analysis to determine the best time for vaccination.

The main reason why kennels stay heavily contaminated is that each new litter of pups, as it becomes infected, picks up a little virus but produces an enormous amount in its faeces. Only if this continual cycle of infection can be broken (by stopping breeding for a few months, by selling pups early before they become susceptible to infection or by finding temporary housing for pups away from the kennel) is it usually possible to clean up the kennel to a point where vaccination programmes are likely to succeed. Incidentally, infected dogs only excrete virus in their faeces for a short period of time (usually a few days and not more than 1–2 weeks). The main risk from recovered dogs (or any dog from an infected kennel) is virus carried on their coats – it is an excellent idea to bath them before introducing them to a clean environment.

When parvovirus occurs in a house, it is impractical to eliminate infection by disinfection before acquiring a new dog – there are too many nooks and crannies and valuable pieces of furniture. It is more sensible to ensure that the new dog is already immune to parvovirus. This can be done by buying an animal which has been vaccinated and shown to be immune by a blood test – most responsible dog breeders will arrange this if the problem is explained – none like the thought of their pups being infected with parvovirus after they have carefully reared them.

Parvovirus myocarditis is now, luckily, an *extremely* rare condition. Most bitches are immune and pass on enough maternal antibody to prevent infection of their pups in the first few days of life, which is the only time when infection will damage the heart. The only pups affected are those of unvaccinated non-immune bitches, which, for some reason, are taken into an infected area at whelping – e.g., an isolated bitch which comes into a kennel to whelp. The routine vaccination programme will prevent myocarditis.

Parvovirus infection, and even vaccination against it (particularly where attenuated live vaccines have been used), has sometimes been blamed for infertility or subfertility in both dogs and bitches and even for neonatal deaths in pups. Careful investigations have failed to reveal any evidence that either parvovirus infection or parvovirus vaccination causes either reproductive problems in the dog or neonatal puppy deaths. Unfortunately, the cause of both these syndromes is often unknown and parvovirus has often been unjustly blamed simply because the real cause has not been identified.

INFECTIOUS CANINE HEPATITIS – CANINE ADENOVIRUS TYPE 1 INFECTION

There are two canine adenoviruses (CAV), CAV-1 AND CAV-2. Both contribute to the respiratory disease known as kennel cough and this is dealt with later. However, CAV-1 also causes the serious liver disease known as Infectious Canine Hepatitis (ICH) or Rubarth's disease. This is much less common than parvovirus or distemper, but still results in death in a significant number of usually young or adolescent unvaccinated dogs.

CAV-1 is a medium-sized DNA virus which is more resistant than distemper but much less so than parvovirus. It is transmitted mainly by contact with contaminated urine.

Development of disease

Infection occurs by ingestion of virus which enters the tonsils and spreads to other lymphoid tissues in the body. After multiplying there for a few days, virus spreads in the bloodstream to the liver, where it grows in and destroys liver cells, resulting in liver inflammation or hepatitis. The spreading virus also damages the lining of small blood vessels throughout the body, resulting in many small haemorrhages. Severely affected dogs may die at this stage (about 7–8 days after infection).

In less severe cases, the dog's immune system then eliminates virus from most parts of the body (10 days after infection) and the dog recovers. Virus does, however, continue to grow in the kidney and is excreted in urine for 6–9 months. Immune reactions in the eyes of recovering dogs may result in opacity or cloudiness of the cornea (the front of the eye) about two weeks after infection; this 'blue-eye' is usually temporary.

Clinical signs

Dogs with ICH are acutely ill with a high fever (up to 106°F), and swollen tonsils and lymph nodes. Liver swelling causes severe anterior abdominal

Figure 174   Canine adenovirus infection (infectious canine hepatitis) – this pup developed 'blue-eye' (clouding or oedema of the cornea) as it recovered from infection. The opacity of the front of the eye resolved spontaneously over a week or so

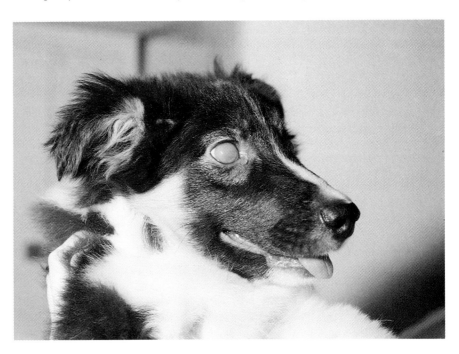

pain. Dogs are restless or may lie groaning with pain, especially if touched over the ribs. They are usually thirsty, vomit frequently and pass a scanty blood-tinged diarrhoea. Breathing is often fast and shallow and the pulse is usually rapid. The linings (mucosae) of the mouth and eyes are often pale due to shock, and small haemorrhages (petechiae) may be seen on the mucosae or the thin skin of the abdomen. Jaundice (a yellow colour) develops in some cases and the occurrence of 'blue-eye' often heralds recovery, since it indicates a good immune response (Fig. 174).

In the most severe cases, collapse and death occurs so fast (within 24 hours) that poisoning is sometimes suspected. In very mild cases, a sudden 'blue-eye' may be the only indication of infection. Most infections are probably inapparent but the majority of dogs which develop diagnosable signs of ICH will die.

Treatment

Only supportive treatment is possible. Intensive care with intravenous fluids is often needed to combat the serious liver disturbances, collapse and shock which kill the dog. Even with the best care, many die. Recovering cases need careful nursing. Steroids are often used in animals with 'blue-eye' but most resolve spontaneously.

Control

Vaccines against ICH are highly effective and are usually given (with distemper and parvovirus) as part of the standard puppy vaccination course. The usual maternal antibody problems apply. Booster vaccinations are given at intervals to adult dogs. Vaccines prepared from both CAV-1 and CAV-2 protect against ICH because the viruses are very closely related. Live attenuated CAV-1 vaccines can cause 'blue-eye' in a small proportion of dogs and most live vaccines these days are CAV-2 types which do not have this effect. Inactivated vaccines do not cause 'blue-eye'.

If infection occurs in a kennel, the accommodation which housed affected dogs must be cleaned and disinfected (ICH is resistant to quaternary ammonium disinfectants like Savlon or Roccal but is killed by most others). In addition, remember that recovered dogs excrete virus in urine for up to 9 months. Special care must be taken to prevent contact between such animals (and their urine) and new pups until 1–2 weeks after successful vaccination.

LEPTOSPIROSIS

Of the many different bacteria of the Leptospira group, two commonly cause disease in dogs. *Leptospira icterohaemorrhagiae* is mainly an infection of rats, but it can affect dogs as well as man and other animals. *Leptospira canicola*, in contrast, is mainly a dog infection, but it can also spread to other animals, including man. Both infections are relatively uncommon, but they are important because they regularly kill affected dogs and can cause serious human disease.

The Leptospirae are quite sensitive bacteria and are destroyed by sunlight, drying and virtually all disinfectants; they survive best in moist conditions. The main source of infection is the urine of infected animals. *L. canicola* infection occurs mainly in urban areas where there is a reservoir in unvaccinated dogs, but *L. icterohaemorrhagiae* occurs in any town or country area where there is contact with rats.

Development of disease

Infection with Leptospirae usually follows ingestion of bacteria in urine or urine-contaminated material. The bacteria penetrate the lining of the mouth and enter the blood. Bacteria can also enter the blood through cuts or grazes on the feet if a dog walks in infected urine. The Leptospirae start to multiply and spread through the body.

With *L. icterohaemorrhagiae*, multiplying bacteria destroy cells in the liver and damage small blood vessels throughout the body. The dog may die at this stage (about 7 days after infection), but if it survives slightly longer, liver and blood vessel damage become obvious as jaundice (icterus) and widespread haemorrhage (hence 'icterohaemorrhagiae'). There is often inflammation in muscle, brain and kidneys. In dogs that recover, a developing immune response eliminates infection from most of the body by 10–12 days after infection, but small numbers of bacteria survive in kidneys for many months and are excreted in urine.

With *L. canicola*, damage to liver and blood vessels during the multiplication stage is less marked and jaundice and haemorrhages are unusual. Once again, the dog's immune response eliminates the Leptospirae from most of the body by 10–12 days after infection, but large numbers can remain in the kidney. Cells of the immune system invade the kidneys to destroy the bacteria and so many cells may invade that normal kidney function is destroyed and the dog dies of kidney failure. In less severe cases, the bacteria are destroyed and the dog recovers, but some Leptospirae usually remain to be passed with urine for several months.

Clinical signs

In dogs with *L. icterohaemorrhagiae* infection, the first signs are usually dullness, loss of appetite and fever. The most severe cases collapse and die rapidly without showing more distinct signs. Less severe cases usually start to vomit (this may contain blood), have a scanty black diarrhoea, become jaundiced and develop haemorrhagic patches on the skin and in the linings of the mouth and eyes. Liver swelling causes severe abdominal pain and the dog may moan in distress. It usually resents being handled and is very stiff and sore. Severe dehydration and shock are likely to result in death.

With *L. canicola*, there is also often a phase of dullness, loss of appetite and fever while the bacteria are multiplying in the blood. This may disappear, only for the dog to develop signs of kidney failure a week or two later. Dullness, loss of appetite, thirst and vomiting are common. In the most severe cases, no urine at all is passed, but milder cases may produce more than normal. The back is often arched because of pain in the kidneys. As kidney failure develops, the dog vomits more often, develops ulcers in the mouth and an ammoniacal smell to the breath, becomes dehydrated and collapses.

Treatment

There are two parts to treatment of Leptospiral infections: antibiotics to kill off the bacteria and supportive therapy to counter the effects of liver or kidney failure. Antibiotics given when the dog is first dull and fevered usually prevent the development of more serious signs. Acute liver and kidney failure usually need intensive care and hospitalisation. Even with dogs which make a fast recovery, it is essential to complete the antibiotic course as prescribed so that infection is totally and speedily eliminated from the kidneys and urine. Remember that Leptospirosis is a serious and sometimes fatal disease in man – great care and scrupulous hygiene is needed when handling actual or suspected cases.

Control

Vaccines against both types of Leptospirae are usually included as part of the standard puppy vaccination programme. These are killed inactivated vaccines and two doses are required to give immunity. Interference by maternal antibody is uncommon since antibody levels in bitches are usually very low. Regular revaccination throughout life is recomended.

Many countries require that imported dogs are free from evidence of leptospiral infection (as measured by antibody in the blood). Recent vaccination may interfere with this test, so it is essential to check with your vet (and the country to which a dog is going) before having dogs due for export vaccinated.

If *L. icterohaemorrhagiae* occurs in a kennel, then there is almost certainly a problem with rats, either in the dog accommodation or a food store, and this needs urgent attention.

RABIES

Rabies is, arguably, the most horrendous disease to afflict man or animals. All warm-blooded animals can be affected and the disease is almost always transmitted by the bite of an infected animal. The danger of a bite from a 'mad' dog was known as long ago as the 23rd century BC. Rabies occurs worldwide with the exception of the continents of Australia and Antarctica. Most countries are affected, with the exception of a few that are islands or almost islands such as Britain, Ireland, Japan, Norway and Sweden or the Iberian Peninsula. In Europe and North America, reservoirs of infection usually exist in wildlife (e.g., the fox); infection spreads from wildlife into domestic animals such as dogs and cats and from them to man. In parts of Asia, Africa and Latin America, the main reservoir is not wildlife but free-living or stray dogs and infection of man is more common.

Rabies is caused by a rhabdovirus – a large enveloped bullet-shaped DNA virus. It is very sensitive to heat, light, detergents (including ordinary soaps) and disinfectants and cannot survive for long outside the body of an infected animal.

Development of disease

Rabies is almost always acquired from the bite of a rabid animal, since the virus, which is present in saliva, cannot penetrate intact skin (a lick from a rabid animal on a cut or graze could also be infective). The virus multiplies in muscle at the site of the wound and then spreads, not in blood, but along nerve fibres into the spinal cord and brain. Growth in the brain and cord cause severe nervous disease and death. The incubation period (from the initial bite to signs of disease) varies from 10 days to 6 months. Virus also spreads *from* the brain along other nerves to organs including the salivary glands – large amounts of virus are produced and excreted in saliva.

The rare exception to infection by bites is found (mainly in America) in caves containing many rabid bats. In these confined, dark, damp places, virus secreted as an aerosol of saliva can survive long enough to be inhaled by, and infect, men or animals entering the cave.

Clinical signs

The first sign of rabies is usually a change in behaviour – friendly dogs become shy and nervous, reserved animals become affectionate. The dog may chew or scratch at the site of the original wound. The next stage is usually 'furious rabies', in which the dog is hyperirritable and aggressive and wanders aimlessly, attacking anything, real or imagined, in its path. It may eat unusual objects or show bizarre sexual behaviour. The voice is often altered (high pitched or hysterical) and the eyes have a glazed expression. The lower jaw often hangs partly open and drips saliva. 'Furious' cases may progress to 'dumb' or 'paralytic rabies', where the dog stands almost stupefied, is less actively aggressive, and becomes increasingly paralysed. The drooping jaw, salivation and glazed expression are usually marked.

Some dogs never show true 'furious' signs and some cases are less typical than others, but, ultimately (within 10–14 days of first being ill), *all* infected animals collapse, become comatose and die.

Treatment

There is no treatment for dogs with rabies. Even in man, with the best of intensive care, the disease can be regarded as invariably fatal.

Control

Most human deaths from rabies still follow dog bites, even when the main reservoir of infection is wildlife, so that control of infection in dogs is essential. In rabies-infected areas, dogs with signs of the disease are killed and the diagnosis confirmed by laboratory examination. Unvaccinated dogs bitten by a rabid animal are often also destroyed, while vaccinated dogs are isolated and observed for several months to ensure they do not develop the disease. Apparently normal dogs (vaccinated or not) which bite people are quarantined for 10–21 days to see whether they develop signs of rabies.

In rabies-infected developed countries, there is usually a strict (often compulsory) dog vaccination programme: an initial inoculation is given at three months of age and boosters are required every 1–3 years. Restrictions on the movement of dogs outside their owner's property and strict muzzling and leashing requirements may also be enforced.

The most essential step if bitten by a potentially rabid animal is to wash the wound *vigorously* with soap and water – remember rabies virus is very sensitive to detergents. Depending on circumstances, a series of inoculations of antisera and vaccines may then be given, but, undoubtedly, the bitten person faces an agonising six months' wait before being sure that he or she has not contracted the disease.

Rabies was eliminated from Britain in 1903 by strict quarantine, muzzling of pets and destruction of strays – wildlife rabies did not occur. Britain has since remained rabies free with the exception of an outbreak after the First World War (caused by soldiers smuggling in pets) and two cases (in 1969 and 1970) which occurred in dogs newly released from quarantine (regulations for quarantine kennels were strengthened). The pain, distress and expense of rabies should convince all British dog owners that strict quarantine regulations are essential for vaccinated as well as unvaccinated dogs – rabies does sometimes occur in vaccinated animals. The rise of the urban fox means that if rabies were introduced into Britain today, infection of wildlife would be a distinct possibility. So if you suspect that an animal has been smuggled into the country, report it to the police!

Editor's note: I am delighted that the author has put the case for continuing quarantine regulations so strongly. Rabies is one of the worst diseases known to man. Many countries (developed and undeveloped) have to live with this risk and we can only extend our sympathy to them. In the UK we are at present rabies free and it is in everyone's interest, especially that of dog owners, that we remain so.

Infectious enteritis

Infectious enteritis is a general term used for episodes of diarrhoea which are clearly transmissible between dogs. Obviously, infectious enteritis is commonest in kennels, but individual dogs can pick up infection indirectly (from faecal contamination of the local common, for example) or, occasionally, from food. Dogs of any age can be affected, but infectious enteritis is more common and usually more severe in pups. Parvovirus is the most likely cause of severe infectious enteritis, but a number of other agents (Table 22) cause similar, though usually less severe, disease. Mixed infections also occur.

Coronavirus infection is widespread, but generally causes only mild enteritis with slight diarrhoea – severe diarrhoea, dehydration and death are very unusual. Other viruses (rotavirus, astrovirus, calcivirus) have been found in canine diarrhoea, but do not appear to be important (except possibly for rotavirus in very young pups up to one week old). The Salmonellae and Campylobacter bacteria are particularly important because they have the potential to cause disease in people as well as dogs. Campylobacter infection in dogs is usually mild or inapparent, but Salmonellae can cause severe diarrhoea. Infection with Salmonella in young pups can often cause death due to spread of infection through the body (septicaemia) rather than simple diarrhoea. Other bacteria probably also give rise to infectious enteritis, but their importance is not really known.

Parasites are often overlooked in infectious enteritis. Intestinal coccidia (often considered harmless) do appear to contribute to diarrhoea problems in pups in particular kennels. Two other protozoa, Giardia and Cryptosporidia, have also been found in some dogs with infectious enteritis – these do not appear to cause serious illness but should be borne in mind as they can also infect man. These and helminth infections (such as roundworms and hookworms) are dealt with elsewhere.

All these organisms are spread mainly by direct contact (hence their occurrence in kennels) or by indirect contact via faecal contamination. Salmonellae and Campylobacter can also be introduced by contaminated or poorly prepared food.

Development of disease

All these infections are taken in by mouth and pass through the stomach to the intestines, where they invade cells at the top of the intestinal lining,

Table 22   Agents involved in canine infectious enteritis

VIRAL	PARASITIC
Canine coronavirus	Coccidia species
Canine rotavirus	Giardia?
(Other viruses?)	Cryptosporidia?
	Roundworms?
BACTERIAL	Hookworms?
Salmonella species	
Campylobacter species	
(other bacteria?)	

unlike parvovirus which attacks the bottom layer of cells of the intestinal lining. Cell destruction and associated inflammation interfere with absorption of food and fluid, resulting in diarrhoea, usually within 2–3 days of infection. Luckily, the multiplying cells at the *bottom* of the lining are unaffected and replace the cells lost from the top in a few days so that normal function is restored and diarrhoea stops. Many infections are asymptomatic. Coronavirus is excreted in faeces for 10–14 days, while the various bacteria can be excreted for several weeks. Immunity to these superficial intestinal infections is relatively short-lived.

Clinical signs

Diarrhoea is the main (often the only) sign of illness with faeces which vary in consistency from soft and pasty to profuse and watery. Severely affected dogs may lose their appetite, vomit, be fevered or have spots of blood in faeces. Very severe cases develop bloody diarrhoea or become severely dehydrated with sunken eyes and an inelastic coat.

Most cases are self-limiting and difficult, if not impossible, to differentiate, especially in individual dogs, from non-infectious diarrhoea, such as dietary upset. Even if spread through a kennel makes an infectious cause obvious, it is almost impossible to be sure which agent, or mixture of agents, is responsible without laboratory tests.

Treatment

Treatment is symptomatic – most cases respond well to 24–48 hours without solid food but with ready access to small amounts of fluid. Urgent veterinary attention must be sought for any animals, but especially pups, which vomit repeatedly or show signs of dehydration or bloody diarrhoea. These will require more intensive fluid therapy, possibly with intravenous drips. Antibiotics are often unnecessary and should only be used on veterinary advice – remember they can upset normal intestinal flora and exacerbate or prolong diarrhoea. If coccidia or other parasites are identified as a problem, then appropriate antiprotozoals or anthelminthics will be needed.

Control

Control of infectious enteritis depends largely on good hygiene and kennel management to prevent the introduction and spread of infection. Vaccines against the various agents known to be involved have not been developed and, since there are so many possible causes and immunity is short-lived, are probably not feasible. In kennels, control measures against canine parvovirus (thorough cleaning and disinfection, batching of groups of dogs) will also control the agents mentioned above, since none of them are as resistant as canine parvovirus. Special care must be taken not to introduce Salmonella or Campylobacter infections in food.

Remember that several of the organisms that cause infectious enteritis in dogs do cause diarrhoea in man. In the home, diarrhoeic pups or dogs should, ideally, be confined to an easily cleaned and disinfected area. Anyone handling or nursing diarrhoeic animals must be very strict about personal hygiene and young children should not be allowed to play with, or handle, sick dogs.

Kennel cough

Kennel cough, like infectious enteritis, is not a single specific disease but a general term given to a group of clinical signs which can be caused by any one, or indeed a mixture, of several different infections. Kennel cough, as the name implies, is characterised by coughing and commonest in dogs which are in, or have recently been in, kennels. However, it is also transmitted anywhere where dogs are gathered together (shows, training clubs, race meetings), and small local outbreaks often follow the return of an infected animal from its 'holidays' in a boarding kennel.

The infections associated with kennel cough are shown in Table 23. The most important agents are thought to be the bacterium *Bordetella bronchiseptica* and canine parainfluenzavirus. Both canine adenoviruses (CAV-1 and CAV-2) can cause kennel cough, but, luckily, vaccination against infectious canine hepatitis (also caused by CAV-1) also protects against respiratory infection with the adenoviruses. Herpesvirus and reovirus infections are uncommon and usually inapparent, while mycoplasmas appear to complicate other infections rather than cause disease on their own. The infectious agents responsible are spread by direct contact or by aerosol transmission – most of the agents are fairly sensitive to environmental conditions and disinfectants.

Development of disease

The infectious agents are inhaled and multiply in (with viruses) or on (with *Bordetella*) the cells lining the nose and airways to the lungs. These tissues become inflamed and usually, within 4–5 days, sneezing and coughing

Table 23 Agents involved in kennel cough

IMPORTANT
    Bordetella bronchiseptica
    Canine parainfluenzavirus

LESS IMPORTANT
    Canine adenovirus (type 1)
    Canine adenovirus (type 2)
    Canine herpesvirus
    Reovirus
    Mycoplasma

results. In severe cases, infection may spread into the lung itself with resulting pneumonia. Recovery, even in severe cases, is usually complete within 2–3 weeks and many infections are inapparent. Viruses are usually only excreted for 10-14 days after infection, but *Bordetella* can remain in the respiratory tract of infected dogs for up to 12 weeks after infection – long after clinical recovery. Immunity to these infections is relatively short-lived.

Clinical signs

The classical clinical sign is a harsh cough which may be dry and irritating or moist and productive. The cough may last for only a few days or for three weeks or more. Coughing is often brought on by excitement or exercise and severely affected dogs have bouts of coughing which end in the dog gagging or retching – a dog which has recently fed may vomit and the retching may be so severe that the dog sounds as if something is stuck in its throat.

Sneezing is common in the early stages, sometimes with a watery nasal discharge which may become thick and mucoid. Most dogs with kennel cough are otherwise bright with clear eyes and a good appetite. A small proportion (usually pups, elderly dogs or dogs with chronic disease problems) develop pneumonia with laboured breathing, fever and loss of appetite. Spread to very young pups may result in severe pneumonia and death. A few dogs with kennel cough never really clear up, but develop a chronic bronchitis.

Treatment

Most cases of kennel cough resolve spontaneously with no need for treatment. Antibiotics are usually only required in severe cases or where there is a risk of pneumonia or spread of infection to other animals. Good management is important to avoid undue excitement and exercise which would precipitate severe coughing spasms – dogs which pull on their collars may be better in a shoulder harness. In dogs with a productive cough, a moist atmosphere will often help loosen and expel mucus from the airways and antitussives (cough medicines) similar to those used in man may help ease an irritating cough.

Control

It is as difficult to control kennel cough in dogs as it is to control the common cold in man. Responsible dog owners should not knowingly take animals with kennel cough to shows – kennel cough may be merely a nuisance in adult dogs but it can be fatal if carried home to young pups. Probably the most important factor in control in kennels is good design and management. Small airy kennel blocks with separate air spaces and good ventilation are much less likely to have problems than long kennel ranges with a common airspace and stuffy or no ventilation. Where possible, kennels should be allocated on a rota basis so that new arrivals are not placed next to dogs which have been in for some time and may be infected. If an outbreak does occur, then the affected kennel block should be emptied, thoroughly cleaned and disinfected (most disinfectants would be suitable) and left empty for 1–2 weeks before admitting new animals.

Vaccines against both *Bordetella* and parainfluenzavirus are available, although immunity to respiratory infections is difficult to induce and of relatively short duration. The most suitable kennel cough vaccine would be a combined *Bordetella* – parainfluenzavirus product. This could be given a few weeks before kennelling so that dogs would have the maximum immunity against the two most important agents at the time of greatest risk. Unfortunately, although there is a single *Bordetella* vaccine (given by instillation directly into the nose) the parainfluenzavirus vaccines available in Britain are produced only in combination with vaccines against distemper and the other killer diseases. It is hoped that more suitable vaccine combinations will become available, but, even so, it is unlikely that kennel cough will be eliminated.

Neonatal infections

As many as 20 per cent of pups which are born alive die in the first fortnight of life, most in the first week. The majority die from non-infectious causes such as hypothermia, starvation, trauma or congenital defects, but some deaths, probably around one-fifth of the total, are due to infections.

Viruses, though often thought to cause death in newborn pups, are very uncommon at this age. The major exception, canine herpesvirus, is dealt with below. Rotavirus has also been reported as causing diarrhoea in pups in the first week of life, but distemper, adenovirus and parvovirus infections are all *extremely* unusual. Bacterial infections are more common, since pups are born into an environment full of bacteria, which, though often harmless in adults, are capable of invading the tissues of newborn animals to cause localised infections or septicaemia. A number of bacteria (e.g., Salmonellae, Leptospirae) and viruses, e.g., Distemper, herpesvirus) can, in theory, cross the placenta and infect pups in the womb. In practice, certainly in Britain, it is uncommon to isolate infectious agents from pups which are born dead or aborted. The main specific cause of canine abortion, *Brucella canis* infection, is dealt with in Chapter 11, page 187.

Canine herpesvirus infection

Canine herpesvirus is a large enveloped DNA virus which causes mild or inapparent respiratory disease in adult dogs – it is one of the less important causes of kennel cough. Occasionally, it also causes small pock-like lesions on the vagina and penis of adult bitches and dogs. Herpesvirus grows best at 37°C and only very poorly at 39°C, so in adult dogs which have a deep body temperature of 39°C, virus growth occurs only at cool superficial sites such as the upper respiratory or external genital tracts. However, the deep body temperature in pups in the first 1–2 weeks of life is only just over 37°C and drops rapidly with chilling, since neonate pups cannot maintain temperature; so in pups infected at this early age, especially if chilled, herpesvirus spreads throughout the body causing widespread tissue destruction and death.

Neonatal septicaemia

Many bacteria are able to invade newborn pups and cause localised problems such as enteritis and pneumonia or more generalised infection (septicaemia). Bacteria commonly isolated from such infections include types of *Streptococci*, *Staphylococci* and *Escherichia coli*, which are relatively harmless in adults, as well as more generally recognised pathogens such as *Salmonella* and *Leptospira* and more uncommon organisms such as *Bacillus piliformis* and *Yersinia*. Bacteria invade through the mouth or nose or through the navel (umbilicus) or abrasions on the skin.

Two main factors combine to make newborn pups particularly susceptible to such infections. First, pups are, to all intents, bacteriologically sterile at birth and only acquire their normal bacterial flora from their dam and the environment in the first few days of life – in these few days, potentially harmful bacteria can multiply freely without competition from the normal flora, which usually help resist such infections. Second, newborn pups have extremely poor resistance to *any* harmful organisms until they have suckled and absorbed the special first milk or colostrum produced by their dam in the 24 hours after birth – remember colostrum contains antibodies which provide temporary protection for the pups until they can develop their own resistance. The risk of bacterial infections is increased, obviously, if the environment is not clean.

Clinical signs

Pups with neonatal infections show similar signs whatever the cause. Weight loss, or failure to gain weight, is often the earliest sign. The pup then stops suckling, cries restlessly and becomes dehydrated. Breathing is often laboured, and, as the pup deteriorates, it stops crying and becomes noticeably cold. Legs may paddle weakly or the body may become rigid with the head thrown back. Breathing may seem to stop for minutes at a time before the pup finally dies. More specific signs are occasionally seen – diarrhoea, navel discharge, abdominal swelling. Small raised red or black sores under the chin and on the backs of the feet are often present in pups with Staphylococcal dermatitis and septicaemia.

Pups which become ill and die in the first week of life are often termed 'fading pups'. Many such pups do *not* have infections but a non-infectious problem, such as immaturity, hypothermia or starvation, which produces identical signs. Post-mortem examination and laboratory tests by your vet are usually needed to determine if infection is involved and, if so, which one.

Treatment

Early detection and good nursing are essential if sick pups are to have any chance of recovery. Pups must be kept dry and warm (environmental temperature of 90°F) and will probably need to be hand fed with bitch milk substitute or glucose and water (5–10 per cent glucose solution). If they are very dehydrated, your vet may adminster subcutaneous fluids. Pups which cannot suck can be fed by stomach tube, but this needs skill to avoid damaging the gullet or stomach and you should ask your vet's advice. Gentle massage of the anogenital region with warm wet cotton wool is needed to stimulate the pups to pass urine and faeces. Antibiotics are usually given by injection or by mouth. Unfortunately, even with prompt and intensive treatment, the majority of neonatal pups which become ill will die.

Control

A number of general measures will reduce the likelihood of neonatal infections. First, and most obvious, the whelping area should be as clean as possible. Second, pups should be encouraged to suckle as soon as possible after birth – the more colostrum they get and the sooner they get it, the better. Do not artificially feed the first pups born to help the bitch – the pups need the bitch's *colostrum*, not simply a milk substitute. Third, ensure pups are kept warm – remember newborn pups cannot maintain their body temperature and can die from simple hypothermia as well as being more at risk from herpesvirus if chilled. Heat lamps must be used with care as too much heat will make the pups, and especially the bitch, uncomfortable. Draughts are particularly likely to cause chilling and are not always obvious – cold air will fall into open-topped whelping boxes placed beneath even a closed window. Fourth, avoid direct or indirect contact between the bitch and pups and other dogs which may be carrying even minor infections – for example, kennel cough in a boarding kennel is a nuisance, but if it spreads into a whelping area it will kill baby pups. Finally, ensure that the umbilical cord and any cuts (e.g., from dewclaw removal) are clean, and that rough flooring does not cause abrasions on the pups' skin.

More specific measures can be used in particular circumstances. Where pups do not receive colostrum (e.g., if the bitch has no milk) your vet can give injections of hyperimmune serum which will have a similar effect. When herpesvirus is a problem, temperature control is particularly important, although it is unusual for a bitch to lose more than one litter from herpes. Where neonatal septicaemia is diagnosed, your vet may arrange appropriate antibiotic treatment of the bitch in the few days around whelping and for the pups in the first few days of life.

Other viral infections

The most important and common viral infections of the dog are dealt with above. It is possible, even likely, that others will be discovered. Two other viruses that occasionally cause disease in dogs are dealt with here.

AUJESZKY'S DISEASE

Aujeszky's Disease, or pseudorabies, is a rare infection of dogs caused by a herpesvirus (Aujeszky's Disease Virus) of which the pig is the natural host. In pigs, infection causes a wide range of clinical signs from inapparent infection to respiratory, reproductive and nervous disorders, but in the dog infection is invariably fatal owing to nervous disease. Infection of man probably does not occur. Aujeszky's Disease Virus is unrelated to the canine herpesvirus which causes deaths in neonatal pups.

Dogs are infected with Aujeszky's Disease by close contact with infected pigs or by eating infected raw pig meat or offal. Dog-to-dog transmission does not occur. The virus passes from the alimentary tract along nerves to the brain, where inflammation causes nervous disease. There may be a change in behaviour, diarrhoea, hypersalivation or difficulty in breathing, but the most typical clinical sign is severe pruritus or itching. The head is most usually affected and the dog rubs or scratches at the area so much that there is severe swelling or even ulceration and tearing of the skin and underlying tissues. Scratching becomes increasingly frantic and, as the dog deteriorates, it becomes ataxic and paralysed. Convulsions usually occur before an inevitable coma and death. The incubation period varies from

1–6 days, but actual illness is very short – most dogs die within 1–2 days. There is no treatment, but infection can be prevented by avoiding contact with infected pigs and ensuring that any pig meat, and especially offal, fed to dogs is thoroughly cooked.

VIRAL PAPILLOMATOSIS

Papillomaviruses are a group of DNA viruses which cause epithelial proliferation and the development of papillomas or warts. There are probably at least two dog papillomaviruses, one causing warts in the mouth and conjunctiva, and the other producing skin warts. Those on the skin are usually solitary or few in number and cause problems only if they occur at a site, such as the feet, where they become damaged and secondarily infected. Oral warts are usually more trouble because they are easily traumatised by teeth or food and can develop in large numbers – 50 or more. Oral papillomas start off as smooth, white, seed-like lumps, 1–2 mm across. They are usually found on the lips, tongue or roof of the mouth. They enlarge rapidly over a few weeks to cauliflower-like masses up to 0.1–1.0 cm in size. Damage and infection result in bleeding and severe halitosis.

Most viral papillomas disappear spontaneously over a few weeks or months. If trauma or infection causes discomfort, especially in the oral form, the warts can be removed surgically or by freezing or burning them off. In very severe cases, your vet may consider chemotherapy or even having a special vaccine prepared from the warts to be given to the affected dog. It is unusual to have more than one dog affected and, although there may be spread between dogs, there is no risk to man.

Other bacterial infections

Several bacteria which are normally considered part of the normal flora do occasionally cause non-specific inflammation in various parts of the body; examples include *E. coli*, *Staphylococci*, and *Streptococci* in the lower urinary tract or on the skin. These infections are dealt with elsewhere. However, a few other bacteria do cause quite specific syndromes in the dog and these are now considered.

BRUCELLOSIS

Canine brucellosis, caused by the bacterium *Brucella canis*, results in infertility with abortion in bitches and testicular degeneration in male dogs. Brucellosis is well recognised in America (especially the southern United States and Central and South America) and parts of Europe, but has not been identified as a problem in the United Kingdom. Infection occurs by venereal transmission at mating or by exposure to the many bacteria present in vaginal discharges of aborting bitches.

Bacteria can persist in the blood of infected animals for up to three years, but settle out mainly in the reproductive tracts. Severe illness is uncommon (there may be lymph node enlargement) and the main effects are on reproductive performance. Pregnant bitches usually abort, often about two weeks before expected whelping. Abortions in bitches can be difficult to spot, especially if they occur early in pregnancy, because the bitch normally eats aborted material – a vaginal discharge may be the only clue. Very early in pregnancy, embryos may be resorbed rather than aborted. Less commonly, an infected bitch will carry to term but produce pups which are born dead or are weak and die within a few days. In the male dog, either swelling or atrophy of the testes can occur; licking at the scrotum may cause a dermatitis. The sperm produced are abnormal and fertility is reduced although libido is not. Infected semen is a major source of infection for bitches.

Treatment of canine brucellosis is difficult because *Brucella canis*, unlike most bacteria, lives *inside* cells and can survive there for many months, even in treated dogs. Elimination of disease from a kennel requires careful blood testing and removal of infected animals. Vaccines have not been effective. *Brucella canis* can infect man to give a chronic flu-like illness. Canine brucellosis does not yet appear to be a problem in Britain, so breeders importing new stock from abroad should enquire whether the disease occurs in the area where they are buying. If necessary, blood tests can be carried out to reduce the risk of importing infected animals.

ACTINOMYCOSIS AND NOCARDIOSIS

Actinomyces and Nocardia are long, branching bacteria. Actinomyces are found in the mouths of normal animals while Nocardia are common in soil. Infection with either most often follows penetrating wounds and two main syndromes are seen: first, subcutaneous infections with localised abscesses or more diffuse cellulitis; second, and more seriously, infection of internal body cavities. Infection of body cavities (the thorax or chest is more commonly affected than the abdomen) results in severe inflammation with massive accumulation of thick purulent blood-stained fluid. Fluid in the thorax causes difficulty in breathing and collapse on exercise; dogs are dull, fevered and off food. Especially where Nocardia is responsible, there may be spread of infection to other parts of the body, such as the bones, liver or lungs.

Both infections are uncommon but seem rather more frequent in rural areas. Usually only one dog is affected, but, occasionally a small cluster of cases occurs over a short period in kennels of hounds or gundogs. Although the thick blood-stained fluid is easily recognisable by your vet, only isolation of the bacteria will show whether Actinomyces or Nocardia is responsible. This can be important, since they usually respond to different antibiotics. Treatment can be difficult, even with laboratory guidance on a choice of antibiotic. Subcutaneous infections may need surgical drainage and drainage is usually essentially for cases with thoracic or abdominal fluid accumulation. Treatment may take several weeks or months – Actinomyces infections respond better than Nocardia.

MYCOBACTERIAL INFECTIONS

Mycobacteria are very resistant organisms. Some are highly pathogenic and cause severe disease, particularly tuberculosis, in man and animals; others, the atypical mycobacteria, are normally present in the environment and rarely cause illness.

Tuberculosis, caused by *Mycobacterium tuberculosis* (mainly in man) and *Mycobacterium bovis* (mainly in cattle), is still an important disease in many parts of the world. Even in Britain, where bovine tuberculosis has largely been eliminated and the incidence in man is much reduced, human tuberculosis still exists, usually in deprived areas or within certain ethnic minorities. Dogs can suffer from tuberculosis, but, in developed countries, infection of the dog is almost always caused by spread from an infected person – an excellent example of a zoonosis in reverse. The rare dog with human tuberculosis usually develops chronic respiratory disease with coughing, weight loss and persistent fever similar to the disease in man. The even rarer cow tuberculosis occurs where dogs are fed on unpasteurised milk from infected cows; vomiting, diarrhoea and weight loss are more likely than respiratory disease. If tuberculosis is diagnosed in a dog, treatment is seldom undertaken because of the risk to human health. The public health authorities will usually screen people associated with the dog to try to trace the source of the infection.

Infection with atypical mycobacteria present in the environment is uncommon and usually follows introduction of infection via a penetrating wound. Growth of the bacteria in subcutaenous tissues results in a discrete, tumour-like swelling. Infection is usually localised, but there can be spread to other organs, especially if the animal is immunosuppressed. Treatment of localised lesions is usually by surgical excision – many are only diagnosed when, as suspected tumours, they are sent for pathological examination. If the infection recurs or there is spread to other organs, antibiotics can be used, but laboratory investigation to determine the most appropriate antibiotic may be necessary.

TETANUS

Tetanus is an uncommon disease of dogs caused by the bacterium *Clostridium tetani*. Spores of this bacterium are present in the soil and in the faeces of many animals. Disease occurs when the spores contaminate wounds, especially deep, penetrating injuries which provide conditions favourable for bacterial growth. As the bacteria multiply, they produce a powerful toxin which has special affinity for nerves and spreads along them through the rest of the nervous system. Tetanus toxin interferes with the transmission of normal nerve impulses, especially those controlling muscle activity, such that the muscles of affected animals go into spasm and become stiff and rigid. Clinical signs develop up to a week or more after the original wound.

Dogs are quite resistant to the effects of tetanus toxin and stiffness can be localised to the area near the original wound, but in severe cases the whole body becomes affected. Dogs with generalised tetanus have a stiff, stilted gait and a 'rocking-horse' stance. The tail is outstretched and spasms of the head muscles give erect ears and a wrinkled forehead. The lips may be drawn back into a grimace (the original sardonic grin) and there may be lockjaw. Light or noise may provoke generalised muscle spasms with the head stretched over the back. Paralysis of breathing causes death.

Treatment of severe tetanus is difficult, time-consuming and expensive, needing extreme intensive care to maintain breathing and other normal functions. Various drugs and antitoxin are given to control spasms and counteract the toxin. Complete recovery may take over a month. Early cases are more easily treated with antibiotics and antitoxin. Prevention is achieved by thorough cleaning of wounds and, especially with deep wounds, antibiotics to prevent bacterial growth.

BOTULISM

Botulism is a very uncommon disease. It is caused by the bacterium *Clostridium botulinum*, which, like tetanus, is widespread in the environment in the form of spores. Contamination of foodstuffs leads, under suitable conditions, to bacterial multiplication and the formation of the most powerful biological toxins known to man. Disease is caused by the animal eating material which contains the *preformed* toxin. The toxin is absorbed from the stomach and intestines and acts by blocking the ability of nerves to stimulate muscles. This results, within a few days, in flaccid paralysis (the opposite of the rigidity seen in tetanus). There is progressive weakness and paralysis with the hindlimbs usually affected first. Ultimately, there is total muscle paralysis and death is caused by interference with breathing. The severity of disease is directly related to the amount of toxin ingested.

Treatment is limited to supportive care to maintain vital functions. Antitoxin may 'mop up' free toxin but does not reverse the effects on nerves which have already been attacked – these gradually recover spontaneously. Antibiotics have no effect on the toxin, but are often given to prevent any complicating secondary infections. Good nursing is essential to keep the paralysed dog comfortable – pain can still be felt although the animal cannot respond to it. Most cases of canine botulism have followed access to carrion or feeding of raw contaminated meat. Botulism can be prevented by stopping dogs scavenging and by thorough cooking of food to destroy the heat-sensitive toxin.

23

ENDOPARASITES IN THE DOG

Amongst the many endoparasites infecting the dog are the roundworms *Toxocara canis* and *Toxascaris leonina*, the tapeworm *Dipylidium caninum* and the protozoan *Toxoplasma gondii*. They are ubiquitous parasites, common to all breeds, and can occur in domestic, working, racing and hunting dogs. Other endoparasites occurring in dogs in Britain are associated with special circumstances in which the dog may feed on raw meat containing the intermediate stage of development of the parasite.

The remaining parasites are associated with imported dogs. The mandatory six months quarantine period imposed on all dogs entering the United Kingdom is applicable to the control of rabies, and although useful in preventing many 'foreign' endoparasites from gaining a foothold in this country it is not sufficient in itself to ensure freedom from all endoparasitic infection, as these parasites may remain in the host beyond the six-month period.

It is intended to discuss the development and significance of our common indigenous endoparasites together with their public health importance where applicable and to refer to some of the endoparasites found in other countries and explain how our temperate climate and environmental differences help to prevent them becoming established in the United Kingdom.

Life cycles of the parasites discussed have been briefly outlined both in the case of roundworms (nematodes) and tapeworms (cestodes) and microscopic organisms called protozoa in order that the veterinary advice often given regarding control becomes more meaningful.

Helminths

Helminths are the phylum (great subdivision) of worms, which include a certain number of parasitic forms found in dogs. It includes the roundworms (nematodes), tapeworms (cestodes) and flukes (trematodes). All worms that are parasitic in the dog spend part of their life cycle in the host and part outside, either in the environment or inside another host, referred to as the intermediate host. This can be a flea, a mosquito, a fish or another mammal, etc. In other words there is a wide range.

NEMATODES (roundworms)

The commonest roundworms found in the dog are *Toxocara canis* and *Toxascaris leonina*.

Toxocara canis and *Toxascaris leonina* are large nematodes which measure from 3–8 in (7–18 cm) as adults. They consist of both males and females and they inhabit the small intestine of the host. In heavily infected puppies, immature worms as well as adults may be vomited or passed through the anus, but normally only microscopic eggs are passed in the faeces, so that you normally do not see the worms in the stools.

Signs in the puppy

Puppies up to 12 days old may show noisy breathing accompanied by nasal discharge, especially when suckling. There is often also retarded growth.

Puppies of 2 weeks of age may show vomiting, abdominal discomfort, particularly after suckling, diarrhoea and lack of growth.

Puppies 6–12 weeks old may show chronic diarrhoea, vomiting, distended abdomen and a characteristic vocal cry rather like a cross between a whimper and a shriek. They may adopt a straddle position of the hindlegs because of the big abdomen. Sometimes not only light but moderately heavy infection may show no clinical signs.

Toxocara canis

While appreciating the fact that puppies can suffer from the effects of *Toxocara canis* it is important to realise that humans can also become infected by ingesting the infective eggs and occasional medical conditions can arise which are of public health importance. This is particularly important with children.

Life cycles

The life cycle of *Toxocara canis* is complicated, since there are a number of alternative migratory routes for the developing worm in the dog.

The fertilised eggs shed from the female worm pass down the intestinal tract and are passed out with the dog's faeces. These eggs require a period of time on the ground in order to become infective. This period can vary from a few weeks in summer to several months in winter. When an infective egg is eaten by a susceptible dog and reaches the small intestine, a larva then hatches. This larva can undergo one of two forms of

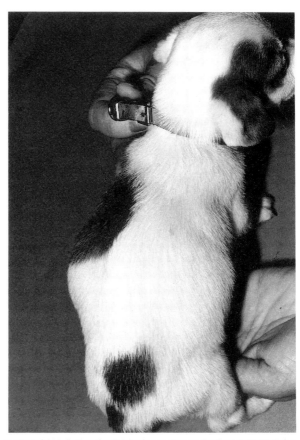

Figure 175 (Right)
Puppies of six–twelve
weeks old with
roundworms may have a
distended abdomen and
adopt a characteristic,
straggle-legged position of
the hind legs

Figure 176 (Below)
Roundworms may be
vomited by affected
puppies

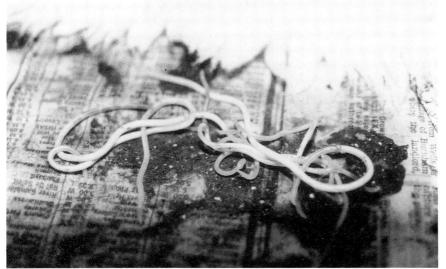

migration. In older dogs larvae do not mature to adults as a general rule but enter the bloodstream, where they are carried to various tissues in which they can become encysted. In puppies, particularly those under the age of one month, the larvae go into the bloodstream and migrate via the liver and the lungs, where they will leave the bloodstream and migrate to the air passages, from where they will finally be coughed up from the trachea or windpipe. They are then swallowed and finally end up in the small intestine, where they mature to produce male and female worms, which in turn mate and result in the production of fertile eggs.

The main method of infection in puppies occurs while they are still in the womb. The bitch, either during or before pregnancy, may acquire infection, in which case the larvae will become encysted in the tissues. When a bitch becomes pregnant some of the larvae in the tissues become active on about the 42nd day of pregnancy. They cross the placenta to reach the foetal pup, so that the pup is born already infected. This activation of larvae may be due to the influence of hormones. During lactation the bitch may shed larvae in the colostrum or fore-milk and also in the milk proper – this is another source of infection for the suckling puppy, which, when infected by this means, may start shedding eggs in its faeces as early as the third week of life with maximum numbers occurring after a further 3–5 weeks. To complicate matters further the bitch may also have intestinal forms of the worms re-established during the period around whelping, which recent work has shown can be associated with a partial suppression of immunity which occurs at this time. Thus she may also be shedding infected eggs and contaminating the environment. Some larvae may fail to remain in the puppy's intestine and are carried out in the faeces to be picked up by the bitch while cleaning her puppies, and these can mature in the bitch and produce even more eggs.

Roundworm infections are complicated!

Other sources of infection

If this were not complicated enough there are also certain other hosts that can result in sources of infection. Hosts other than the dog are referred to as *paratenic hosts*. These animals may eat infected eggs, in which case the larvae will hatch and enter the bloodstream and become encysted in various tissues, just as they will in an adult dog. Paratenic hosts include mice, rats, rabbits, chickens, sheep, pigs or man. If a dog eats an infected mouse or rat then the larvae in the tissues will be released and develop to become adult worms capable of producing eggs which pass on to the ground.

A broad understanding of these complicated life cycles is important for several reasons. Puppies infected in the uterus and during the suckling period are the source of the greatest contamination to the environment. Eggs appear in the faeces from the third week and increase in numbers for a further 3–5 weeks. The bitch may also be shedding microscopic eggs and be a source of contamination of the environment during this period.

A lesser source of contamination may be the adult dogs, which may have eaten an infected rodent containing encysted infective larvae, which are released by the digestive juices of the dog and develop into adult worms. The female worm will soon be shedding *Toxocara canis* eggs.

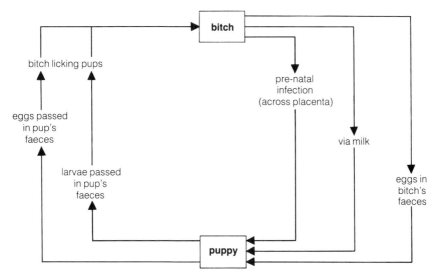

Figure 177   Toxocara canis – the relationship between bitch and puppy

Public health

If the infective eggs of *Toxocara canis* are ingested by man then the larvae will invade the tissues and become encysted in various organs – humans act like any other paratenic host. If a large number of infective eggs are ingested, then clinical disease may become evident. This is particularly important where children are concerned. Soil in some areas, for example public parks, can become heavily contaminated with *Toxocara canis* eggs and toddlers do have a habit of eating earth. In extreme cases the infective larvae can cause fever or affect the liver. A rare occurrence, but one that has received much publicity, is the case of larvae reaching the retina of the eye and thus causing impairment of vision or even the loss of the eye.

Control

The objects of control are to prevent any illness or ill effects in the puppy, to stop the area becoming contaminated and thus cut down the risk of spread of infection and, associated with this, to reduce any associated public health risk.

The methods of control are hygiene and treatment with suitable drugs called anthelmintics, which eradicate the worms. As the main source of infection is the bitch, ideally an anthelmintic to remove the larvae in the tissues would be an ideal method of control. Such an anthelmintic is available, but it is expensive and has to be given daily for a fairly protracted period and is therefore not at present widely used. This leaves us with anthelmintics which are effective against the worms established in the small intestine. These can be used with bitches as well as the puppies. Veterinary advice should be sought on when and at what intervals to dose, particularly in the case of the puppies. Ideally pups should commence being dosed from about two weeks of age up to weaning and beyond at frequent intervals. Children should be kept away from areas where the dogs defaecate as the elimination of eggs in and on the soil is almost impossible to achieve. The worm eggs are very resistant to environmental variations and strong chemicals, being almost indestructible. The removal and safe disposal of faeces, however, will reduce the risk of *Toxocara canis* infection.

Toxascaris leonina – life cycle

In this case the life cycle is comparatively simple as there is no migration of larvae to the tissues. Larvae are not found in the milk as in the case of *Toxocara canis*. Infection takes place only via two routes, either by the host eating infected eggs or through eating a paratenic host in which the larvae have developed.

Control

This tends to be concentrated on the 6–12 month-old dog. As development takes place in the stomach and lumen of the digestive tract, control is not difficult. The strategic use of an efficient anthelmintic should be sufficient to eliminate the worms present.

Piperazine is a cheap and effective anthelmintic that is available without prescription from both pharmacies and pet shops, but if you are in any doubt at all consult your veterinary surgeon regarding control.

CESTODES (tapeworms)

Dipylidium caninum

This is the most common tapeworm of the dog. All the cestodes found in the dog require a main host, the dog, and a second or intermediate host. The tapeworm consists of a head attached to the wall of the small intestine. From this head grows a series of greyish-white segments which are shed singly or in short chains at irregular intervals. They pass along the alimentary tract, finally being passed out through the anus.

Life cycle

When the tapeworm segments reach the outside they can sometimes be seen attached around the anus or on the tail, looking like small rice grains. Eventually they drop to the ground and break up, shedding the eggs which have formed inside the segment. If the dog has fleas or lice, these eggs may be picked up by either the larvae of the flea or the adult louse. Once inside the larval stage of the flea the egg then develops to become infective inside the adult stage of the flea. During natural grooming or biting to allay the irritation caused by the flea, the dog can ingest the flea and become infected with the tapeworm.

In heavy infestations the dog may show signs of anal irritation. This can be one of the causes of 'scooting' or dragging the bottom along the ground, although there are of course other causes of this condition, such as impacted anal sacs. Again, with heavy infestations the dog may appear thin and poor, but usually the tapeworm does not cause too many problems in the dog – it is mainly the appearance of these mobile segments crawling around the anus, that causes the owner to consult the veterinary surgeon regarding treatment.

Control

This consists of giving the dog a suitable anthelmintic and the elimination of the flea or louse intermediate host by the use of a parasiticide both on the animal and also in the environment, since fleas, unlike lice, will live and develop away from the host animal.

Figure 178   Dipylidium caninum

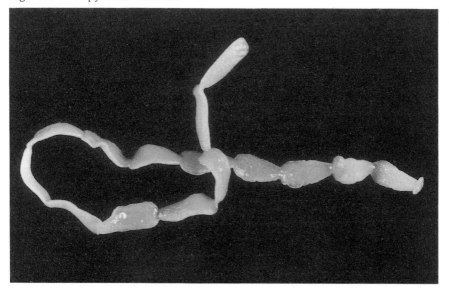

Public health

On rare occasions it is possible for a child to ingest a flea containing the intermediate stage of this parasite and become infected with the mature tapeworm, but this is unusual.

Protozoa

The phylum, or great subdivision protozoa, includes a great variety of organisms whose bodies usually consist of a single cell.

A suitable example is the microscopic *Amoeba proteus*, which we all learn about at school.

Most protozoa are harmless, free-living organisms and many that live in the intestinal tracts of higher animals are only associated with disease under certain circumstances. Nevertheless, some forms are the cause of distinct disease both in man and animals. Amongst these are the coccidias, malarias and blood sporozoans (haemosporidias), the organisms referred to as haemoflagellates, which are the cause of 'sleeping sickness' in man (trypanosomiasis and leishmaniasis). Although more commonly found in warmer climates, protozoan parasites are found in the dog in the UK. These include *Toxoplasma gondii*, *Sarcocystis*, *Coccidia* spp. and *Giardia* spp. The other protozoans will be referred to in connection with imported dogs which have introduced parasites from tropical or subtropical countries.

Toxoplasma gondii

This is a coccidian parasite of the cat from which the oocysts or protozoan eggs are passed in the faeces. The life cycle of a coccidium is complicated because development takes place within the hosts' cells as well as in the environment.

Toxoplasma gondii, when it becomes infective in the cat, completes its life cycle in the epithelium of the small intestine and sheds oocysts in the faeces for about two weeks. After this period oocysts are no longer shed and the cat becomes refractory to further infection, but after a time this immunity may become less. One of the ways in which a dog can become infected is by eating a cat's faeces which contain the developed, infected oocysts. When taken in by mouth these tend after a time to encyst in various tissues such as the liver, lung, muscles and brain.

The cysts of *Toxoplasma gondii* are sometimes found during the post-mortem examinations of the brains of dogs which in life have shown so-called 'distemper syndromes'.

There are three ways in which the dog can become infected:

1. By ingesting infective oocysts from the faeces of a cat as previously mentioned.

2. By eating undercooked meat or the carcase of an already infected prey in which the encysted forms are present, e.g., rat, mouse, rabbit, etc.
3. A bitch infected with *Toxoplasma gondii* can pass the parasite on to the puppies during pregnancy, since the organism can be transmitted across the placenta.

In all these cases the dog is acting as an intermediate host. The cat is the only final host in which a sexual cycle can take place in the intestine and so shed oocysts.

Public health

Humans may become infected with toxoplasmosis either by eating the infective stage of the oocysts or by eating undercooked or raw meat containing the cyst forms. The dog, as an intermediate host, is unlikely to pass oocysts in the faeces and therefore the risk of *Toxoplasma gondii* being transferred from canine sources to man is remote. However, there is the risk that a person can become infected by taking in infected oocysts from the faeces of an infected cat which is the final host. In the case of a pregnant woman who becomes infected, transplacental infection of the baby can occur. The amount of malformation and damage caused will depend on the virulence of the strain of the organism and the time of the infection during pregnancy. Probably hundreds of thousands of cases of human toxoplasmosis go unrecognised, since mild illness characterised by a slight fever, and slight enlargement of the lymph nodes are the only signs.

Control

The control of toxoplasmosis is not easy because the final host, the cat, can stray and shed oocysts over a wide area. Thus toxoplasmosis can infect sheep and cause abortion in this host, as well as infecting dogs, man and wild animals. The preventive measures consist of scrupulous hygiene. Removal of cat faeces from the litter tray by someone other than a pregnant woman is sensible. All meat should be adequately cooked, and drugs should be administered only under veterinary supervision.

Endoparasites found in kennels and working dogs

HELMINTHS

Hookworm (*Uncinaria stenocephala*)

This is the 'temperate climate' hookworm and it measures less than 12 mm (⅜ in.) long. Adult worms are found in the small intestine of the dog and produce eggs which are passed out with the faeces. These microscopic eggs hatch larvae whilst on the ground. Although some of these larvae may affect the feet and cause a pedal dermatitis, the majority are taken in by mouth and may cause diarrhoea as well as loss of condition. These hookworms do not cause the anaemia seen with infections of the tropical hookworm *Ancylostoma caninum*.

Uncinaria stenocephala is found most commonly in Greyhounds, dogs hunting in packs (e.g., Foxhounds, Harriers and Beagles) and sheepdogs. It can be prevalent in fact wherever dogs are exercised on grass.

Control

The replacement of grass runs with concrete and regular dosing with a suitable anthelmintic.

Whipworm (*Trichuris vulpis*)

The 'whipworm' is so called because the adult worms found in the caecum have the appearance of a stockwhip and measure up to 7 cm (3 in.) in length. The microscopic egg is very slow to develop to the infective stage, which contains a larva. In the United Kingdom they can be prevalent in hot summers, when grass runs are used as exercising areas. Under these conditions the eggs can survive for up to 5 years. Not all infected dogs show clinical signs, but in some cases intermittent diarrhoea is present. This is again a condition seen in dogs exercised mainly in confined areas of grass.

Control

This is very difficult and requires the replacement of the grass runs with concrete areas. Veterinary advice is required on the use of anthelmintics.

Filaroides osleri

This is a worm which is found in the lungs of the dog. It is located at the bifurcation of the trachea (windpipe) and along the bronchi. The worms are found curled up in nodules which can be seen on bronchoscopic examination of the anaesthetised dog. They produce microscopic larvae which are coughed up and swallowed, passing out with the faeces. Infection is mainly associated with dogs bred in kennels. Transmission is thought to be from bitch to pups during cleansing, when the larvae are transferred in the sputum. Clinical signs are not always present, but a dog showing the presence of a persistent dry cough should receive veterinary examination.

Control

Anthelmintics are available for the eradication of this worm, but veterinary advice must of course be sought.

CESTODES

Although *Dipylidium* species do occur in kennel and working dogs, other cestodes are also important.

Taenia species

These are tapeworms that the dog acquires when eating prey or offal containing the infective cystic stage. All the *Taenia* species are large tapeworms with distinctive segments which collectively can grow up to 1 metre (36 in.) in length. There are two species that the dog can obtain by eating the cystic stage in the rabbit, hare and also some rodents. The cysts themselves are located either in the peritoneum (lining of the abdomen) or between the muscles of the intermediate host (rabbit or hare). These animals become infected in the first place by either eating segments containing eggs or the eggs themselves, which have become dispersed on the ground due to the disintegration of the ripe (or gravid) segment, which has been passed from the anus of a dog.

Other *Taenia* species infecting the dog are acquired from carcases of sheep or being fed infected uncooked meat from a slaughterhouse. The cystic stages are situated in the brain, the offal or muscle of the intermediate host sheep.

The effect of these tapeworms in the dog does not appear to be of great clinical significance other than that they may occasionally cause anal irritation. The main effect is the aesthetic and undesirable sign of moving segments seen in the surroundings. The condition is seen mostly in country dogs, hounds and sheepdogs.

Control

This is a matter of hygiene and meat inspection and the prevention of dogs getting access to infected carcases. Very efficient anthelmintics are available.

Echinococcus species

These are very small tapeworms that consist of only three or four segments and are less than 1 cm (³⁄₈ in.) in length. There are two strains of *Echinococcus*. One forms cysts in the livers of sheep when they ingest eggs from ripe (gravid) segments shed by an infected dog. The other strain similarly forms cysts in the liver of the horse. The cyst is referred to as an hydatid cyst and the condition is hydatidosis.

A single cyst can grow up to 10 cm (4 in.) in diameter. The sheep form of hydatid cyst is mostly picked up by farm and sheepdogs as well as the fox. The horse form is mostly associated with foxhounds that have been fed raw horse meat or offal.

Public health – hydatidosis in man

Man can become infected by ingesting eggs that have originated from the faeces of dogs or foxes harbouring the adult tapeworm.

Although investigations have been carried out with the horse strain there seems to be little evidence that man becomes infected with this strain. The reported cases are all associated with the sheep strain. Hydatidosis in the UK is most prevalent where there is an association with dogs and extensively grazed sheep, particularly in Wales. The prevalence of hydatidosis in humans in Britain is therefore mostly confined to hill and mountainous sheep grazing areas where dogs and foxes scavenge on dead carcases.

In other parts of the world the disease is of much greater significance. Certain countries (see below) have successfully eradicated the problem.

Control

National control schemes have been introduced with considerable success in New Zealand, Iceland, Cyprus and Uruguay. The method of control consists of registration of certain categories of dogs, regular treatment with an effective anthelmintic, educating the dog-owning public of the risks and legislation to ensure that untreated offal is not fed to dogs. In this way the risk to man has been greatly reduced if not completely eliminated.

PROTOZOA

Coccidia species

When young puppies kept in breeding kennels have diarrhoea, in certain cases they may be considered to be suffering from '*coccidiosis*,' and this is occasionally a veterinary diagnosis. The reason for this is that oocysts of a certain genus of *coccidia* which develop in the small intestine of the host are found to be present in very large numbers when faecal droppings are examined under the microscope. However, as mentioned previously (page 390), many protozoa multiply in conditions of diarrhoea. The condition usually clears up spontaneously or with the help of certain so-called coccidiocidal or coccidiostatic drugs which your veterinary surgeon will prescribe.

Sarcocystis

Sarcocystis is the genus of parasitic protozoa, very similar to coccidia. *Sarcocystis* spp. form cysts in the muscles of various intermediate hosts. The dog is the final host and if it consumes the flesh of cattle, sheep, goat or swine which has cysts in the muscles, it becomes infected. The digestive juices of the dog release the immature forms called bradyzoites, which invade the wall of the small intestine but do not migrate to the muscles in the dog. Instead the parasite develops in the wall of the small intestine to produce so-called sporocysts, which pass out with the faeces, and when ingested by other non-canine hosts the cycle is completed. Any clinical effects in the dog are usually transient and may involve diarrhoea. The public health aspect is not considered sufficiently important to document.

Giardia species

Infection with this microscopic flagelleted pear-shaped protozoan is known as giardiasis. The parasite can be found in the small intestine of the dog. Passed in the faeces it forms a cyst on the ground which can be ingested by other hosts, including many other species of animal as well as man. It is known that *Giardia* can produce a severe type of enteritis in chinchillas. How much significance it has in cases of diarrhoea and dysentery in dogs and humans is at present unclear, although there is a lot of investigative work presently under way.

Public health

There is some evidence that cross-infection may occur between man and dog, but the extent to which this protozoan can be transmitted to humans by other hosts is unclear.

Endoparasites that may enter the United Kingdom via imported dogs

Dogs entering the United Kingdom and Republic of Ireland are subject to the 'Rabies (Importation of Dogs, Cats and other Mammals) Order (1974) (Amendment) Order (1977)'. This involves restriction to a licensed quarantine kennel for a period of six months, during which time the animals are under constant veterinary supervision. This does not involve a routine examination for the presence of endoparasites, but if signs of disease are apparent naturally blood and faecal examinations are likely to be carried out as part of the diagnostic work-up. Examinations of these dogs have demonstrated the presence of all or any of the parasites already mentioned. In addition to the above, dogs may enter the United Kingdom and Republic of Ireland with *Dirofilaria immitis, Ancylostoma* spp., *Babesia canis* and *Leishmania* spp.

Heartworm disease in the dog

Dirofilaria immitis is a roundworm (nematode) which causes heartworm disease in the dog. It is a parasite of tropical and sub-tropical regions. It does not occur in Great Britain except in imported animals. They are large worms, adult males reaching 16 cm (5½ in.) and females 25–30 cm (10–12 in.) in length. They are slender and white in colour and are chiefly located in the right ventricle of the heart and the adjacent blood vessels.

Heartworm disease is considered to be one of the most important conditions seen in small animal practice in the United States. Prevalent in the eastern United States, especially Florida, it is also present in parts of southern Europe and eastern Australia. The larval form of the nematode is transmitted by mosquitoes and is referred to as a microfilaria. Microfilariae are found in the bloodstreams of infected dogs and can only develop further when ingested by a mosquito after it has bitten the dog. They develop in the mosquito to become infective and are transmitted to the dog host when it is again bitten by an infected mosquito.

Although heartworm does not occur in British dogs, imported dogs are a source of infection, and as the period of development to the adult stage is about six months after infection it is possible that clinical signs of disease may not show until after the dog has been released from the statutory six months' quarantine. Dogs with typical heartworm disease show fatigue on exercise, cough and appear rough and unthrifty.

Although mosquitoes of a suitable species are found in this country, it is believed that temperatures in the UK are unsuitable for development of the parasite in the intermediate host.

Control and treatment

This is difficult as the adult stages have to be eliminated as well as the microfilariae in the bloodstream. The veterinary policy is:

1. Improve the condition of the animal before administering the necessary drugs.
2. Eliminate the adult forms while the patient is hospitalised.
3. Eliminate the microfilariae.

Ancylostoma species

Three species of this hookworm can be found in dogs undergoing the statutory period of quarantine, of which *Ancylostoma caninum* is the most common. The adult forms of this tropical hookworm are about 1–2 cm (½–1 in.) long and are found in the small intestine, where they attach themselves to the lining of the bowel (mucosal wall) and where they suck blood and can cause severe anaemia. The eggs pass out in the faeces on to the ground and eventually larvae hatch from the eggs in a similar manner to that of the eggs of the temperate climate hookworm *Uncinaria stenocephala*. The larvae of *Ancylostoma caninum* can enter the host either by the mouth, skin or from the colostrum in the milk in the case of suckling pups. *Ancylostoma caninum* will not normally survive in the United Kingdom because the ground temperature is generally too low for development of the larvae. An immunity to the disease may occur, but breaks down if the dogs become underfed. The methods of control are similar to those used for the temperate climate hookworm.

Babesia canis

This is a protozoan parasite which has a widespread distribution. It is most troublesome in the southern States of the USA, South Africa and Asia, and is transmitted principally by the tick *Rhipicephalus sanguineus*. Although this tick may enter the United Kingdom, it requires a high climatic temperature for its survival. The protozoans called piroplasms enter the red blood cells when the infected tick bites the host. The resultant clinical signs are a febrile disease with progressive anaemia and jaundice. Imported dogs need to be treated under veterinary supervision.

Leishmania species

This is a protozoan parasite found in man, dogs and certain rodents in many parts of the world, but not Australia, and is transmitted by the sandfly (*Phlebotomus* species). It is the cause of visceral and cutaneous leishmaniasis in the dog and may remain latent until long after the quarantine period, but when it shows itself clinically it is very serious. The disease originates in endemic areas such as Brazil, China, southern Europe and the Mediterranean regions. The infected sandfly containing the flagellate forms bite the host and inject into the blood vessels organisms which become engulfed by blood cells. These cells, called macrophages, may be found in many tissues, but mainly the bone marrow, spleen, liver and lymph nodes. The last three enlarge as the protozoans multiply. Any imported dog showing enlarged lymph nodes, lack of appetite, wasting, skin lesions or diarrhoea needs to be considered for veterinary treatment. Treatment of dogs imported into the United Kingdom with leishmaniasis has to be considered very carefully, since there is a public health risk, particularly when handling infected specimens, e.g., blood samples from infected dogs. In man, visceral leishmaniasis is known as Kala-azar.

Some parasites occurring outside the United Kingdom

Strongyloides stercoralis

This nematode is found in dogs in the Far East (India, China, the Philippines), Africa, North and South America and parts of Europe, but has not been reported in the UK. A very similar parasite is found in man in the same areas. The life cycle is complicated as it is altered by changes in environmental conditions. Infective larvae enter the host via either the skin or the mouth. Clinical signs are seen in puppies which show lack of appetite, bronchopneumonia, diarrhoea and, in severe cases, death. The dog may act as a reservoir for human infection, but generally the chance of it spreading from dogs to man is low.

Dioctophyma renale

This is the largest nematode to be found in the dog, the adult female possibly reaching up to 103 cm (40 in.) in length. The adult forms are located in the kidney, frequently the right kidney, and the organ may be destroyed. The parasite is found in North and South America, Europe, Russia, Japan and Africa, but not in the United Kingdom. The eggs laid by the female worm are expelled in the urine and are swallowed by annelid worms which are parasitic on crayfish. When infected crayfish are eaten by other fish the parasites become encysted in the mesentery and liver. It is at this stage that the dog can become infected by eating infected raw fish.

Diphyllobothrium latum

This is a tapeworm (cestode) which can parasitise the small intestine of dog and man. It is referred to as the broad fish tapeworm and often exceeds 2 metres (6·5 ft) in length. It has been found in Europe, the USSR, the Baltic States, Canada, Chile, Japan and, extensively, in the Far East. It has not been found in the United Kingdom except possibly in Northern Ireland. The parasites require the presence of a freshwater crustacean and a freshwater fish, so the existence of freshwater lakes is required. Dog and man become infected by eating raw or undercooked fish containing the parasite.

These are just a few of the vast number of endoparasites found in dogs outside the United Kingdom and this limited number is included in order to highlight the diversity of life cycles to be found among the parasites of the dog.

Medical and Surgical

24

VETERINARY NURSING

During the last two decades the dog-owning public have become more and more aware of the Veterinary Nurse, the professionally trained person at the clinic or surgery who does so much to help the owner, the animal and the veterinary surgeon.

In times gone by the person who helped the vet was probably the parlour maid, the housemaid or the vet's wife. This is not sexist; remember female vets are from the relatively recent past – the first qualified in the late 1930s. In the 19th century very few pet animals received veterinary attention. Cats were kept as pets, but spent most of their lives outdoors in 'outhouses' and dogs kept as pets were also often kennelled outside, receiving scant veterinary attention. With the popularity of the 'lapdog' so beloved by society ladies in the last century things began to change. It was perhaps these animals that formed the basis for small animal (pet animal) practice as we know it today. Assistance with treatment, holding the dog for example, was often the task of the lady's maid, as was any subsequent treatment ordered by the veterinary surgeon.

Over the years small animal practice started to develop. There were definite efforts at nursing 'small animals', i.e., those other than horses, cattle and sheep. A Canine Hospital is recorded as having existed in Neasden, London, at the end of the last century, with facilities for 200 canine patients, quite remarkable when one considers few veterinary surgeons in Britain today hospitalise more than 30 dogs and even large boarding and quarantine kennels seldom exceed 200 animals. This Neasden hospital was run on similar lines to a general hospital and there were even male and female wards, according to an article in a magazine called *Homechat* in January 1899. A dog bathing pool was provided and the magazine published a photograph of two dogs swimming complete with three men in attendance. Were these the first male veterinary nurses?

An eminent veterinary surgeon at the beginning of this century, Sir William Hobday, had a practice in Kensington, London. Reference is made in his book, *Surgical Diseases of the Dog and Cat*, published in 1906, to his small 'infirmary' at the practice. However, personnel are not mentioned.

It is on record that a Canine Nurses Institute was in existence prior to the First World War and the nurses employed by this Institute wore uniforms and a CNI badge embroidered in red on a white ground. At this time nursing sick dogs was considered a means of 'opening up a new line of work to women'. Remarkably, the rules of conduct of the Canine Nurses Institute are very similar to those we present-day veterinary nurses follow and which appear in our contracts of employment, particularly those relating to professional conduct towards both the animal patients and the owner.

This Institute would provide qualified nurses when required for the sum of £1 5s 0d per week (£1.25) plus board, lodging and travelling. We do not know the training or how they were considered qualified. Obviously they were considerably better paid than many other employees at that time and one wonders whether they priced themselves out of business, since no further references can be found to the Canine Nurses Institute. Training, we know, covered treatment of sick animals, setting and bandaging broken limbs and giving medication. Tuition on coat care and even showing was included, together with care of cats.

It seems that the South of England was undoubtedly the place for these forerunners of our veterinary nursing scheme, for in Middlesex the Ruislip Dog Sanatorium published an illustrated brochure in 1913 with what appears to be a 'lady nurse' sitting outside a door labelled 'Surgery and Office'. The Sanatorium was under the direct supervision of a veterinary surgeon, William Kirk. One can only guess the whereabouts of the exact site of this sanatorium today, since the site is occupied by a modern housing estate.

In 1938 a cigarette card in a series issued by Churchman's cigarettes depicted Mrs. Florence Bell, the Head Nurse at the Royal Veterinary College, in London's Camden Town. Speaking with two veterinary surgeons who were on the staff at the College at the time, I was told she was very respected and even feared by some members of the staff. They recall her as a very dedicated person who most definitely cared for her patients often rather more than their owners on occasion!

A book entirely on canine nursing was published by veterinary surgeon David Wilkinson in 1938. Throughout this book reference is made to the unpleasantness of the tasks, the strong disinfectants needed and the necessity for wearing thick gloves to protect the nurse. At that time few small animal diseases could be positively cured and only devoted nursing could help the fortunate ones.

Prior to the Second World War an attempt was made by two veterinary surgeons in small animal practice in Mayfair, in London's West End, to 'train women nurses for dogs'. They approached the Royal College of Veterinary Surgeons, the governing body for veterinary education in Great Britain, with a request to recognise the status of canine nurses, after they had passed appropriate examinations based on study of a syllabus to be approved by the Royal College.

This approach to the Royal College was the first serious attempt to establish a national veterinary nursing course as we know it today. It was nearly 30 years before it came to fruition, for it was in 1961 that the Royal College of Veterinary Surgeons inaugurated the veterinary nursing scheme. Small animal practice had by this time become an established part of the veterinary scene and in 1957 the British Small Animal Veterinary Association (BSAVA) had been established by a group of veterinary surgeons particularly interested in 'specialising' in small animal matters. Those forward-looking veterinary surgeons were aware of the need for staff, trained to a basic standard, who could assist and support them in their work. Thus only four years after formation of the BSAVA a scheme to train people who later were to become known as veterinary nurses was commenced officially by the Royal College of Veterinary Surgeons.

Early years presented many problems. A syllabus was organised but the difficulties lay in determining the level of knowledge required and the standard to set. Many people had been working for veterinary surgeons for years and were considered very competent. Many veterinarians held the view that their home-trained staff were better than any 'outside trained' personnel and why should their staff not be considered 'qualified'?

There was the problem of the name – the simple, elegant, descriptive title, 'veterinary nurse', could not be used. The title 'nurse' was protected by the Royal College of Nursing and could only apply to a person trained in human nursing. Difficulties were encountered in the use of the term 'veterinary', so the title Registered Animal Nursing Auxiliary (RANA) was agreed as a compromise and RANAs we remained until 1984.

The Nurses, Midwives and Health Visitors Act of 1979 and the Nurses Act of 1957 were due for repeal in July 1983 and this opened the way for the official recognition of the title Veterinary Nurse. The Royal College of Veterinary Surgeons moved swiftly and effected the necessary changes, so with effect from 1 November, 1984, those qualifying could legally use the term Veterinary Nurse and bear the letters VN after their name. Those of us who qualified as RANAs were able to convert from 1 November, 1984, so many of us possess two certificates, one as a RANA and the other as a VN, and two similar badges, inscribed VN and RANA.

A Statutory Register for Veterinary Nurses, giving them official recognition as a professional body, is still in the future, since this will have to be incorporated into a new Veterinary Surgeons Act.

In 1990 the academic requirements for enrolment as a veterinary nursing trainee are four GCSE passes at Grades of A, B or C. The subjects must

THE ROYAL COLLEGE OF VETERINARY SURGEONS

This is to Certify

that, by virtue of having completed the course of training and passed
the necessary examinations,

Jean Margaret Turner

has been registered as an Animal Nursing Auxiliary.

Chairman, Animal Nursing Auxiliaries Committee

Registrar, Royal College of Veterinary Surgeons

Certificate No. 419

Date of Issue 10 November 1971

Figure 179a   Original Registered Animal Nursing Auxiliary Certificate

THE ROYAL COLLEGE OF VETERINARY SURGEONS

This is to Certify

that, by virtue of having completed the course of training and passed

the necessary examinations

.......................JEAN MARGARET TURNER.............................

is declared to have qualified as a Veterinary Nurse, and has been placed on the list of

Veterinary Nurses maintained by the Royal College of Veterinary Surgeons.

....

Chairman, Veterinary Nursing Committee

....

Registrar, Royal College of Veterinary Surgeons

Certificate No. ....419................

Date of Issue .....1 NOVEMBER 1984........

Figure 179b   In 1984 RANAs became Veterinary Nurses

include English Language and a Science subject, preferably a physical science or mathematics. Acceptable alternatives are GCE passes in O level examinations at grades of A, B or C or a Certificate in Secondary Education at grade 1. The minimum age for enrolment is 17, but there is no upper age limit for training. The trainee must be employed for a minimum of 35 hours a week at a training centre approved by the Royal College of Veterinary Surgeons. Approved training centres (ATCs) are usually established practices with a high component of small animal work, although certain other establishments such as the Dogs' Home Battersea, London Zoo and the Royal Army Veterinary Corps are also approved training centres. The trainee has to work for at least two years in an approved training centre before qualifying as a VN and in addition must be successful in the two professional examinations. The preliminary examination is taken at the end of the first year's training and deals basically with anatomy, physiology, kennel and cattery management and first aid. The successful candidate then embarks upon the syllabus for the final examination, which many regard as veterinary nursing proper, with subjects such as radiography, surgical and medical nursing as well as intensive care, anaesthesia and laboratory work.

The veterinary nursing qualification is not easily won. It requires tremendous dedication to study subjects superficially unrelated to the day-to-day work, particularly after a hard day's toil. This is particularly apparent in the case of the preliminary syllabus, when the finer aspects of anatomy and physiology are hard to reconcile with a day spent scrubbing out a ward of dogs with enteritis!

There are currently over 800 approved training centres in Great Britain. Some employ several trainees, others may engage one at a time. In addition to the minimum entry requirements, some training centres require trainees to be 18 years of age or over, especially if they are living away from home. Others demand a higher academic level of entry. There are many qualified veterinary nurses who commenced training with several A levels. Many of us have trained as mature students.

Training methods vary, but all follow the guidelines published by RCVS in the current *Guide for Persons wishing to train as Veterinary Nurses*. This is obtainable from the Veterinary Nursing Secretariat, Royal College of Veterinary Surgeons, 32 Belgrave Square, London SW1X 8QP.

The aim of the course is to produce practical veterinary nurses trained to a minimum standard, so therefore much of the training is covered by normal day-to-day duties in the ATC with additional formal tuition. Some ATCs provide this in the form of lectures at the practice, given by the staff and sometimes outside lecturers. There are various part-time courses, some in the form of day-release courses and others run as evening classes. Full-time residential courses are also available at several agricultural colleges as well as block release courses. In addition the BSAVA run day and weekend courses for trainees on various parts of the syllabus and the British Veterinary Nursing Association (BVNA) arranges meetings, which are often of use to trainees.

A correspondence course is available to those who are unable to travel to formal lectures and this has veterinary surgeons and veterinary nurses as tutors.

Both the preliminary and final examinations consist of two written papers plus oral and practical examinations covering the appropriate parts of the syllabus. Examiners are veterinary surgeons and veterinary nurses and are appointed by the RCVS Veterinary Nursing Committee.

The scope of the work open to veterinary nurses is today widening, but the majority are still employed by veterinary surgeons in small animal practice. The Veterinary Surgeons Act of 1966 makes it illegal for anyone other than a veterinary surgeon to treat animals or carry out the 'practice of veterinary medicine and surgery', except in very limited circumstances. Veterinary nurses therefore are restricted in their duties and can only carry out procedures under the direct supervision of a veterinary surgeon. However, carrying out our work entails considerable responsibility and it is recognised that our training allows us to carry out our nursing duties more competently and efficiently than someone untrained.

There are many Veterinary Nurses employed in commerce, working as veterinary representatives, managing drug wholesalers' warehouses, or working as product managers for drug companies. Many of us are also involved in practice management. Here we undertake stock control, ordering and running practice laboratories. Veterinary nurses with business qualifications are increasingly in demand as practice managers.

Figure 180 Laboratory procedures are part of the Veterinary Nurse's everyday work

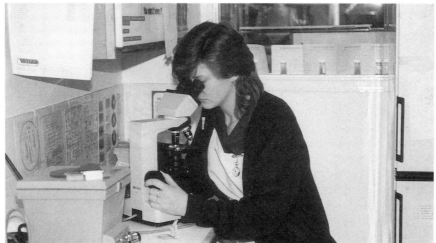

Veterinary nurses are employed as kennel managers in boarding, breeding and quarantine kennels; as lecturers on veterinary nursing and related courses at agricultural colleges, as well as nurses, administrators and counsellors in small animal practices and welfare organisations. Several dog wardens have veterinary nursing qualifications. The opportunities are endless. Thus criticism that there is no career structure is clearly unfounded.

Responsibility in general practice can vary from head nurse over two or three others to part of a senior nursing team in a larger practice with responsibilities in one area only, such as the operating theatre, client counselling or, if your interest lies in laboratory work, you may find your metier in charge of the practice laboratory. It is impossible to accurately define a career structure in such a wide range of practice situations. Promotion in the accepted term of the word is often impossible, but a change in jobs is possible and with the variety of openings mentioned previously, a more senior position is attainable.

In 1989 the introduction of the Diploma in Advanced Veterinary Nursing (Surgical) was introduced. This is a further qualification for those qualified two or more years. The Diploma course covers two years, and details of this are available from the Royal College of Veterinary Surgeons, whose address is given earlier in this chapter.

British Veterinary Nursing Association

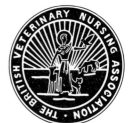

In 1965, two years after the first final examination, there were 46 qualified nurses, or RANAs to use the official but hated title. The scheme was a success. The next logical step was the formation of an official Veterinary Nursing Association and this came into being on 13 March of that year as the result of the efforts of a group of RANAs considerably aided by a minority of veterinary surgeons committed to the concept. The name selected by the original committee was the British Veterinary Nursing

Figure 181 Members of the British Veterinary Nursing Association have their own badge

Association, another sign of the distaste for the officially assigned designation. The aims of that original committee were commendable and should be acknowledged. Sadly, the establishment prevailed and before long the association's name was changed to British Animal Nursing Auxiliaries Association (BANAA). The President was, until 1984, a veterinary surgeon. Subsequently a Veterinary Nurse was elected to this office.

The early development was similar to that of all new and numerically small associations. Newsletters were typed, duplicated and issued sporadically. Meetings were few and far between. Membership grew, however, and before long BANAA was invited to attend BSAVA's annual congress. Uniforms were organised and approved and exhibited at veterinary congresses. The image of the veterinary nurse was becoming established.

After the title VN was approved and the demeaning title 'auxiliary' lost, so the Association was able to revert to its proper title of BVNA, which marked a tremendous increase in membership.

Today BVNA publishes its own Journal to members every two months. This has scientific articles, news items, details of forthcoming meetings, branches, etc. There are over 30 BVNA branches around the country with meetings arranged approximately every two months by each branch. Support for the branch comes from BVNA members and anyone else interested in veterinary nursing.

The Association flourished even before its change of name. During the 1970s the first all-day scientific meeting was held to coincide with the AGM. This became an annual congress. Its popularity led to its outgrowing the long-standing venue at the Berkshire College of Agriculture and in 1987 it moved to the National Agricultural Centre at Stoneleigh. With a capacity for 325, nearly 100 potential delegates were turned away. In consequence a larger facility was booked at Stoneleigh in 1988 and nearly 500 delegates attended. Particularly impressive was the large trade exhibition. In 1989, for the first time, a dual presentation took place with simultaneous lectures in two different lecture rooms. With a present BVNA membership of around 1,200 it was anticipated this would be the best congress ever and final figures available at the time of writing confirmed the number of delegates at 633, with nearly 100 trade stands.

The association is now established as the voice of the veterinary nursing profession and is self-supporting. Support for the BVNA from the veterinary profession as a whole continues with consistent support from 'the trade', those drug companies, pet food suppliers, equipment manufacturers and pet insurance houses who realise that it is the veterinary nurse in practice they must contact to generate business.

Until 1988, BVNA, like so many other associations, was run by its Council Members, who met at a central venue every six to eight weeks but carried out most of their work from their homes. As membership increased so the need for an established office was apparent. Various options were explored, and help came from many quarters. One past president of the Association, the last veterinary surgeon to hold that office, offered free office space in order to allow the Association to find its way. BSAVA was supportive with unstinting advice and once more friends in the trade were ready to help wherever needed. Legal advice was taken and a decision made to establish an independent office in Essex.

All BVNA Council business is conducted there. In less than a year the office was being used to its capacity. The decision was justified.

Much of the office equipment was donated by commercial companies

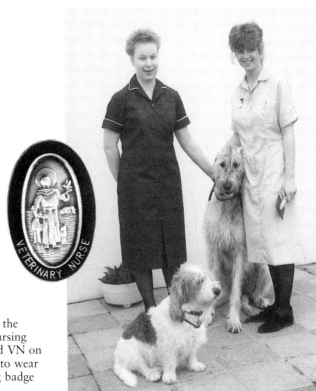

Figure 182   These are the approved veterinary nursing uniforms. The qualified VN on the left is also entitled to wear the Veterinary Nursing badge (*inset*)

and other veterinary organisations. A small plaque affixed to each item of equipment indicates its source.

The approved uniform for veterinary nurses was suggested by the BSAVA. Qualified VNs wear a bottle green dress, with a bottle green belt and white apron. Trainees' dresses are green and white striped with a black or grey belt, depending on whether they are in the first or second year of the course, plus a similar white apron. In the early days of the scheme a white cap was also worn, but this has been discontinued; in the practical job the hat was not very suitable. Similarly uniform cuffs are seldom seen today.

In 1986 a booklet *Veterinary Nursing, the First Twenty Five Years* was published by BVNA and this is available from the BVNA Office at The Seedbed Centre, Coldharbour Road, Harlow, Essex, CM19 5AF, cost £1.50, including postage and packing.

Membership details of the Association are available from the office. There are several membership categories, ranging from the qualified VNs to trainees, and associate membership for those working in veterinary practice or allied fields and for supporters of the Association.

25
NURSING THE SICK DOG

An awareness of the differing needs of the sick dog is required before nursing can be correctly undertaken. Owners are frequently too emotionally involved with their pets to realise the need for certain instructions to be carried out precisely. In such situations, it is often preferable for the dog to be nursed in the veterinary practice, and it is for this reason that it is advised.

The condition of the dog dictates the care that is needed and here guidance from the veterinary practice is important. Specific conditions will be mentioned in this chapter only as necessary and when an example is required. Nursing of the many conditions from which dogs may suffer will not be covered individually nor in detail since the object of this chapter is to give general outlines only of the common methods employed when nursing the 'sick' dog.

There is a marked difference between nursing a dog in the home environment and in the veterinary practice. At home the dog is in familiar surroundings, with the family coming and going, the television or radio on, noises from the vacuum cleaner, traffic outside the house, etc. In the practice it is in a cage or kennel, surrounded by strange people and noises. Even stranger smells come from disinfectants, medication and other animals. Surprisingly, perhaps, most dogs do well under these circumstances, probably due in no small part to the social nature of the animal itself and the dedicated attention received from the veterinary personnel. The majority of dogs hospitalised are pets and so respond to voice and touch, as they do with their owners at home. One of the main functions of the veterinary nursing team is to provide this stimulus to get well via 'touch and talk', although early in the course of treatment and hospitalisation in some cases, with very ill dogs, the veterinary surgeon may decide that even this stimulation must be denied. However, in the majority of cases this is, compared with us, only for a very short period.

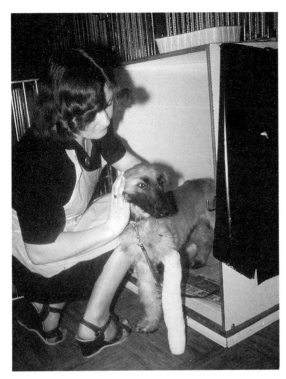

Figure 183 (Left) 'Touch and talk' is an important part of veterinary nursing

Figure 184 (Right) Dogs on intravenous drip require constant attention

It is a matter for the attending veterinary surgeon to decide where best the animal should be nursed. It makes sense that the dog returns home as soon as possible because, as with people, recovery is that much more rapid in familiar surroundings. However, there are some situations where home nursing is just not possible. For example, if the dog has to be placed on fluid therapy, i.e., an intravenous drip, treatment would be very difficult at home since the dog must be in an environment where movement is strictly curtailed and trained personnel are immediately available to adjust flow rates, change solutions and ensure complete comfort. The dog must be confined in a kennel, where little movement is possible, so that the intravenous line is not dislodged. Within the practice there are various methods to hand to ensure the drip remains in place, but even so a determined dog can sometimes remove the drip, and could cause damage to the vein in the process if this went unnoticed. Intravenous fluids are often administered into the cephalic vein in the foreleg; this is achieved by the insertion of a plastic or metal tube or catheter into the vein. This is then carefully strapped or bandaged in place. Sometimes, if it is not possible to use the vein in the leg for any reason, i.e., a dog with multiple lacerations or fractures following a road traffic accident, the jugular vein in the neck is used to receive the catheter.

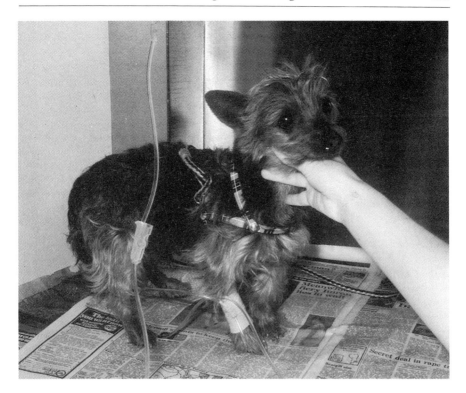

While very ill the dog will not care that these catheters are conveying life-giving fluids to the bloodstream, but once they have done their job and the dog feels better the order of the day will be very much that this strange object must be removed at all costs. Even an owner with some medical training would find it difficult to cope in such circumstances.

The administration of medication, in tablet or capsule form, can be undertaken by most owners. A little bit of encouragement or bribery works well. Owners should follow instructions carefully and ensure all medication is given as instructed. If in doubt, do not be afraid of asking. Tablets to be given three times a day should be equally spaced out, i.e., at approximately eight-hourly intervals, to provide a correct level of the drug for maximum effect. This is why modern labels do not say twice daily but at 12-hourly intervals, for example. Instructions for giving medication before meals or after meals are important. Different drugs need different regimes. Be guided by your veterinary surgeon and follow instructions precisely.

Some drugs have to be given by injection and most owners cannot cope unless some training has been given, e.g., insulin for the diabetic animal. Depending on the animal's condition, the drugs can be given on an out-patient basis, i.e., you attend the practice with the dog. If frequent

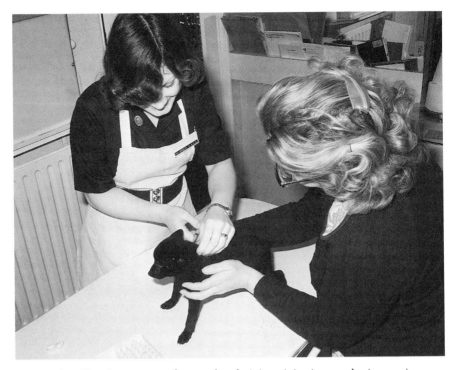

Figure 185 Veterinary nurses frequently administer injections under instructions from the veterinary surgeon

injections are needed the veterinary surgeon may decide to 'keep the dog in'. This is always worrying, but remember it often leads to speedier recovery. Some injections other than drips need to be given intravenously. These may sometimes be given on an outpatient basis, but again if frequent dosage is required, an intravenous line, as with fluid therapy, may be set up and the catheter, which is inserted into the vein, may be capped between injections. If the dog goes home with the catheter *in situ* care is necessary to ensure that it is not pulled out, since dogs are adept at destroying even copious dressings and the same problems arise as discussed previously.

Should your dog have received an intravenous injection, e.g., a general anaesthetic, it is likely that a small quantity of hair may have been clipped from one or both forelegs. This is done to expose the skin over the vein into which the intravenous injection is to be made and ensures the site can be aseptically prepared. Remember an intravenous injection is really a surgical operation and surgical cleanliness is most important.

In practice we are often requested that the leg of a dog about to receive an intravenous injection is not clipped 'because he is a show dog'. In a relatively smooth-coated dog this may not be a problem, but in a heavy- or long-coated animal it is sometimes impossible to locate the vein if the hair is not removed and then it is possible for the drug to go perivascularly, i.e., outside the vein. This can cause tremendous irritation with some drugs. The dog can worry at the leg and end up with more problems due to self-inflicted damage than if the minimal amount of clipping required for the procedure had been carried out. It will be obvious to any judge in the show ring that the leg had been clipped for an intravenous injection and the dog should not be penalised for this.

Your veterinary surgeon may decide to admit your dog to restrict movement. This is especially so where any orthopaedic procedures are involved. In the practice the dog will be confined in a kennel with sufficient room to stretch out, stand up and turn around, but little more than this. He will be taken out frequently in order to perform his natural functions, but will receive no more exercise than this. Think of what will happen at home. Your dog will perhaps be put in the kitchen. Compare the size of your kitchen with the size of the dog and relate this to the size of the kennel at the practice. He will be in an area several times larger, which means more movement. In the practice the surrounding noises will have little effect, but at home . . . Just think of it – Mum comes home from the shops, always an exciting moment for the dog because that is where the supply of food comes from; Johnny comes home from school and he always plays with his pet before doing anything else; the neighbour calls, the postman, the milkman . . . the distractions are endless and the dog is up and down the whole time. You may have a relatively small garden, but still it will be an area considerably bigger than that at the practice when the dog needs to defecate or urinate. Remember this when the vet asks to keep the dog in. The enforced rest will aid a more rapid recovery. Hospitalisation makes sense in many situations. The veterinary surgeon wants your dog restored to normality just as soon as you do!

Sometimes bandages or a dressing are applied to an injured part of the dog's body. Care needs to be taken to ensure these do not get wet and they are not too tight or uncomfortable. The additional amount of movement at home compared with the practice can cause problems with dressings, so your veterinary surgeon may decide to keep the dog in for a day or so.

If, for example, your dog has sustained a cut paw and is sent home with a dressing, do follow instructions regarding redressing and returning the dog for the necessary check-ups. It is important that the healing of the wound can be assessed.

I would recommend you have a first-aid box in the home with a separate section for the dog. The majority of first-aid dressings apply equally to people and dogs, but people leave dressings alone, dogs often do not. Therefore the addition of elastic adhesive plaster and some form of wound dressing powder would be useful.

Except in the emergency situation, dressings should not be applied unless you have been instructed to do so. For example, in summertime dogs can

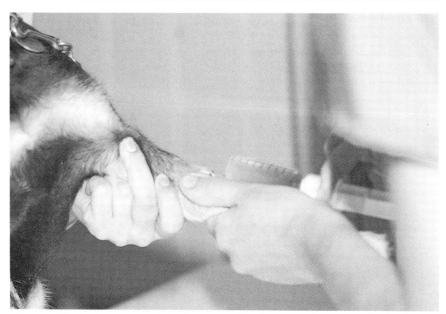

Figure 186   An intravenous injection is usually given into the vein of the foreleg

Figure 187   Hospitalisation may be necessary to restrict movement to a minimum

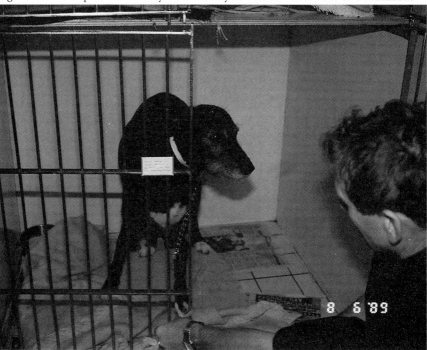

suffer from 'hot spot' eczema and owners will often try to apply plasters over these sore areas. These will usually only irritate the dog and make him scratch more. However, it is sensible to restrict bleeding from a badly cut foot and a dressing in this situation will prevent contamination of the wound. You will be very welcome at your veterinary surgeon's if your dog has a dressing on the badly cut, bleeding foot so that the nurse on duty does not have to wash the floors, the entrance paths and your route to the practice. Equally, you will be more popular at home if the car is not covered with blood! It can take a long time and a lot of effort to remove the evidence of a cut foot from the surgery premises and just as long to clean your car, in fact both may take longer than it takes the veterinary surgeon to treat the wound! A deep wound can bleed quite profusely and a firm bandage can reduce blood loss considerably, to the benefit of your dog and a more rapid return to normal.

In an emergency situation a towel, piece of sheeting or similar can be wrapped round a bleeding foot and a plastic bag round it will prevent a lot of mess and can assist in reducing the amount of blood lost. Never use an elastic band to secure this, it gets hidden in the hair and the poor dog can end up with a serious restriction to blood flow or even another wound where the band has become embedded in the skin. Incidentally, the rule about never using an elastic band applies to all animals, at all times, particularly when children are around. Try to remember to telephone your veterinary surgeon to advise you are on your way with such an injury; it is possible there will be no one free to attend to you if you arrive unannounced. Although your injured dog is quite rightly your prime concern, the practice could be just as occupied with other people's animals. Prior warning will help everyone, including the injured pet.

It will depend on the policy at your practice whether the dog will be sent home following major orthopaedic surgery or kept in for a few days. Your veterinary surgeon will consider the type of surgery that has been carried out, the breed and temperament of the dog and your wishes, but the needs of the dog must come before the wishes of the owner, sorry!

If your dog has been sent home with a dressing on an orthopaedic wound, perhaps following the repair of a ruptured ligament or a broken bone, it is imperative to follow your veterinary surgeon's instructions. Do not hesitate to ring the practice if you are at all worried. Signs to cause concern are loss of movement, heat around the area of the dressing, any odour, swelling or any discharges, restlessness or lack of appetite. Your veterinary surgeon will be happy to advise you and would prefer to know of any problems, however minor they may appear to you, before they become major.

When nursing your dog at home you will often be requested to restrict exercise or allow lead exercise only. This really is important. If you have another dog in the home, make the veterinary surgeon aware of this fact;

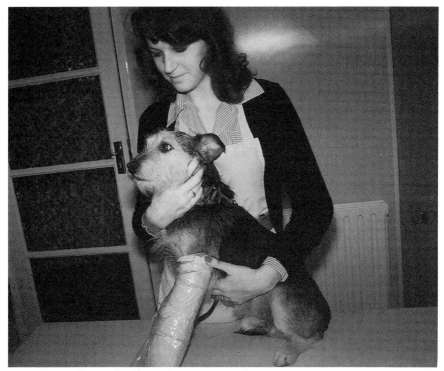

Figure 188 If your dog has a dressing on his limbs it is important that veterinary instructions are carefully followed

it may influence his decision on when a dog should go home. Two dogs together exercise themselves a great deal, which is not ideal if your veterinary surgeon has ordered exercise to be restricted. Think of the dog in the practice. As mentioned earlier he will be confined in a kennel and let out for a limited period, under supervision. Take him home, and there is your kitchen and a garden which is a relatively large space. By lead exercise we do mean the dog is taken out to be clean, on a lead, and then immediately brought back indoors. In orthopaedic cases it is of particular importance that there must be NO STEPS OR STAIRS for the dog to navigate and that NO JUMPING ON FURNITURE OR BEDS is permitted. This can be a problem if you live in a flat or your dog is used to sleeping on the furniture. Under these circumstances it may be better that the dog remains with the veterinary surgeon for a few days longer. Even once up and down the stairs can spell disaster in some cases.

Grooming as part of the normal care of your dog becomes more important when he is sick. The dog needs the reassurance of a familiar touch with the brush and comb, the comforting and close presence of the owner while grooming takes place. Stroking, brushing and combing imparts a sense of well-being. Normal equipment is all that is needed plus

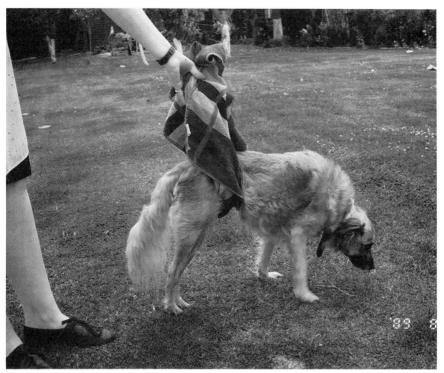

Figure 189   A paraplegic still needs to go out to be clean. A towel makes a useful support

some first-aid items such as cotton wool. This is used for bathing eyes and wiping around the mouth with plain water or any solutions advised by the veterinary surgeon.

No matter how incapacitated your pet may be, he will be even more distressed if he is unable to fulfil his natural functions. All his life you have trained him to go outside to be clean and he will be most upset if he soils himself or the surroundings. A sick dog will not be as quick to request to be let out as when healthy and you should anticipate his needs. Carrying him outside may be necessary. A big dog can be supported with a towel under his middle in the form of a sling and will soon learn how to move without too much discomfort. Watch for signs of constipation or diarrhoea and report this to your veterinary surgeon.

Feeding will depend on the animal's condition. If there has been a bowel upset or the dog has had surgery performed to the intestinal tract, then an adjustment to diet will be necessary until recovery is complete. The veterinary surgeon will instruct you on the type of diet needed. These days we are fortunate in having commercial, scientifically prepared diets available for many conditions. There are diets that assist dogs with impaired hearts or kidneys or recovering from operations. There are diets to build him up and also help him lose weight, if necessary. Your veterinary surgeon will supply these as appropriate.

Whatever the reason that the dog needs nursing, do always liaise with your veterinary practice. The qualified veterinary nurse will be of great help to you. He or she has been trained to support the veterinary surgeon and can reassure you on your pet's progress or help when needed. It is important to have a rapport with the practice as well as the pet.

The biggest factor in the restoration of your dog to its normal healthy lifestyle is a matter of common sense; of carrying out your veterinary surgeon's instructions and ensuring you keep the follow-up visits requested. Put yourself in your dog's position, think how you would like to be treated and you will not go far wrong.

26

FIRST AID

First aid is the care and treatment given to an individual in an emergency, and this is usually directly after a serious injury or the sudden onset of illness. Its principal purpose is to preserve the life of the patient, but other important aims are to reduce pain and discomfort (i.e., to alleviate suffering) and to minimise the risk of permanent disability or disfigurement by preventing further damage to the already injured tissues. In the context of first aid, an *emergency* can be defined as a situation, usually unforeseen and rapid in onset, which requires immediate attention. Emergencies which are a prime cause of concern are:

1. The absence of breathing, or severe difficulty in breathing,
2. severe bleeding, and
3. signs of severe shock.

Signs which *might* have equally serious consequences are:

1. Unconsciousness and/or convulsions, and
2. signs of poisoning.

The latter are dealt with in more detail in Chapter 27.

In these emergency situations it is essential that assistance be given promptly and maintained until the professional help of a veterinary surgeon is available. It might subsequently be the opinion of a veterinary surgeon that euthanasia of the injured animal would be the most humane course of action, but this is not a decision for others to take and first-aid efforts should be directed towards keeping the animal alive until a professional opinion can be obtained.

Road accidents are the most common emergencies in which dogs are involved, especially in urban areas, as a consequence of allowing them to wander freely. Many different types of injury can be caused and multiple injuries are common. One in every eight dogs dies from a road accident, in most instances either immediately or within the next 24 hours – the highest mortality rate for any of the common causes of injury. Of those that die, 95 per cent have suffered damage to their chest or abdomen.

PRIORITIES

With all emergencies it is important first of all not to panic, and to approach the problem calmly. Also, with all injured animals, before help can be provided it is necessary for them to be *adequately restrained*. The approach to and restraint of the injured dog is a vital preliminary, although animals that have suffered the most damage are usually the least likely to offer any serious resistance.

The *ABC approach* is a useful way of remembering the priorities in giving first-aid treatment. These are:

1. *Airway* – ensure that the animal's airway is not obstructed so that its breathing is unimpaired.
2. *Bleeding* – control major, and therefore life-threatening, haemorrhage, and
3. *Collapse, convulsions and lack of consciousness* – in these situations treatment for shock may be required and it becomes particularly important to make sure that the animal is in a place where it will not suffer further injury.

The treatment of these life-threatening signs must receive priority; always leave the cleaning of wounds and other non-essential procedures until afterwards and concentrate on saving the animal's life.

The help and advice of a veterinary surgeon is essential in virtually all emergencies and professional assistance should be obtained as soon as possible. The first-aid measures described subsequently are therefore designed to precede, not to replace, proper veterinary attention. The initial contact with a veterinary surgeon is best made by telephone to avoid any possible confusion about the reception of the injured dog.

RESTRAINT

After a major injury an animal, unless unconscious, will be extremely bewildered and frightened and it may resent handling and be aggressive. However, handling will be essential for its examination and subsequent treatment. Restraint also avoids the animal inflicting further damage to itself and injuring those trying to help it.

It is, of course, imperative that if the animal is in a dangerous position, e.g., in the roadway after an accident, it should first be removed to a safer, and preferably sheltered, position.

The approach to such a dog should be calm, quiet and yet purposeful. It is valuable to have the help of two or three sensible people, but noisy and hysterical onlookers should be asked to leave. By talking to the animal in a quiet, reassuring voice you may be able to get close enough to restrain it, at least temporarily. Be cautious if the animal is above ground level, or is cornered, because it may try to attack. If a dog has a lead attached to its collar or harness, attempt to take hold of that first; it is useful to put your foot on to the end of the lead before picking it up, to prevent the animal moving away. However, collars and leads are not always securely attached, and if old they may break, and so whether you have managed to secure the lead or not, the next step is to make a few preliminary stroking movements and then if possible to take a firm grasp of the scruff of the neck. Don't place your hands near the animal's mouth and avoid touching any obviously injured part. Watch the animal all the time and be prepared for it to struggle. Don't let go unless you absolutely have to because second attempts at securing it are usually much less successful.

If you are unable to gain the animal's confidence sufficiently to allow you to do this you may be able to apply a 'slip noose' made from a strong, flexible dog lead by passing the end with the clip through the looped end. Without sudden movements the slip noose should be dangled in front of the animal's head and slowly manipulated backwards to a position around its neck. A quick pull will then tighten it, and the lead should be held high to prevent the animal biting through it (Fig. 190). In an emergency a similar slip noose can be made by running a narrow trouser belt or dress belt through the buckle.

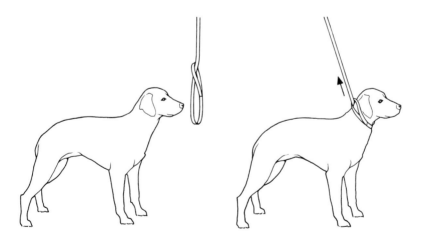

Figure 190 Applying a slip noose. A 'slip noose', made by passing the clip-end of a flexible dog lead through its loop, is dangled in front of the dog until it can be passed over the head. The 'slip noose' is then tightened round the neck by a quick pull on the lead. Keep the lead held high to prevent the dog from biting at or even through it

If all attempts at catching the animal fail, it may be necessary to telephone for professional assistance, e.g. from an animal welfare society, veterinary surgeon or the police. Then devices specially developed for catching stray animals will probably have to be employed.

Throughout this procedure do not chase the animal, which will be counter-productive, and do not bother to tempt it with food or drink since this wastes time. Animals seldom want to eat or drink in this situation and if they do so it may well interfere with subsequent treatment. Above all, do not trust the animal; if it is frightened, and even if you are the owner, it may still bite or try to escape.

The application of a muzzle, a purpose-made one if available, but otherwise an improvised tape muzzle, will allow a nervous and/or injured dog to be examined and treated without the risk of being bitten. A tape muzzle can be made from a 3–4-foot length of 2–3-inch wide tape or gauze bandage, or in an emergency from a tie or dress belt. The method of applying it is shown in Fig. 191.

AIRWAY – PROBLEMS WITH BREATHING

If a dog is breathing irregularly or with difficulty it is important to first ensure that its airway is unobstructed, and if it is not, or if clearing it produces no improvement, artificial respiration must be applied.

If breathing appears to have stopped completely and yet the animal is still alive, as determined by checking for its heartbeat, etc., artificial respiration is essential.

When breathing ceases, all the body organs, including the brain and the heart, are deprived of their normal continuous supply of oxygen. After a few minutes they will be unable to function normally, and then the animal will become unconscious and eventually die. Depriving the brain of oxygen for longer than four minutes produces irreversible damage. For this reason, in an emergency *artificial respiration should take precedence over every other procedure*. Once it is under way, attention can be directed towards other problems.

Ensuring a clear airway

Any foreign material in the air passage (respiratory tract) or in the lungs must first be removed. If the dog has drowned (usually because steep walls prevent its escape from the water in swimming pools, canal locks or even a rainwater butt) it is important to first wipe away any oil or mud from the mouth and nostrils and then to allow as much water as possible to drain from the lungs by holding the dog upside-down by its thighs. Check that there is nothing around the neck (e.g., collar, choke chain, rubber band) that is causing compression. Obstructions in the throat usually produce choking, coughing or gulping. Foreign bodies such as balls, bones

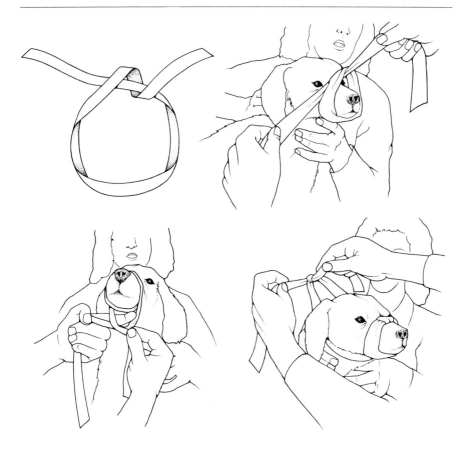

Figure 191 Applying a tape muzzle. First tie a half-hitch in a length of gauze bandage or strong tape, keeping the ends fairly long.

Then, with the dog firmly restrained, place the loop of tape around the dog's nose. By pulling the ends sideways draw the loop tight, closing the dog's jaws.

Immediately bring the ends downwards and cross the right to left and left to right underneath the lower jaw. Keep the tape tight and draw the ends backwards.

Finally, tie a tight bow at the back of the dog's head, making sure that the knot is in front of the dog's collar. Check that the tape-muzzle is secure

or broken teeth should, where possible, be quickly removed with the fingers or a pair of pliers, and if the problem is vomit, mucus or blood at the back of the throat it should be carefully wiped away. After opening the jaws and pulling the tongue well forward, the throat can be checked with a torch. In snub-nosed (brachycephalic) breeds of dog the soft palate can interfere with breathing, so the tongue should be pulled forward and the soft palate lifted.

Artificial respiration will be ineffective if there is a penetrating chest wound. Usually if this is present air can be heard passing through the opening and frothy blood appears from the wound. Blood-stained froth is also coughed up and appears at the mouth and nostrils. The wound in the chest must quickly be sealed by plugging the opening with a clean (and preferably sterile) piece of gauze or cotton wool, but in an emergency any other clean piece of material (e.g., a handkerchief) will suffice. Ideally this plug should then be covered by a further thick pad which is bandaged in place. However, the immediate aim is to obtain an airtight seal.

Checking for signs of life

If breathing appears to have stopped completely, i.e., there is no obvious rhythmical rise and fall of the chest in an animal which is showing no other sign of life, it is sensible to check for the heartbeat, because clearly artificial respiration will be of no value if the dog is already dead.

The normal heartbeat can be felt by placing the fingertips on the lower part of the chest wall on the left side, just behind the front leg (Fig. 192). In the case of a very small dog, the beat can be detected by placing a hand around the lower part of the chest between, or just behind, the forelegs. With fingers and thumb on opposite sides of the chest the heartbeat can be felt between them.

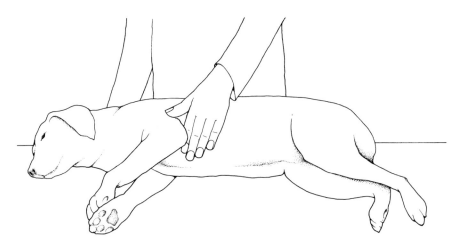

Figure 192 Finding the heartbeat. To detect the beat of your dog's heart, place your fingertips on the lower part of its chest wall, on the left side, just behind its front leg. In most non-obese animals the beat can be felt. If not, alter the position of the fingers slightly and try again

If a heartbeat can be felt, proceed immediately with artificial respiration.

The cessation of breathing may be caused by an existing lack of oxygen to the brain (asphyxia), as can occur if the animal is obliged to breathe smoke or carbon dioxide or suffers from an obstructed airway (as above). Also, following electrocution, the respiratory muscles can be paralysed.

Bear in mind that an unconscious animal can resemble a dead one in that there may be no movement for a long period, and during this time it may not respond to such stimuli as noise or movement. It should be appreciated that in death the eyes do not close automatically, so this cannot be used as a sign to distinguish it from unconsciousness. In both conditions the muscles relax and become limp, and relaxation of the sphincters of the bladder and the anus may permit urine and motions to be passed. Of course, in cases of death the body gradually becomes colder and after three to seven hours the muscles become rigid (rigor mortis).

Performing artificial respiration

With the dog lying flat on its side, remove its collar and make sure that its head and neck are stretched well forward. In the case of a drowned animal the head should be lower than the rest of the body, and if the animal has any wound that should be uppermost. Then both hands should be placed on the chest wall over the ribs, and firm downward pressure applied to expel the air from the lungs (Fig. 193). Excessive pressure should not be applied in a small dog because it is easy to produce crush injuries. The pressure is then immediately released, allowing the chest wall to expand again and the lungs to fill with air. This procedure should be repeated at approximately five-second intervals. Applying pressure more rapidly will not allow the oxygen to remain in the lungs sufficiently long for it to diffuse into the blood.

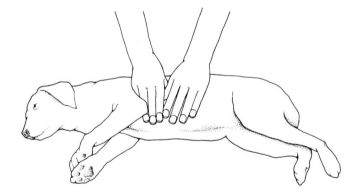

Figure 193 Artificial respiration. Remove any collar and, with the dog lying on its side, stretch the head and neck forwards. Place both hands over the rib-cage and press down firmly every five seconds, releasing the pressure immediately afterwards

Provided that the heart continues beating (at intervals a check should be made on the heartbeat and to ensure that the airway is still clear) artificial respiration can keep the animal alive almost indefinitely, certainly long enough for veterinary help to be obtained. If the dog is being transported to the veterinary surgeon's premises it will need to be continued throughout the journey.

Mouth-to-mouth resuscitation ('kiss of life') has been attempted in the dog, but because of the shape and size of its mouth it is usually not very effective. A better procedure is to close the animal's mouth with your hands and to blow firmly and regularly into its nose with your lips closely applied to the dog's nostrils. It is recommended that blowing should occupy about three seconds, followed by a two-second pause, and that this should be repeated continuously.

BLEEDING – CONTROLLING SEVERE HAEMORRHAGE

When a large blood vessel is severed the flow of blood is so considerable that any clot which begins to form is quickly washed away. This is especially likely when an artery is damaged, since it carries blood under high pressure, and indeed a separate spurt of blood can be seen with each heartbeat. The recommended method for controlling severe haemorrhage is to apply pressure to the cut end of the blood vessel using a *pressure bandage* (pressure pad, pressure wrap). A half-inch thick pad of clean (preferably sterile) absorbent material, e.g., cotton wool, or in an emergency a clean handkerchief, is positioned over the end of the blood vessel and firmly bandaged in place. The rough surface facilitates clot formation. A crêpe bandage, which gives more certain, even pressure, is preferred, but in an emergency a scarf, dress belt, handkerchief, etc., can be used. It is difficult to apply pressure pads too tightly except where the wound is around the neck. If a pad becomes soaked with blood another should be applied, usually tighter and on top of the original, until a veterinary surgeon can examine the animal. As an alternative, if no materials are readily available, the sides of a large wound can be tightly pressed together. Care should be taken not to push fragments of foreign bodies, such as fragments of glass, further into the wound and any obvious pieces should be removed.

To control severe haemorrhage while these materials are being found and the pressure bandage is being put on, direct pressure should be applied to the cut end of the bleeding vessel, or alternatively pressure applied to specific pressure points (Fig. 194). The three major pressure points are:

- On the inside of the thigh at the point where the femoral artery crosses the bone, to control bleeding from the lower part of the hind limb;
- On the inside of the foreleg just above the elbow joint, where the brachial artery crosses the humerus, to control bleeding from the lower part of the forelimb; and
- On the underside of the tail, where the coccygeal artery passes beneath the vertebrae to control bleeding from the tail.

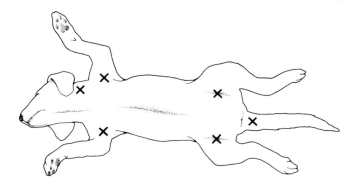

Figure 194 Pressure points. Temporary control of severe haemorrhage can be obtained by pressing with the fingers at the points illustrated, i.e., when there is bleeding from the tail, hind leg, foreleg and the head region

The use of a *tourniquet* to stop bleeding is not recommended for routine use because totally cutting off the blood supply to tissues can result in their death. For this reason applying pressure to pressure points, or the use of a tourniquet, should be for a maximum of 15 minutes at a time. An emergency tourniquet can be made from a narrow strip of cloth, 1–2 inches wide (e.g., a handkerchief or tie) or a supple dog lead or a thick rubber band, which is then firmly tied or clipped around a limb or the tail, *nearer* to the body of the animal than the wound. The efficiency of the tourniquet can be improved by tying a short stick (e.g., pencil, ruler) on top of the first knot and then twisting it round several times until the bleeding stops.

Special first-aid treatment is needed to arrest bleeding from sites around the head, although in all cases it is best if the animal is restrained lying down, with the site of haemorrhage uppermost, and is kept quiet. If bleeding is from the eyeball or from the nostrils, a pad of lint or cotton wool soaked in clean, cold water should be applied and held in place. Bandaging is not successful here, and attempts should not be made to insert materials into the nostrils. If the bleeding is around the mouth the head should be kept low to prevent clots forming at the back of the throat, and if the animal is unconscious blood and clots should be regularly wiped out of the mouth and throat. Haemorrhage on the inside of the lips or cheek may be controlled by squeezing the part between fingers and thumb. With bleeding from the ear flap, a pad of cotton wool should be placed either side of the flap, rather like a sandwich, and the ear flap then folded flat across the top of the head so that the ear tip points towards the opposite side. Then the flap should be firmly bandaged in position using a crêpe bandage passing around the head (not too tight). The same procedure can be used where there is bleeding from the ear canal, but it is advisable to place a small piece of cotton wool in the canal first to assist clotting. In all such cases the animal should be prevented from rubbing or pawing at the lesion or shaking its head. There is a pressure point on the carotid artery at the lower part of the neck in front of the foreleg which may help control bleeding from the head and neck, but it is difficult to find and control is often unsatisfactory.

Internal haemorrhage (i.e., bleeding into the chest or abdominal cavities or into hollow organs) may produce no visible sign until shock develops, unless blood is seen to pass out of the mouth or nostrils, or appears in the urine, vomit or motions. It usually follows crushing or severe impact injuries such as falls or kicks (e.g., by horses), and especially road traffic accidents. There is little that the lay person can do to control internal haemorrhage apart from keeping the animal quiet, treating for signs of shock if they appear (see later in this chapter) and wiping away any blood that might appear in the mouth or nostrils to keep the airway clear.

Minor haemorrhage, even if extensive (e.g., with abrasions – 'scrape' injuries), will stop on its own after a while as a blood clot forms. It can be facilitated by applying a fine powder such as talcum powder or flour, but clots which have already formed should not be disturbed because this may initiate fresh bleeding.

COLLAPSE, CONVULSIONS AND LOSS OF CONSCIOUSNESS (COMA)

Collapse is a non-specific term, but it encompasses conditions in which the animal is usually unconscious as well as some in which it is not.

Collapse follows the sudden onset of complete unconsciousness, as occurs in the following examples:

- Physical damage to the brain, i.e., with head injuries
- Heart failure, e.g. after exercise
- Stroke, i.e., blockage of blood supply to the brain by a blood clot
- Certain types of poisoning and snake bite (see Chapter 27)
- The effects of 'natural poisons' such as bacterial toxins and accumulated waste products, as occurs in cases of advanced renal disease or diabetes mellitus
- Heat stroke
- Hypothermia (exceptionally low body temperature)
- Asphyxia (interference with breathing)
- Most forms of severe shock, e.g., electrocution
- Convulsions, including those due to epilepsy.

Animals may also collapse but remain conscious in varying degrees when the same causes are present to a lesser extent, and also when animals are extremely weak (as with anaemia or with severe fluid losses) or are unable or unwilling to move because of great pain or mechanical difficulty, as with fractures, arthritis, spinal lesions and extensive muscle wasting.

Collapse

If possible, the dog should be left where it has collapsed, provided that it is not in a dangerous situation (e.g., in a roadway or an area full of gas, fumes or smoke) and that it will not become too cold. Otherwise the animal should be moved to a safe, sheltered place where there is plenty of fresh air, to avoid further injury. This should be done gently and carefully, especially if there are head or back injuries. It is best not to raise the animal's head or to prop it up, e.g., by putting a cushion under it, because saliva and possibly also blood and vomit can pass to the back of the throat and block the airway. Check that the animal is breathing satisfactorily (as above) and treat for haemorrhage, and for shock (see later), if necessary.

Loss of consciousness (coma)

It is important to check the dog's breathing; clearing the airway and applying artificial respiration if there appears to be difficulty or if breathing has temporarily stopped.

Where breathing appears to have ceased completely, other signs of life should be checked for as described earlier. Dogs that remain unconscious for 48 hours after an accident rarely recover.

Convulsions (seizures)

A convulsion (fit or seizure) is a series of violent, uncontrolled spasms of the muscles, accompanied by partial or complete loss of consciousness. It begins with a series of muscle tremors followed by muscle contractions – the animal falls to the ground and shows 'paddling' movements and champing of the jaws. Often the dog will salivate and froth at the mouth and pass motions and urine. The eyes are open and have a fixed stare. Upon recovery the dog may be dazed, confused and unable to see properly. Most convulsions last around three minutes (and no more than ten), but at times the convulsions can be continuous (*status epilepticus*).

The causes include:

- Convulsive poisons, e.g., organochlorines, lead and metaldehyde
- Brain tumours
- Head injuries
- Encephalitis and meningitis – inflammation of the brain (encephalitis) and its covering membranes (meningitis) can result from infection with canine distemper, rabies or pseudorabies
- Tetanus
- Diseases of the liver and kidneys, where there is accumulation of toxic substances in the body
- Low levels of blood sugar or calcium

An abnormally low blood calcium level (hypocalcaemia) may occur in the nursing bitch, and the convulsive state which develops is termed eclampsia.

The condition popularly known as *epilepsy* (responsible for epileptic fits) is believed to be due to an inherited defect in the metabolism of the nerve cells in the brain and is particularly common in Miniature and Toy Poodles and in Spaniels. The recurrent convulsions often appear when an animal is lying quietly or is waking from sleep. Usually they first appear between the ages of 6 and 18 months and attacks may be so short, mild or infrequent as not to justify continuous treatment with drugs.

A convulsing animal is best left where it has collapsed, unless it is in a dangerous situation (e.g., near to a fire), when it is best to lift or carefully pull the animal to safety. However, to avoid getting bitten in the process it is best to throw a blanket or coat over the dog first. The dog should be kept as quiet as possible and not disturbed; certainly do not attempt to hold it or give it anything by mouth. At home, objects (e.g., small pieces of furniture) should be moved away from the animal, the curtains drawn, gas or electric fires and the radio, television or hi-fi turned off.

Veterinary treatment should be arranged as soon as possible, and if the fit turns out to be continuous (as with poisons) there may be no alternative but to transport the animal in the convulsing state. This is best done by picking it up in a blanket and, still covered, restraining it as best you can on the back seat of a car. If, as is more usual, the fit ends spontaneously, the animal should remain confined in the same cool, dark room until sufficiently recovered to be taken to the veterinary surgeon or until a domicillary visit has been arranged. Any urine or faeces on the coat and any froth round the mouth can then be cleaned up. Usually animals will sleep for some time afterwards.

Often a warning that a fit is imminent is given by the animal showing a staring expression, salivation and licking of the lips, twitching and restlessness and jumping when handled or in response to a noise. Sometimes animals will hide or seek affection and at times *hysteria* precedes convulsions, in which the dog begins violent howling or barking and runs wildly about in a semi-conscious state, banging into objects and often passing urine and motions. Such behaviour may last for between a few minutes and several hours before the dog goes into convulsions, although at times the exhausted animal may simply go to sleep. Because the animal is frightened and does not recognise people it may easily bite in defence. It should therefore be confined to a quiet, darkened room or other area (e.g., garage or shed) where it can do minimum damage until the attack is over and then a veterinarian should be contacted.

SHOCK AND ITS TREATMENT

Shock is a clinical state in which there is an inadequate blood flow to the body tissues, which leads to a lack of oxygen, an accumulation of acids (acidosis) and ultimately death of the cells.

There are three major causes:

1. *Hypovolaemic shock*, resulting from a severely reduced volume of blood in the circulation. This occurs due to:

   Acute blood loss, i.e. severe haemorrhage
   The loss of large amounts of fluid from the body, e.g., diarrhoea and vomiting
   The movement of massive amounts of fluid from the circulation that occurs following crushing injuries, electrocution and the effects of corrosive poisons and burns

Internal bleeding can result in 'secondary shock' occurring some 4–6 hours after an injury.

2. *Cardiogenic shock*, due to reduced output of blood as occurs with many types of heart disease.
3. *Vasculogenic shock*, caused by the dilation of blood vessels. This may be the result of either
   (a) local release of toxic substances:
       Septic shock, as occurs in peritonitis or pyometra
       Anaphylactic shock, as occurs following insect stings, e.g., wasp stings or
   (b) effects on the autonomic nervous system following damage or depression, such as very deep anaesthesia (neurogenic shock); this type is rare in animals

Tell-tale signs of shock are as follows:

1. The animal is weak, collapsed and almost always lies down. It is often only semi-conscious and does not respond to stimulation.
2. Breathing is rapid (more than 15–20 breaths per minute in the case of a large dog and more than 30–40 per minute for a toy breed) and also shallow (panting).
3. The lips, gums and tongue appear pale and greyish and feel cold and clammy; the only exception being septic shock, when they may appear reddened.
4. The paws feel cold, even though the animal may be in warm surroundings, and it often trembles or shivers. The temperature, when taken, is found to be below normal. (Again, the only exception to this general rule is in septic shock, where fever may exist.)
5. The heart beats more rapidly (i.e., more than 80 beats per minute for a large breed and more than 140 beats per minute in a small one).
6. The pupils are dilated (i.e., wide open) and the eyes appear glazed and unseeing.
7. The dog *may* vomit.

Treatment of shock

Any problems with breathing or haemorrhage should be attended to first, as described previously. The dog should be maintained horizontal if possible to ensure effective blood circulation and it should be kept warm. If the animal is wet it should be dried and not allowed to lie directly on a cold or wet surface. Body heat should be conserved by covering it with blankets and giving it a *warm*-water bottle, but it should *not* be subjected to direct heating in front of a fire or a radiator, or on a heating pad. Although the aim is to maintain normal body temperature, animals survive moderate hypothermia better than overheating.

Generally a dog should be kept quiet and undisturbed, but if it is sufficiently conscious to drink and wishes to do so it can be given small amounts of warmed fluids (e.g., milk or water, possibly with added glucose). However, withhold liquids if the animal begins to vomit and never force them upon it. Certainly *avoid* giving any form of alcohol (e.g., brandy); this can prove beneficial in some types of shock, but it is also extremely harmful in others.

Shock is a serious condition and veterinary attention should be obtained quickly. An important part of treatment is fluid therapy, preferably given intravenously, to restore the circulating blood volume plus, in some cases, the use of specialised stimulant drugs.

SPECIFIC PROBLEMS IN FIRST AID

The general principles, as described above, apply in all cases, but at times there may be specific problems.

Fractures

A fracture is a break or crack in a bone caused by the application of physical force. Most fractures are the result of road accidents and in the dog the bones most often affected are the radius and ulna in the foreleg and the femur (thigh-bone) in the hind leg, but fractures of the pelvis and of the tibia and fibula (lower hind leg) are almost as common.

Fractures are described as 'open' or 'closed', depending on whether or not the skin surface is also disrupted and sometimes the broken end of the bone protrudes through the skin. Such 'open fractures' are more likely to become infected.

Fractures are also classified on the basis of the number of breaks, on the fragments of bone or on the damage done to the surrounding tissues, but from a first-aid point of view such classification is unimportant, the only type worth special mention being a '*greenstick fracture*', in which the bone is not completely broken but merely cracked and bent. This type usually occurs in young animals, where the bones are still flexible.

The six major signs of a fracture (not all of which need necessarily be present) are:

- Pain at the fracture site, which can make the animal resent handling and lead to shock,
- Swelling due to bleeding and bruising,
- An unnatural degree of movement of the lower part of a limb, or the tail, which may swing freely or even be dragged along,
- A loss of function so that the animal may be unable to move or to use the fractured part normally; consequently it may appear lame,
- Some deformity which may be obvious (e.g., shortening or twisting of a limb) or which may only become apparent when felt (such as a protrusion or sharp edge along the bone), *and*
- A grating noise (crepitus), which may be heard when the animal moves or is handled, due to the roughened broken ends of the bones moving against each other. This noise of course will be absent from a greenstick fracture.

If you are uncertain whether the shape of a bone is abnormal or whether there is undue movement present, it is always valuable to compare it with the same part on the other side of the body.

Treatment In addition to applying general principles of treatment, movement of the fractured bone should be limited to minimise pain and prevent further damage to surrounding tissues. The animal's movements should be severely restricted and the limb or other affected part not handled unnecessarily. It should be supported and immobilised as far as is possible, especially if the animal is being transported. A small dog may be carried in your arms or in a suitable container (e.g., a cardboard box); a large dog which is unable to walk should be lifted/pulled with the help of at least one other person on to an old coat or rug, moving the body first so that the legs trail, and without bending the spine. The animal can then be lifted and carried on this makeshift stretcher by two people holding opposite ends.

Fractures and dislocations of the spine may result in paralysis of the hindquarters, demonstrated by the animal's inability to move its hind legs. To avoid further damage it is important that such animals are lifted with the spine kept perfectly straight, e.g. on a flat board (an ironing board can be useful for this purpose). Regrettably the long-term outlook for such cases is poor.

Dislocations

A dislocation (luxation) occurs when one of the bones which forms a joint moves out of place. Usually considerable force is required for this to happen; it frequently follows a road accident, and dislocation of the hip joint is the most common example. Also the lower jaw can be dislocated so that the mouth will not close properly.

In some dogs a congenital defect in the stifle joint allows the patella (knee-cap) to dislocate very easily without undue force, especially in small breeds such as Miniature Poodles. However, dislocation of the patella can also occur if the animal twists suddenly when running at high speed. The patella slips to the inside of the leg, causing considerable pain and making the animal hold its leg up off the ground.

Although there are many features in common with fractures, useful distinguishing signs are that pain and swelling is usually confined to the region of a joint, movement is more restricted rather than increased and there is no grating sound or penetration of the skin. However, it can be difficult to make a complete distinction, especially when fractures occur near joints, and of course at times they may occur together. In general the same basic advice applies as in cases of fracture.

Burns and scalds

Burns are caused by dry heat (a flame or a hot surface) and scalds by hot liquids (boiling water or hot fat), but for practical purposes there is no need for this distinction – both can be described as *thermal burns*. Also, because blistering of the skin is not a feature in dogs, they are best not classified as first-, second- and third-degree burns but as superficial, partial-thickness and full-thickness burns. A major burn is a partial-thickness or full-thickness injury, which involves more than 20 per cent of the total body area.

Burns are painful, produce shock and later exude plasma. They may become infected and cause contraction of the skin due to scar formation.

Their immediate treatment involves dousing any flames and then applying cold water liberally to remove residual heat. Occasionally animals are actually on fire, sometimes as a result of a malicious act, and the flames should be smothered by covering the dog with a blanket, rug or coat. Water should be applied liberally for 5–10 minutes, and as soon as possible, using a spray attachment or hose, or simply poured or sponged over the area. Any constriction around the site (e.g., a collar) should be removed because the area will swell, but any burned material which is adherent to the skin should be cut away (if there is a large mass do this 3–4 inches away from the skin surface) and not simply pulled, which will also remove skin layers.

Old-fashioned remedies such as applying grease should be avoided.

It is not necessary to have a very high temperature to destroy skin cells; 70°C for one minute will suffice, and the cause can be apparently trivial, such as holding a hot hair clipper or hair dryer too close to the skin or contact with a hot-water bottle, something which is a risk if the animal is unconscious.

Sometimes when hot liquids have been splashed on to the back of a dog in the kitchen, it is not appreciated that scalding has occurred until a day or so later, when one or more scabs are felt when stroking or grooming the animal. In all cases the help of a veterinary surgeon should be sought, and obviously in cases of major burns this should be done immediately.

In addition to thermal burns, there are also freezer burns, chemical burns, electrical burns, sunburn, radiation burns and frictional burns (due to the heat of friction in addition to abrasion of the skin surface, e.g., when an animal is dragged along the ground or contacts a rapidly moving wheel).

Electrical burns are reputed to occur most often when puppies chew through a live flex. Also dogs occasionally fall on to the live conductor rail of an electric railway. The important general point is to ensure that the current is switched off before handling the animal, but with relatively low-voltage domestic supplies, i.e., up to 250 volts, use some dry material (e.g., a dry coat, blanket or rug) to cover the animal and provide insulation before pulling or pushing it away from the source of current. However, this should not be attempted with a high-voltage supply that is still functioning, as you may be electrocuted as well. In severe cases of electrocution, artificial respiration is essential to enable breathing to recommence.

Heatstroke

Heatstroke will affect dogs kept for a long period in extremely hot, poorly ventilated surroundings, especially if they are also without water. It most commonly arises when dogs are left in cars parked in direct sunlight during the summer, but it can also occur in dogs chained up in direct sunlight (i.e., without shade) or in small, enclosed rooms or buildings in hot weather.

The dog becomes unable to regulate its body temperature and this gradually rises. The dog becomes increasingly distressed and weak, panting rapidly and drooling saliva, with its tongue and lips initially appearing bright red. Eventually the animal will collapse, go into a coma and subsequently die.

Treatment First-aid treatment should attempt to lower the body temperature promptly by the application of cold water to the skin. The animal can be carefully placed in a bath or paddling pool, provided its head is kept above water, or water can be sprayed from a hose, or simply poured or sponged over the animal. Successful treatment is rewarded by an obvious improvement in breathing and the dog's appreciation of its surroundings within 5–10 minutes.

There is a danger of overdoing the cooling process because the normal temperature-regulating mechanism of the brain has been severely impaired and once the body temperature has begun to fall it may continue to do so.

In some cases it may be necessary to apply artificial respiration.

After cooling, the dog should be dried and left to rest in a cool place with adequate drinking water, but it is usually advisable to seek veterinary advice to ensure that there are no complicating factors.

Protrusion/prolapse of organs

In all cases where body organs are displaced and appear externally they should be covered with a suitably large piece of clean (preferably sterile) cloth that has been soaked in clean, cold water and wrung out. This should be held or bandaged in position to prevent further injury to, and drying out of, the organs until veterinary assistance is available. Do not apply any dry material which will stick and cause damage when removed. Fortunately such situations seldom arise, but when they do they appear very dramatic and frightening.

Following damage to the abdominal wall (usually in a road accident) the intestines may protrude. No attempt to push the contents back should be made, but the dog should be restrained, ideally on its back, otherwise on its side, and the organs covered as described above and then held in place with a wide bandage.

At times the eyeball may be forced out of its socket due to increased pressure behind it. This is more common in the short-nosed breeds of dogs after fights or accidents and may even happen in some breeds, e.g., the Pekingese, if the scruff of the neck is grasped too tightly. After prolapse the eyeball rapidly swells and cannot easily be replaced in its socket. Do not try to replace the displaced eyeball yourself, or allow the animal to rub it on the ground or with its paw. Hold the damp pad in position and try to keep the animal calm until it receives treatment.

On rare occasions other organs may protrude through normal body openings, usually as a result of excessive straining. These are:

- the rectum through the anus, usually in puppies with diarrhoea;
- the uterus through the vulva, in bitches during or after whelping;
- the urethra from the end of the penis in males, usually following masturbation; and
- the bladder through the vulva of bitches.

In all these cases the prolapsed organ appears as a reddish mass at the respective body opening, often with some degree of bleeding. Again the organ should be covered with a damp cloth, and the animal prevented from interfering with the area while veterinary attention is obtained.

27

POISONING

A poison is regarded as any substance which, after entering an animal's body in sufficient quantity, will injure the animal's health and even cause its death. Fortunately poisoning is not common in the dog; it has been estimated that only one in a thousand dogs presented for treatment has been poisoned and that only one dog in every 2,500 will be poisoned at some time during its life, most often before it reaches two years old. Unfortunately about one in eight of such cases end fatally.

Many illnesses that owners suspect are due to poisoning are subsequently found to have another cause, in particular the early stage of an infectious disease. Nevertheless, when a pet animal suddenly develops signs of illness many owners suspect that it is being deliberately poisoned by someone bearing a grudge. Deliberate malicious poisoning of pets does, of course, occur from time to time, often as a series of cases in one particular area, but then the dog usually consumes far more poison (disguised in some tasty morsel) than is commonly the case with accidental poisoning. As a result the signs that appear do so much earlier, are of greater intensity, and are more likely to be fatal.

In Britain, dogs may also eat poisoned bait laid illegally to kill birds of prey, crows and other wildlife. The practice is widespread, with alpha-chloralose, mevinphos (Phosdrin) strychnine and paraquat being the poisons most commonly used. In Britain, where strychnine is intended to be limited to the destruction of moles by farmers, its sale is restricted. But in those countries, e.g., France, the Netherlands, Mexico and the USA, where it is freely available as a rodenticide it has been far and away the most important single cause of poisoning, although recently other pesticides have become more important in developed countries.

SOURCES AND ROUTES OF POISONING

There are several thousand poisonous substance in existence, including such commonly used items as disinfectants, herbicides (weedkillers), fungicides and pesticides (rat poisons, and slug and insect killers, including moth balls), coloured pencils and crayons, anti-freeze, lead preparations (putty, solder, linoleum), paint thinners, fuel oils, shoe polish, creosote, oven cleaners and most drugs in excessive amounts (including patent medicines). Poisoning can also be due to snake and toad venoms and to bee, wasp and hornet stings and to plants and bulbs.

Most poisons are taken orally by dogs because they are often greedy and inclined to scavenge; because of their hunting instinct, which causes them to catch and eat animals (rodents and birds) which have themselves been poisoned (*secondary poisoning*); and, particularly in the case of puppies, because they ingest material out of curiosity. Some animals even develop a liking for certain substances, e.g., slug pellets, searching them out to eat them. Sometimes dogs will chew at a plastic container which is holding, or used to contain, a toxic substance. Where drinking water is not provided they may resort to consuming water containing a poison, e.g., from a bucket containing a diluted phenolic disinfectant, such as Jeyes Fluid, or water containing antifreeze (ethylene glycol), which has been drained from a car radiator. Also, having picked up a toxic substance on their coat (e.g., a herbicide from long grass or an insecticide deliberately applied by the owner), or on their paws (e.g., having walked through creosote or paraffin splashes) they may, in grooming themselves, consume a dangerous amount.

Occasionally a poisonous gas or vapour may be inhaled, most commonly carbon monoxide. Usually this is produced by a solid fuel- or oil-burning stove which is not combusting properly in the area (usually a kitchen) where the dog sleeps. Carbon monoxide is also present in the exhaust gases of motor vehicles and may poison a dog hiding in a garage if the garage doors are closed and the vehicle's engine is kept running. Natural gas contains *no* carbon monoxide, unlike coal gas (town gas), which it has entirely replaced in Great Britain. Also toxic are the vapours of organic solvents (e.g., in glues, dry cleaning fluids or fire extinguishers) used in poorly ventilated areas, and the smoke and fumes from burning materials, including fat (producing acrolein), but especially furniture foam, which releases many dangerous chemicals.

Very rarely a poison may be absorbed through the skin.

ESTABLISHING THAT POISONING HAS OCCURRED

At times the evidence for poisoning is beyond dispute; the dog may actually be seen consuming material which is known, or subsequently discovered, to be poisonous. Knowing the nature of the poison may greatly assist in the subsequent treatment.

Alternatively there may be strong circumstantial evidence if the dog develops signs of poisoning and could have access to a poison; a toxic spray might have been used in the neighbourhood or a rat bait laid.

Animals that are allowed to wander freely have a greater opportunity for contacting poisons without their owners' knowledge. It may be that the dog has been dosed with a drug or its coat treated with an insecticide, or drugs used by members of the household may have been interfered with. Examination of the dog may show signs consistent with poisoning, such as burning and blistering around the lips and in the mouth caused by a corrosive poison, a strange smell on the breath, a residue of material around the mouth and, especially important, the dribbling of coloured saliva. Many rat and slug baits are coloured, and this observation may be valuable in identifying the poison (Table 23).

Contrary to popular expectation, the analysis of samples of blood, urine, vomit, etc., from the affected animal may be of limited value, since signs of poisoning are usually of rapid onset and cases resolve within a short time, i.e., a poisoned dog will frequently be dead or better within 24 hours. The unavoidable delay in obtaining the results of a toxicological analysis means that it is usually of little value in treatment, though it may assist the treatment or prevention of poisoning in other animals. Also there is no 'blanket' test for poisoning and each individual test has to be paid for. The cost of estimating the concentration of a single, previously named, common poison (such as metaldehyde or lead) is between £15 and £35 and examination for a more unusual poison can cost £45 or more. The cost of a search for all possible poisonous substances would therefore prove prohibitive and may yield a negative result. Clearly, before an analysis is undertaken, there needs to be more than just a vague suspicion that poisoning has occurred.

SIGNS OF POISONING

Corrosive poisons are a special case because they kill from *shock*, as a result of the enormous amount of damage they inflict on the body tissues, usually the digestive system, and the consequent pain. When, as is usually the case, the poison has been ingested, animals show signs of intense pain, including rubbing or pawing at the mouth, followed by rapid panting and collapse (signs of shock). As mentioned previously, there may be evidence of burning and blistering in and around the mouth and a tell-tale odour of the particular corrosive substance.

Corrosive poisons include substances such as:

Acids and alkalis   Ammonia; quicklime; oven cleaning sticks and other de-greasing agents; paint strippers; dishwashing powder

Phenolic compounds   Creosote; lysol; Jeyes' Fluid and similar types of disinfectant

Table 24 Substances responsible for poisoning in dogs

Poison	Source	digestive signs	breathing difficulty	inco-ordination	convulsions	coma	Notes
		Signs					
Acrolein**	Burning fat			+			
Alphachloralose	Rodenticide			+	+	+	Light green*
Antu**	Rodenticide	+	+				
Arsenic**	Fruit sprays, wood preservatives	+		+			
Barbiturates	Sleeping tablets					+	
Calciferol	Rhodenticide	+				+	Brown*
Carbon monoxide	Faulty stoves, vehicle exhausts			+	+	+	
Chlorate	Weedkiller	+			(+)		
Corrosives	Acids, alkalis, phenols, bleach, petrol products	+		(+)	(+)		
Cyanide	Industrial uses, killing wasps			+	+	+	
Ethylene glycol	Antifreeze	+		+		+	
Fluroacetate	Rodenticide	+	+	+	+	+	
Lead	Paint, putty, solder, weights (curtains & fishing), lino	+		+	+		
Metaldehyde	Slug pellets		+	+	+	(+)	
Organochlorines	Insecticides, rodenticides			+	+	+	Pink*
Organophosphates & carbamates	Herbicides, pesticides parasiticides	+	+	+	+	+	
Paraquet, diquat	Weedkillers	+	+				
Plants	Bulbs, leaves, etc.	+		(+)	(+)		
Strychnine	Mole bait, 'illegal' baits			+	+		
Warfarin, difenacoum bromadiolone, etc.	Rodenticide						Blue* (anticoagulant)
Zinc phosphide**	Rodenticide	+	+	+	(+)	+	
2.4.D. & 2.4.5.T.	Weedkillers	+		+	+	+	

*These colours are used in 'Rentokil' products **Not often encountered

Petroleum products Petrol (gasoline); paraffin (kerosene); diesel oil; white spirit (paint thinners)

Bleach

Other types of poison damage the dog's health by interfering with some essential metabolic function and this may cause the animal's death. They generally produce one of four signs:

1. *Digestive signs*, such as abdominal pain, vomiting and diarrhoea,
2. *Difficulty in breathing*,
3. *Nervous signs*, which can vary in their nature and intensity from staggering, excitement and muscular tremors (twitching), to convulsions, paralysis and coma; *and*
4. *Depression*, including a loss of appetite. Depression also often follows the other signs, and precedes death in the case of slow-acting poisons.

However, the signs produced by a particular poison can vary considerably in different individuals, and in the case of some poisons there is no single sign that occurs in every instance; a fact which greatly complicates diagnosis.

Some rat poisons produce other types of signs; warfarin and similar anticoagulant poisons cause internal haemorrhages and consequently result in anaemia; thallium (seldom used nowadays) can produce hair loss and alphachloralose has an anaesthetic effect and causes the animal to become very cold (hypothermic).

It should be emphasised that *all* of these signs can be produced by conditions *other than* poisoning.

Table 24 lists some of the more common poisons and groups of poisons, together with their sources and the major signs that develop.

Plant poisoning is not common in dogs (compared with farm animals and horses), but a number of plants are toxic and they may be consumed experimentally or out of greed. Generally they irritate the digestive tract, causing vomiting and diarrhoea, but some also, or only, produce nervous signs. Important examples include the bulbs of spring flowers (crocus, daffodil, hyacinth, narcissus, snowdrop and tulip) and of gladiolus, the berries of holly and mistletoe, the leaves and flowers of the delphinium, Christmas daisy, hydrangea and rhododendron, the leaves of box, laurel and yew, the seeds of bluebell, sweet pea and wisteria and the whole plant in the case of clematis, lily-of-the-valley, ivy, lupin and oleander.

Problems can also arise if dogs consume poisonous fungi, i.e., members of the mushroom/toadstool family, or the toxins that are produced by algae blooming on stagnant ponds in hot weather ('blue-green algae') or by moulds growing on foodstuffs (aflatoxins). More often foods contain preformed toxins of *bacterial* origin (true 'food poisoning'), which usually result from contamination with, and growth of, staphylococci, though on rare occasions *Clostridium botulinum* in canned products has been responsible for the fatal disease of botulism. Food may, of course, become contaminated with other poisons, especially those used to protect it from the attentions of rats or insects during storage, but poisoning can also be due to certain preservatives and 'improvers', to the excessive consumption of salt or chocolate (containing theobromine) and to the ingestion of horse-meat from an animal which has been put to sleep and which still contains significant amounts of the anaesthetic agent (barbiturate or chloral hydrate) used for euthanasia.

FIRST AID TREATMENT OF POISONING

Poisoning by mouth

The treatment for oral corrosive poisoning is quite different from that for other types of poisoning in that the animal should *not* be made to vomit. This is to avoid the corrosive causing further tissue damage and shock as it passes back again from the stomach. Unfortunately, however, vomiting *may* arise spontaneously as a result of the irritation produced by the corrosive. Consequently the first thing to do is to look at the animal's mouth for the characteristic signs of corrosive poisoning – burning and blistering (with yellow-grey areas on the lips, gums and tongue), pawing at the mouth, increased salivation and often a characteristic odour (e.g., of creosote or disinfectant).

Corrosive poisons If the signs of corrosive poisoning are present, and the dog is not collapsed or unconscious, as much of the chemical as possible should be washed from around and inside the mouth. In a conscious animal wipe around the mouth with a pad soaked in water and trickle water into the mouth using a disposable syringe, if available, or a small bottle or other utensil such as a jug or a small teapot. It will be beneficial whether the animal splutters the water out or swallows it. Indeed, rather than attempting to neutralise such poisons, the best policy is usually to dilute them in the stomach with plenty of water or milk. One real danger is of causing liquid to pass down into the lungs, resulting in the development of an inhalation pneumonia.

  If the animal is already unconscious and is perhaps showing difficulty in breathing, treat as for shock (page 454) and administer artificial respiration (page 447). The help of a veterinary surgeon should be obtained as soon as possible.

Other poisons In the case of all other consumed poisons, provided that the animal is still conscious and is not having convulsions, the first thing to do is to administer a substance which will make the animal vomit. Ideally this should be done within half an hour of the poison being taken and certainly within two hours if it is to be of any value. As soon as possible, even before the emetic substance has taken effect, the animal should be taken to a veterinary surgeon.

The most reliable method available in the home for making a dog vomit is to administer a crystal of washing soda (sodium carbonate) the size of a hazelnut (thumb-nail size). This should be given in the same way as a tablet (Fig. 195). An alternative is to give a large crystal of rock salt.

Figure 195 Administering solid medication, e.g., tablets, capsules or a crystal of washing soda. Position the dog in a good light, ideally with someone holding it. Place fingers and thumb at either side of the upper jaw.

Press just behind the upper canine teeth while pulling the jaw upwards and the lower jaw down with the hand holding the crystal or tablets etc.

Place the crystal or tablets etc as far back in the throat as possible. Use your fingers or the flat end of a pencil to push it over the back of the tongue.

Then close the dog's mouth and, with its head inclined upwards, gently stroke its throat until it gulps and licks its nose

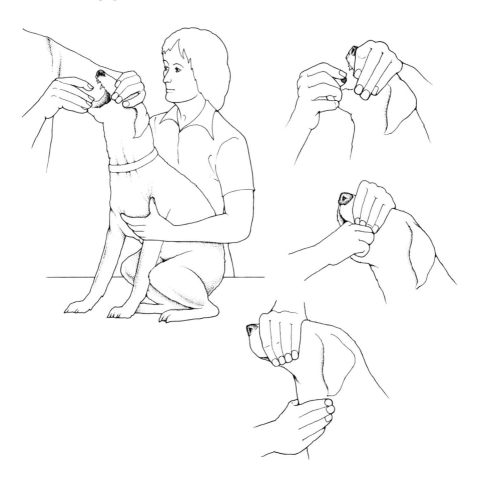

Giving liquids to cause vomiting is often less successful, but the following substances might be tried if they are available and washing soda is not. The doses recommended are for a medium-sized (30–35 lb) dog and should be scaled up or down accordingly.

1. Hydrogen peroxide; half a 5 ml teaspoonful of the usual 6 per cent (20 vol) solution, or one 5 ml teaspoonful of a 3 per cent (10 vol) solution.
2. A strong salt solution; half a level teaspoonful of salt in as little warm water as will dissolve it.
3. Mustard powder (English mustard); half a level teaspoonful of the powder mixed in half a teacup of warm water.
4. Syrup of ipecac; one tablespoonful (15 ml).

In all cases, administration will be simpler using a disposable syringe (Fig. 196) if available, a small plastic bottle or other utensil such as a jug or small teapot. Do *not* try to give an unconscious or convulsing animal *anything* by mouth.

If vomiting is going to occur it usually does so within 10–15 minutes of giving the emetic. It is worth taking a specimen of the vomit to the veterinary surgeon (preferably in a clean glass jar with a lid) *in case* an analysis is judged likely to be useful. If nothing happens after dosing do *not* give further amounts. If the vet is unable to visit and you have to take the animal to his or her premises, it could be that vomiting will take place on the journey. An animal that is very excited may be transported after being securely wrapped in a blanket, or at times even muzzling may be required. If the animal is unconscious you may need to give artificial respiration and/or treatment for shock, and if it is having a fit it should be dealt with as described on page 451. Then you might consider moving it.

If you know the name of the poison or medicinal product that the animal has eaten, tell the vet, and if you have the packet, take that along with you. Poison centres in human hospitals can help identify the poisonous components in various products. Otherwise take a sample of the poison (or suspected poison); it is possible that it can be identified.

Occasionally a dog will consume a quantity of human contraceptive pills but experience has shown that these appear not to produce ill-effects and treatment is not essential. It should, however, be appreciated that drugs that are generally used without problems in humans, e.g., *aspirin* and *paracetamol*, can cause poisoning in dogs, especially small breeds, if the normal human dose is given to them.

Inhaled poisons

If the dog has been poisoned by inhaling toxic fumes, smoke or gases, it is essential to move it immediately into fresh air and if necessary to give artificial respiration while waiting for veterinary attention. Do take care, however, that you are not also overcome by the same toxic vapours.

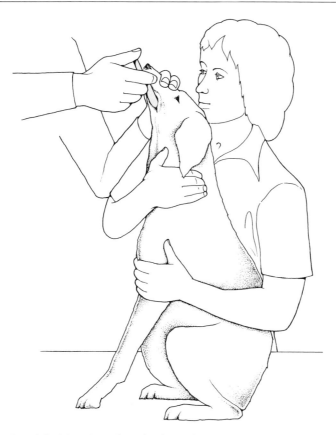

Figure 196 Administering a liquid. This technique is used for liquid medicines such as drug solutions or syrups. Hold the dog's head so that its mouth is shut and its nose is pointed slightly upwards. Place the end of a 5ml syringe between its lips at the side of the mouth and then very slowly drip the liquid out

Corrosive poisons on the skin

Diesel oil, creosote and phenolic disinfectants are corrosive and should be removed quickly. If veterinary assistance is not immediately available, as much of the material as possible should be wiped away with rags or absorbent paper towels and then 'Swarfega', or failing that, cooking fat, applied thoroughly before being washed away using soap or dishwashing liquid plus plenty of warm water. If the eyes or mouth are involved, rinse those areas thoroughly. On no account use liquids such as paint stripper or turpentine on the skin because these are themselves corrosive and will cause further damage.

Small areas of hair covered with tar (which is corrosive) or oil-based paints can be cut off (allow the paint to dry first), but more extensive deposits of tar may need to be softened first with cooking fat, lard, margarine, vegetable oil or liquid paraffin, sometimes for several hours, before being washed out with detergent (dishwashing liquid) and lukewarm water. While this softening process is going on, it is advisable to cover the area with a pad of gauze and to bandage it in place to prevent the animal licking at the toxic material.

A thorough shampooing is required afterwards to remove any residues which might be licked from the coat.

While carrying out these procedures it is desirable that all those involved wear protective gloves.

VETERINARY ATTENTION FOR POISONING

At the vet's, the animal may be given an injection to stimulate vomiting, if this has not already occurred, and/or have the stomach washed out via a stomach tube (gastric lavage). Ideally this should occur within two hours of consuming the poison. To do this effectively the animal, if not already unconscious, will probably need to be anaesthetised. After washing, substances which bind to certain poisons (e.g., activated charcoal or Fuller's earth) can be placed in the stomach to limit the absorption of any residual poison, particularly that which has already passed into the small intestine. Likewise saline laxatives (e.g., Epsom salts) and enemas, by causing the bowel to be evacuated, can reduce absorption of the poison.

Supportive treatment, in the form of fluid therapy and drugs to control particular signs (especially pain and shock), may be administered. If necessary, oxygen will be given and/or artificial respiration applied using an anaesthetic machine and pump.

In some cases of poisoning, though by no means all, there may be a specific *antidote* which can be administered to assist in reversing the effects of the poison. In the case of Warfarin, an injection of vitamin K counteracts its anti-coagulant effect; with alphachloralose, simply keeping the animal warm until its anaesthetic effects wears off is usually all that is required (though initially this poison *may* have an excitement phase).

PREVENTION OF POISONING

To minimise the risk of a dog being poisoned requires attention to the following points.

1. Do not administer any drug which has not been supplied, prescribed, recommended or approved by your veterinary surgeon. Cases are known of owners sharing addictive drugs with their pets, sometimes with disastrous consequences. All preparations for human use should be kept out of the animal's reach.

2. Keep dogs away from poisonous substances. Despite the fact that in Britain repellants have been added to all metaldehyde slug baits since 1980, some dogs can develop a craving for it and seek it out. Easy access to slug and rat poisons should be avoided by siting the poison carefully or covering it. It is recommended that rat poison be placed in the middle of a length of narrow drainpipe or under a heavy paving stone raised a couple of inches above the ground using pieces of brick at each corner.

   Any dead or dying rodents or pigeons should be removed before a dog can find and eat them, and dogs should be kept off areas of the garden and other land during and after treatment with weedkillers. Spilled liquids such as creosote, paraffin, etc., should be cleaned up before the dog walks in them.

   Dogs should be kept well out of the way when spraying with horticultural sprays and care taken that they do not come into contact with open containers of liquid herbicides or pesticides in either a diluted or undiluted form. Diluted solutions of most pesticides deteriorate with storage and it is officially recommended that any surplus spray solution should be disposed of.

   Dogs eating grass sprayed with paraquat are stated not to be at risk since the chemical becomes so tightly bound to plant tissue that it is not removed during digestion. The consumption of concentrated paraquat, usually in the form of illegal poisoned baits intended for foxes, is responsible for most casualties.

3. Do not apply an excessive amount of any anti-parasitic preparation to the coat of the animal in the form of powders or sprays, and try to avoid the dog licking its coat immediately after application. Powders should be brushed out after 30 minutes. *Never* apply fly sprays.

4. Any antiseptic solution applied to the mammary gland of a suckling bitch should be rinsed off before the puppies feed again. Hexachlorophene poisoning has followed failure to do this.

5. Ensure that the dog always has drinking water available to it, otherwise it may seek out other sources containing toxic chemicals.

6. Do not treat any wooden kennels or beds or wickerwork baskets for dogs with wood preservatives or paint them with lead-based paints. All dogs, particularly puppies, are likely to chew at painted woodwork and the sweet taste of lead may encourage them in this habit.

7. Discourage or prevent dogs from eating house plants, flower bulbs and plants and shrubs in the garden.

8. If poisoning has *already* occurred, make sure that the source of the poison is removed or isolated, wherever possible, to avoid the same thing happening again.

VENOMS

Snake bite

In Britain the only naturally occurring poisonous snake is the common adder or viper (*Vipera berus*), which is particuarly common on dry heaths and moors and sunny areas of hills, particularly in the southern part of the country. Usually the snake is basking in the sun and only attacks in self-defence when a dog blunders into it or, more often, begins to investigate or attack it. For this reason dogs generally get bitten on the head and neck, less often on the limbs.

The injected venom causes a severe swelling, in the centre of which are two small puncture wounds where the fangs have penetrated. Because the actual biting by the snake is seldom witnessed, the presence of these signs is significant in an animal which roams the countryside or has been taken for a walk there. The venom produces excitement, trembling, staggering and shock, with the later appearance of depression, collapse and even death. Consequently treatment should be given promptly.

The animal should be taken to a veterinary surgeon as soon as possible for treatment, e.g., administration of antivenom or other drugs. In the meantime the dog should be kept as quiet as possible and exercise reduced to a minimum. In the case of a small dog it would be desirable to carry it rather than have it walk any further. It is helpful for the wound to be cleaned with soap and water (provided this does not introduce an unnecessary delay). Procedures such as applying a light tourniquet around the limb above the bite, applying an ice pack around the site or incising the puncture wounds and sucking out the venom should only be attempted if there is likely to be an excessive delay in obtaining veterinary attention.

Bites from the non-venomous grass snake may occur if it is attacked, but there is little swelling of the bitten part and the clinical signs caused by adder venom do not occur. The bite has a typical U-shaped appearance and the two prominent fang marks are not seen. However, the teeth can be infected with bacteria, so the wound should be cleaned thoroughly.

Toad venom

The common toad in Britain (*Bufo vulgaris*), like other toads, secretes a venom over its skin surface. This passes into the mouth of any dog which picks up the creature to play with it. The venom contains a number of toxic substances (including bufotoxin) which, within a few minutes, produce intense irritation in the mouth and salivation, causing the animal to be distressed and to paw at its mouth. Long 'strings' of thick saliva hang from its jaws.

The mouth should be thoroughly washed with water. A more effective solution, although not essential, is a 2 per cent sodium bicarbonate solution, which can be produced by dissolving one level teaspoonful of sodium bicarbonate in a tumbler of tepid water. Water or sodium bicarbonate solution can be introduced through a number of utensils, e.g. a small bottle or small teapot, but the most convenient to use is a disposable syringe (see Fig. 196). Most animals recover, even without treatment.

Wasp, hornet and bee stings

In most dogs single stings produce intense local pain with some swelling but no serious effect. Many stings are in, or around, the mouth as the animal catches or tries to catch the insect, and the pain results in it pawing at its mouth and showing increased salivation.

Attention is normally drawn to stings on the skin by continual licking of the site. Multiple stings obviously increase the amount of pain and in rare cases of several hundred stings, death may ensue.

Serious consequences can also arise if:
1. the tongue is stung, because it can swell to the extent that it blocks the passage of air through the back of the throat, *or*
2. the individual animal is allergic to the sting and goes into a state of severe shock and collapse (anaphylactic shock) requiring treatment along the lines indicated on page 454.

The site of the sting should be examined and if the sting is still present, looking like a large black splinter, it should be carefully removed with a pair of tweezers. It is usually present following bee stings, but *not* with wasp or hornet stings. The application of an antihistamine cream is valuable. If the sting is in the mouth, the mouth should be washed out with a sodium bicarbonate solution (as above), again best introduced using a disposable syringe.

If there is much swelling in the mouth and/or difficulty in breathing, or if the animal appears shocked and collapsed, a veterinary surgeon should be contacted immediately. A dog that appears to be choking should be laid on its side and the tongue grasped and pulled well forward out of the mouth. Artificial respiration may be required.

28

NOTES ON CANCER IN THE DOG

DEFINITIONS

Cancer in the *Pocket Oxford Dictionary* is defined as a malignant tumour spreading indefinitely and tending to recur when removed. Cancer is also the name of the crab in the zodiac, and the crab with its grasping invasive claws has often been used in illustrations of malignant disease. If we look up 'tumour' in the dictionary, we find it is a swelling in some part of the body due to morbid growth. It is important to recognise that 'morbid' means diseased – there are from time to time swellings in the dog that are perfectly normal and certainly not tumours. Perhaps the most commonly noticeable normal swelling is in the vulva of the bitch at the time of oestrus (coming into season). Some other swellings which are not normal are also not classified as tumours, e.g., umbilical hernias.

Tumours can be benign, when the abnormal new growth often referred to as neoplasia remains local, does not deeply invade the surrounding tissue and does not spread to other parts of the body. Malignant tumours are more virulent and these cancers not only invade locally, but clumps of cells can break off and spread to other parts of the body. When the cells enter the bloodstream they frequently lodge and grow into new tumours in the lungs, but many other organs can also be affected. This process is known as metastasis.

INCIDENCE

Cancer is unfortunately just as common in dogs as it is in people, and it is likely that as many as one in four dogs will develop a benign or malignant neoplasm.

Veterinary surgeons see more cases of cancer now than they did 30 years ago. Because of the development of effective vaccines against many of the major infectious diseases of dogs, such as distemper or parvovirus disease, more dogs are living longer than previously, and as they become older they are more likely to develop cancer. Some cancers such as leukaemia can occur in young dogs as is also the case with children, but the large majority of cases occur in middle aged and older animals.

There is some evidence that pure-bred dogs get slightly more cancer than mongrel dogs. Among the various breeds of dogs the toy breeds are lucky in that they seldom develop bone tumours – these tumours are much more common in the giant breeds such as the Great Dane and the Irish Wolfhound. However, the Dachshund, which is a small breed, appears to have a rather higher incidence of mammary tumours than the average for all breeds. The Bull Mastiff has a very high incidence of lymphosarcoma, a malignant disease of the lymph glands related to leukaemia. In the Boxer a tumour developing from cells in the deeper layers of the skin, the mast cell tumour, is all too common. Flat-coated Retrievers appear to have a higher incidence of skin sarcomas and mouth tumours than the average for all breeds. The generalised form of a skin tumour called intracutaneous cornifying epithelioma is particularly seen in the Norwegian Elkhound.

CANCER PREVENTION

It has been reported that in the USA some strains of St Bernard have a higher incidence of bone tumours (osteosarcoma) than other strains of St Bernard; similar observations have been made for Great Danes in Holland. It may, in time, be possible to breed from low-incidence strains and reduce the cancer incidence.

The most dramatic reduction in cancer which is possible relates to mammary tumours in the bitch. If bitches are spayed (*ovariectomised*) before the first or second season, they will not develop mammary tumours, and even up to two and a half years of age ovariectomy will have a sparing effect on mammary tumours. In older bitches there is no obvious effect. Mammary tumour incidence is falling in the USA, where spaying is common, compared with Britain, where spaying is less common, and Sweden, where spaying is not allowed. Mammary tumours in Guide Dogs for the Blind in Britain are unknown due to early spaying.

SIGNS OF CANCER

Signs of cancer are very variable and diseases other than cancer can produce some similar signs. However, if your dog exhibits any of the following signs it is worthwhile contacting your veterinary surgeon without delay.:

1. Abnormal swellings that continue to grow. The rate of growth of an abnormal swelling may be important. When growth is rapid the tumour is more likely to be malignant and veterinary advice should be sought immediately.

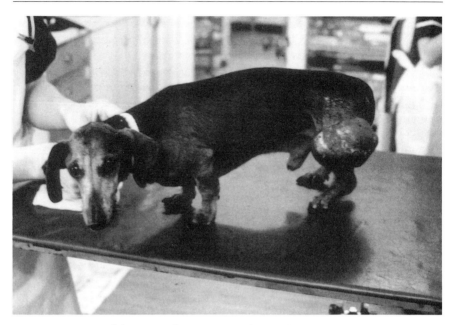

Figure 197 One of the signs of cancer is an abnormal swelling that continues to grow

2. Sores that do not heal.
3. Bleeding from the mouth, nose or rectum.

In advanced cases of cancer the dog may show anaemia, weight loss and a generalised weakness. When a tumour has spread to the lungs, there is frequently an increase in respiratory rate and sometimes a cough.

DIAGNOSIS AND PROGNOSIS

As noted the signs of cancer are very variable and malignancy may not at first be suspected in a sick dog; only after very thorough clinical and radiographical examination plus laboratory tests is a diagnosis obtained. In other cases diagnosis is much easier; a firm, hard swelling in the mammary gland is much more likely to be a tumour than mastitis – tumours are common in the bitch mammary gland and mastitis is rare. It is, however, useful to get an exact diagnosis of the suspected neoplasm, as when this is known more precise and hopefully more successful treatment can be given. With this end in view your veterinary surgeon will attack the problem in one of two ways. Where the swelling to the trained veterinary eye appears to be a tumour, it can be removed surgically without too much difficulty, e.g., in the skin or mammary gland. A representative piece of the tissue is then submitted to a diagnostic laboratory. The cost of the laboratory examination is well worthwhile as without this basic information the prognosis or likely outcome of the case cannot be assessed accurately. Where the suspected tumour is inoperable or very difficult to remove completely, a biopsy is made, i.e., a small piece of the abnormal tissue is excised and examined under the microscope in the laboratory after appropriate staining techniques have been carried out. Specially trained histopathologists will then decide on the tumour type.

Your veterinary surgeon will receive this pathology report usually within one week and the news may be good or bad. Good news would be that your veterinary surgeon thinks that all the tumour has been removed surgically and the laboratory report indicates that it is benign; bad news would be that the tumour is inoperable and the laboratory report indicates that it is very malignant and likely to metastasise, i.e., spread to other parts of the body. Even in this latter event, however, useful therapy can be given in selected cases, in other cases it may be decided that euthanasia may be necessary to prevent further suffering.

SURGERY

Surgery is the main line of attack against cancer, both in people and in animals. Very small skin tumours can be excised under local anaesthesia, but for most cancer surgery a general anaesthetic is required. Modern anaesthetic methods have greatly reduced the risks associated with surgery and old animals can be successfully treated, provided they are in reasonably good health, e.g., heart, lungs and kidney function are satisfactory. Surgery is usually undertaken with the object of cure, that is total removal of the cancer without recurrence or development elsewhere in the body, but in some malignant tumours the chances of complete cure may be poor, and additional to surgery other treatments such as cryotherapy, radiotherapy or chemotherapy may be given.

Whether to operate or not is the question to be discussed with your veterinary surgeon, who will consider the nature of the tumour where known, i.e., benign or malignant, the magnitude of the operation and the general health of the dog. The general health of the dog is much more important than the age of the dog; some dogs look old at nine years and others appear young at 14 years. In general, it is wise to excise suspect tumours soon after diagnosis, especially if they are known to be growing quickly. In the case of malignant tumours of the mammary gland or mouth the larger the tumour the poorer the outlook (prognosis) for the dog. A wait and see policy can often result in serious problems and is only justified on a few occasions. One example would be in the case of an old, fat Labrador with a poor heart and several fat tumours (lipomas), where it would then be sensible to delay operation. Operating would have to be done, however, if one of the tumours was causing a serious problem, e.g., interfering with swallowing or breathing or becoming ulcerated because it was in a position where the dog injured it when moving or lying down.

The operation may be minor, e.g., benign skin tumour or major, e.g., excision of part of the jaw for a malignant tumour. Following major surgery pain-relieving drugs are given, and in general the recovery of animals following surgery is much quicker than in human beings. Not only do they recover from the surgery quicker, but owners frequently notice a marked general improvement in the 'well being' of the dog, e.g., they appear more alert and have a better appetite following the removal of a malignant tumour which has previously had a depressing influence. Following surgery for malignant tumours it is necessary to have a veterinary examination at intervals sometimes for several months, so that possible recurrence or spread to the surrounding lymph nodes can be detected at an early stage and if necessary further surgery or other therapy instituted.

CRYOSURGERY

It is well known that arctic explorers and mountaineers sometimes get frostbite, which kills the ends of the fingers and toes. The same principle is used to kill tumours. Under controlled conditions using liquid nitrogen, which is intensely cold, the tumour tissue can be frozen while the surrounding normal tissue remains unaffected. Usually, to make sure all the tumour cells are dead, the cells are allowed to thaw and are then re-frozen. The method is time-consuming, but can achieve the desired result of a cure in some cases. Success is more likely to be achieved in small tumours which do not invade too deeply rather than the very large, deeply invasive tumours. The larger tumours may indeed have to be given cryosurgery on two or three different occasions. It was hoped, at one time, that the dying tumour cells would produce an immune stimulation, but unfortunately this is now considered unlikely to have worthwhile therapeutic value. Unfortunately, after cryosurgery there is often a very unpleasant odour as the cells die. Many tumours of the mouth treated by cryosurgery are followed by bad breath as the tissue dies. This does not inconvenience the dog, but is unpleasant for the owner.

RADIOTHERAPY

Radiotherapy is used frequently and often very successfully in many tumours affecting people. However, especially with tumours of the lungs and alimentary tract, there are frequently toxic effects. There may be nausea or even vomiting, with weakness and lassitude. Dogs are seldom treated with radiotherapy for lung tumours or tumours of the alimentary tract; most radiotherapy carried out on dogs is for tumours of the skin, mammary glands, mouth and also bone cancer. An important difference between dogs and people is that radiotherapy, when used at the above sites, does not appear to produce radiation sickness in dogs or cats as it does in people. Systemic effects following radiotherapy are uncommon. There is often some local loss of hair, but there is no generalised hair loss, and animals are rarely ill, a rather surprising species difference, but welcome to both dog and owner. Tumours responding well to radiotherapy include some of the skin tumours, e.g., mast-cell tumours and lymphosarcomas as well as mouth tumours, including basal cell tumours, carcinomas and melanomas. In the case of melanomas, however, spread to other parts of the body is a major problem, even though the original mouth tumour reduces in size following irradiation. Tumours of the tonsil often show a poor response to radiotherapy and bone tumours cannot be cured with radiotherapy. However, the dog may live six or even twelve months post radiotherapy without pain before there is tumour recurrence or development of tumours elsewhere. Responses of a few months or a year with good quality of life may not seem a long time to some owners, but a year in the life of a dog is a considerable percentage of its total life span.

Minor side effects can follow radiotherapy, such as soreness of the skin or, following a death of a tumour in the mouth, local infection. These problems are usually readily overcome using minor surgery or such drugs as cortisone and antibiotics.

CHEMOTHERAPY

There is frequently a fear of cancer chemotherapy. Many people have relatives or friends who have had cancer chemotherapy and often they are ill during treatment and may suffer considerable hair loss. For children with leukaemia, intensive care is required so that fatal infections do not occur during therapy and long periods in hospital are often required. The aim in these cases is cure, and cure is indeed obtained in a high percentage of acute lymphatic leukaemia cases.

The treatment of animals using cancer chemotherapy differs from human therapy in that cure is seldom the aim. More important is the control of the cancer, with the dog living a normal and happy life for as long as possible. Very high doses of toxic drugs are therefore seldom used so that unpleasant side affects can be avoided. Thus when used in proper doses vomiting and hair loss seldom occur. A condition called lymphosarcoma, which resembles Hodgkin's disease in man, is a condition most often treated with drugs. One of the drugs used in the treatment regime, Prednisone (a cortisone compound), stimulates appetite and dogs generally appear more lively and active during treatment.

It is usually necessary to have a blood test every four to eight weeks during treatment to ensure that the white cells in the blood, some of which are also destroyed by the drugs, do not fall to very low levels. When low levels of white blood cells occur, infection is more likely. Some of the newer drugs are very expensive, but other useful drugs are now much more reasonably priced than a few years ago, making the treatment of some cases of cancer in the dog with drugs well worthwhile, humane and economically possible. In other cases, e.g., invasive melanoma of the mouth with metastatic spread to the lungs, sadly no drugs of value are available for therapy.

FOOD AND THE CANCER PATIENT

Many dogs with cancer show no loss of appetite or weight loss until the disease is very advanced. In some cases, however, rapid weight loss occurs and the dog has a poorer appetite.

As with other illnesses where appetite is poor, small amounts of food should be fed frequently. Often fish, chicken or cottage cheese will tempt the appetite and warm foods or strong-smelling foods such as pilchards or sardines may be eaten. Today there are specially formulated diets available which your veterinary surgeon may prescribe.

If food intake is poor because of pain or infection, your veterinary surgeon will prescribe the appropriate drugs. A dog should not be fed on the day that surgery or radiotherapy has been planned until after recovery from the general anaesthetic.

Dogs with lymphosarcoma treated with corticosteroids may have a greatly increased appetite, leading to scavenging of dustbins and stealing food, so some additional bulk foods such as cabbage or turnips can be given, but additional biscuits or other food of high calorific value should be avoided.

SKIN TUMOURS

These are the most common tumours in the dog and about 20 different types occur.

Tumours may be of epithelial origin, i.e., originating from the surface layer of the skin. If they originate from the deeper layers they are said to be of mesenchymal origin. An example of a benign epithelial tumour is a papilloma (wart) or, if arising from a gland, an adenoma. Their malignant counterparts are carcinomas – squamous cell carcinoma and adenocarcinoma. Examples of benign mesenchymal tumours are fibroma (arising from fibrous tissue) and lipoma (arising from fatty tissue); when malignant they are called sarcomas, i.e., fibrosarcoma and liposarcoma. Other types of tumour occurring in the skin include melanoma from melanin pigment cells, mast cell tumour from mast cells and lymphomas from lymphoid tissue.

When presented with a dog having abnormal skin in one or more areas, the veterinary surgeon clinically assesses whether this is likely to be due to inflammatory, developmental or neoplastic disease. Sometimes foreign bodies, i.e., thorns or small pieces of glass, can produce skin lesions which appear like tumours. In the case of tumours, further examination is required to ascertain if the tumour is of epithelial or mesenchymal origin. If the lesion is neoplastic the essential information as to whether it is benign or malignant is required. Most benign tumours grow slowly, do not appear inflamed and are well defined. Most malignant tumours grow rapidly. They can ulcerate and frequently invade the adjacent tissues.

Small, single, suspect tumours are best excised completely, but in larger tumours or multiple tumours a biopsy may first be taken. Dependent on the laboratory report the prognosis then becomes more clear and a method of therapy can be determined. In the vast majority of cases surgery is the method of choice.

There are certain breeds which have an excess risk for some types of skin tumours. Mast cell tumours seem to occur especially in Boxers, Boston Terriers and Bulldogs, while melanomas are particularly common in the Scottish Terrier. Squamous cell carcinoma is associated with the Basset Hound, Weimaraner and Scottish Terrier, while Dachshunds and Weimaraners seem more prone to lipomas.

MAMMARY GLAND

Tumours of the mammary gland are common, being second only to skin tumours in numbers occurring. Nearly all occur in female dogs, but about 2 per cent occur in male dogs. The incidence in mongrel dogs is less than in purebred dogs; amongst the high-risk breeds are some of the Pointers, Setters and Spaniels, also the Pyrenean, Miniature and Toy Poodles and Airedales.

Mention has been made of the sparing effect of spaying on the incidence of mammary tumours. On the other hand, long-term administration of some of the progestogen hormones used for the suppression of oestrus (season) can induce both benign and malignant tumours.

The majority of mammary tumours occur in older dogs, 9–13 years of age. Mammary tumours have only rarely been reported in bitches less than two years old. Again, as with skin tumours, the rate of growth can be important; certainly with malignant tumours the size at diagnosis affects the prognosis, i.e., the larger the tumour the more likely it is to recur after surgery or develop in other parts of the body. When the tumours are fixed to the skin or to deeper tissues they are more likely to be malignant than

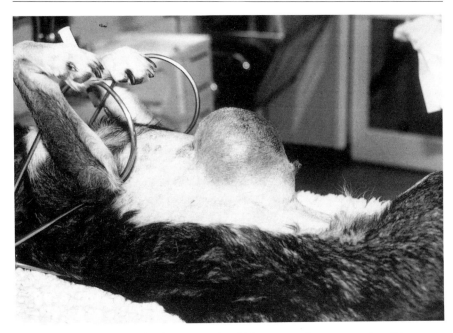

Figure 198 Mammary gland tumours should be removed as soon as possible, otherwise rapid growth or spread (metastasis) may make surgery difficult

benign. Ulceration is also a bad sign, as are tumours showing inflammatory changes – heat, redness and fluid in the tissues.

Tumours can appear in one mammary gland or several and it is possible for a tumour to be malignant in one gland and benign in another. Malignant mammary tumours can spread to the draining lymph nodes, the inguinal and popliteal glands in the case of the posterior glands and axillary in the case of anterior glands. They can also spread to the lungs, so that a chest X-ray may be well worthwhile before embarking on major surgery. If the lungs contain a tumour there is usually little to be gained in excising the primary tumour.

It is generally wise to excise a tumour or suspect tumour in the mammary gland as soon as it becomes apparent. A 'wait and see' policy may result in rapid growth or metastasis. Other factors, however, influence this decision – a prolonged surgical operation in an old bitch with poor heart or kidney function would be unwise. Much discussion occurs among surgeons in this field, be they veterinary surgeons operating on dogs or human surgeons operating on people, about the need to remove only the tumour or the whole breast. Certainly, if only the tumour is removed it is possible for further tumours to develop in the remaining breast tissue at a later date, and cosmetic considerations, which are important in women faced with breast removal, do not apply to the bitch.

The pathological report indicates whether the tumour is benign or malignant. More than half the mammary tumours in the bitch are benign and are unlikely to recur following adequate surgery. The malignant tumours vary in their degree of malignancy – tumours which show invasion in the breast tissue are more likely to recur after surgery, or to metastasise, than are tumours which have a capsule around them, the so-called circumscribed tumour. For malignant tumours, survival times following surgical treatment vary according to the pathology, but about half the carcinomas can be cured by surgery alone.

Following removal of the breast (mastectomy) in women because of a malignant tumour, many hospitals give post-operative radiotherapy to prevent or reduce the incidence of local recurrence; this may also be of value in the more aggressive types of mammary tumour in the bitch as may be the administration of an anti-cancer drug such as cyclophosphamide.

Further research is indicated here, as is the possible value of hormonal therapy. Hormonal therapy for breast cancer in women is of proven value, but additional information is required in the bitch before recommendations can be made. Spaying (ovariectomy), which has a sparing action in the young bitch, has no proven value in preventing tumour recurrence following mastectomy in old bitches, but it may be of value for other reasons. Ovariohysterectomy, where the uterus is removed as well as the ovaries, is a useful operation when the uterus becomes infected (pyometra), which occurs not infrequently in older bitches.

LEUKAEMIA AND LYMPHOSARCOMA

Leukaemia, which is a malignant disease of the white blood cells, occurs in the dog, but much more common is malignancy of the lymph glands and other lymphoid tissue. This resembles lymphosarcoma and the related condition of Hodgkin's disease in man.

Lymphoma or lymphosarcoma, sometimes also called pseudo-Hodgkin's disease in the dog, occurs in several forms and affects different parts of the body. Commonly lymph glands enlarge in the neck as well as in other areas and there may be difficulty in swallowing or the dog may snore.

When the alimentary form occurs in the lymphoid tissue of the small intestine there is often vomiting and diarrhoea, sometimes with blood, and animals show weight loss. When lymph nodes in the chest are affected animals show an increased respiratory rate, sometimes with a cough and difficulty in swallowing.

The clinical signs are, however, very variable as the disease can affect many different organs in the body, including the brain and the eye.

In leukaemia also the clinical signs are very variable. Frequently affected dogs are listless, lose weight, and the appearance of the skin of the lips and inner eyelids is pale due to the anaemia which occurs.

The cause of leukaemia in the dog is not yet known. In the cat many types of leukaemia are caused by a virus and some tumours in man are also of viral origin. There are also genetic influences. Mention has already been made of the high incidence in the Bull Mastiff.

In leukaemia, malignant dividing cells occur in the circulating blood and can easily be detected on microscopic examination of a blood smear. In lymphosarcoma only a small percentage of dogs show malignant cells in the blood and it may be necessary to examine a section from a lymph node before a definite diagnosis can be made. When the chest or abdomen are mainly affected, X-rays help considerably with the diagnosis.

Both lymphosarcoma and leukaemia are fatal conditions in the dog and without treatment nearly all dogs die within three months of diagnosis. Animals with alimentary or chest malignancies often have to be put to sleep on humane grounds soon after diagnosis. The prognosis in dogs where the more superficial lymph glands are mainly affected is better. Even here, however, long-term survivals are rare, although with treatment pain-free life can be extended.

Treatment of leukaemia and related malignancies in man and the dog is different, even though many of the drugs used are the same. In children with acute lymphatic leukaemia, intensive chemotherapy and radiotherapy are given over several months and toxic side-affects can be severe. This is warranted, however, as a high percentage of cures and long-term survivors results. In dogs, simple treatment with corticosteroids often improves the condition for short periods of time without serious side-effects. Additionally, anti-cancer drugs in smaller doses than those used in man can cause useful palliation without toxic effects such as vomiting or diarrhoea. The main toxic effect of these drugs is on the bone marrow. Unfortunately normal white cells are killed as well as malignant cells, leading to the problem of infection. To prevent this occurring to a serious degree, it is usual to examine the blood every four to six weeks and to so adjust the drug dose that the white and red cell numbers do not become too low. Unlike the position in children with acute leukaemia, where cure is the aim, the object of treating dogs with leukaemia is to improve the quality of life and to prolong this for as long as possible without toxicity. When therapy fails, which usually varies in time from three months to a year (occasionally longer), and the dog is no longer enjoying life, euthanasia is the only humane option left.

Treatment which results in good quality life for a year may be considered a success as it is 10 per cent of the dog's life span.

TUMOURS OF THE MOUTH

There are four main tumours which occur in the mouth. They can be sited on the gums, tongue, lips, palate or tonsil. They are:

Plate 16 Bulldog skull showing extreme brachycephalic reverse scissor bite

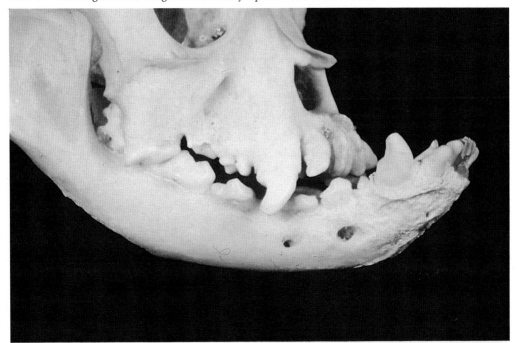

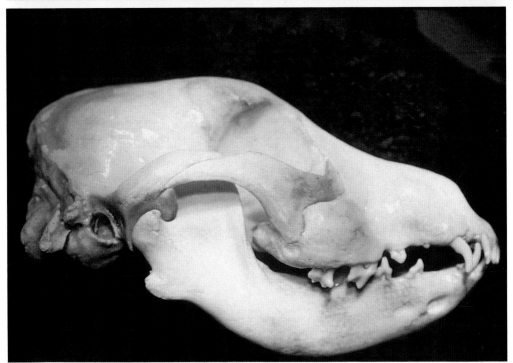

Plate 17 11-week-old Giant Schnauzer skull showing temporary dentition

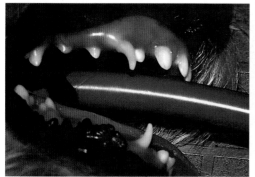

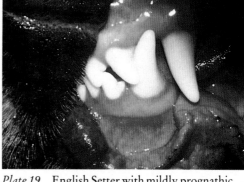

Plate 18 13-week-old West Highland White Terrier with retained upper and lower temporary canines; the right upper canine is seen erupting too rostrally

Plate 19 English Setter with mildly prognathic bite – 'displaced canines'

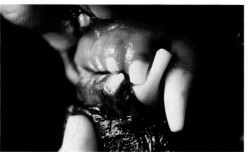

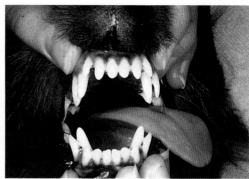

Plate 20 Level bite. Note the excessive wear (attrition) of the incisors and the lower canines as the teeth in contact have worn each other away

Plate 21 Retained temporary upper and lower canines. As the dog's mouth is closed the medially displaced lower canines are driven into the hard palate

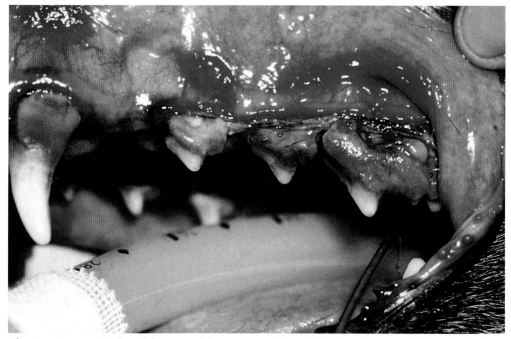

Plate 22 Severe periodontal disease with large accumulation of calculus, plaque and debris, gingival recession and contact ulcers on the alveolar mucosa

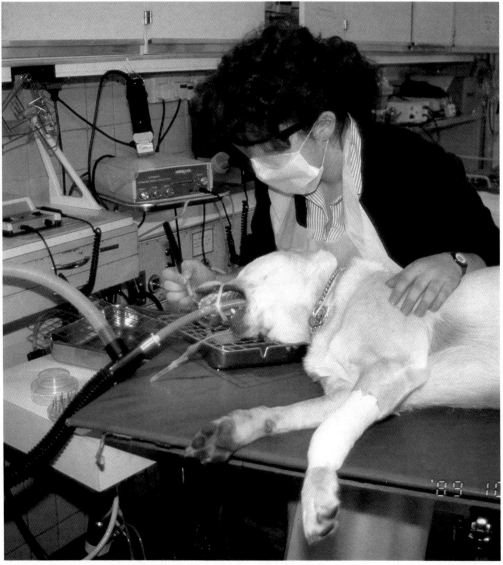

Plate 23   Removal of plaque and calculus using ultrasonic scaler

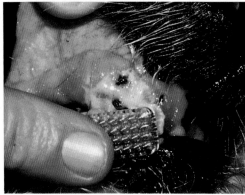

Plate 24   Brushing a dog's teeth

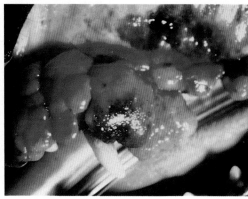

Plate 25   Epulis covering the incisors and premolars and almost growing over the canines

Plate 26 Caries (decay) of the lower first molar

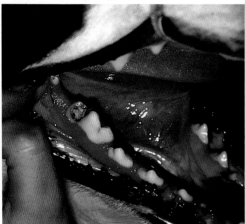

Plate 27 Purple discoloration of a lower canine tooth indicative of pulpal necrosis

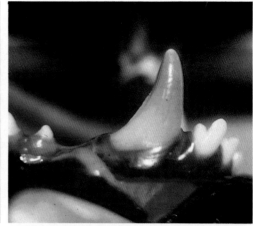

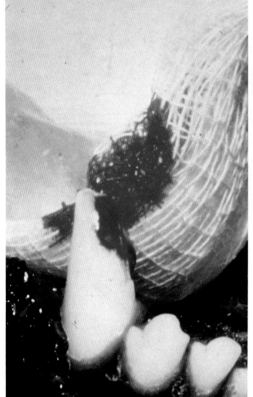

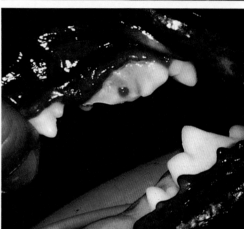

Plate 28 (left) Fresh fracture of a lower canine with pulpal haemorrhage

Plate 29 (right) Slab fracture of an upper fourth premolar exposing the pulp and providing a rough surface on which plaque and calculus have accumulated

1. squamous cell carcinomas;
2. fibrosarcoma;
3. melanoma;
4. basal cell tumours.

(1) Squamous cell carcinomas

These usually occur in older dogs and can often appear as ulcerated swellings which may bleed. Simple surgery or cryosurgery may be successful in small tumours, but usually more complex surgery, perhaps involving the removal of a piece of jaw bone, is required. It may appear to be rather drastic, but in the majority of cases the results are very good, with the dog able to eat and drink without difficulty and the cosmetic result satisfactory. Cures are certainly possible, but in some cases tumour recurs at the operation site or spreads to the draining lymph nodes in the neck. Radiotherapy is also of value in gum squamous cell carcinomas, usually prolonging life for several months or a year and in some cases, which are not too advanced when first seen, cures can be obtained. Tonsil carcinomas have a poorer prognosis. They recur after surgery and often spread elsewhere.

(2) Fibrosarcomas

Similar methods of therapy are used as for carcinomas, but results are usually not as good. Most of the tumours receiving radiotherapy recur after six to twelve months.

(3) Melanomas

The main problem with melanomas is metastasis, whatever method is used to control the primary tumour (surgery, cryosurgery or radiotherapy). The tumour, unfortunately, spreads to the regional lymph nodes, lungs and other organs of the body and after a few weeks or months from diagnosis, and euthanasia is usually necessary.

(4) Basal cell tumours

Many of these originate from developing dental tissue. They can occur at any age, but many occur in young dogs one to three years old and occasionally in very young dogs three or four months old. If they can be resected surgically the prognosis is good, as they do not spread elsewhere. Radiotherapy also gives good results as the tumour is very radiosensitive.

In addition *Dentigerous cysts* can also occur. These cysts occur in the enamel organ of an unerupted tooth and can usually be treated successfully by surgical excision.

BONE TUMOURS

Bone tumours occur mainly in large dogs, particularly giant breeds, and they are nearly always malignant. It is likely that the genetic factors are important, but the exact reasons why bone tumours occur is poorly understood. Tumours can occur in damaged bone, e.g., in fractures where plates or pins have been used or in bony proliferations, but in the majority of cases the bone is apparently normal before tumours occur. Sometimes a bone tumour develops a few weeks after injury, but it is not generally thought that the sole factor producing the tumour is the injury.

The main tumour is the osteosarcoma, which develops from the bone cells (osteoblasts), but other tumours, e.g., fibrosarcomas developing from fibrous tissue and chondrosarcomas developing from cartilage, can occur. The most common site for osteosarcoma is in the radius and ulna just above the carpal (wrist) joint, but it occurs also in other long bones and also in the ribs.

The usual manifestation is swelling of the affected area, sometimes accompanied by pain and lameness. Bone tumours are not one of the common causes of lameness and often the early signs are thought to be due to a sprain or possible arthritis. Some of the tumours can produce a lot of bone destruction, which may result in fracture.

Diagnosis is usually made after the examination of X-rays, but it may be necessary to confirm a suspicious case by taking a biopsy and examining tissue under the microscope.

Bone cancer is one of the worst forms of cancer in the dog and cures are very rare. There are two problems, both of which are so far insoluble. One is the inability to sterilise the primary tumour and the other the development of tumours in other parts of the body, particularly the lungs. Using existing drugs or radiotherapy no cures of the primary tumour have been reported, although with X-irradiation, reduction of pain and prolongation of life for a few months is often possible. As a temporary measure pain-relieving drugs such as phenylbutazone can be of value.

Amputation of the affected limb does not cure the condition, as usually within three or four months metastatic tumours develop in the lungs, and euthanasia is required for this reason.

Research is in progress using limb grafts and new anti-cancer drugs, but at the present time there is no really satisfactory method of treatment.

CANCER IN OTHER SITES

Cancer of the stomach, liver, pancreas, brain and base of the heart are not common, and all have a very poor prognosis. In nearly all cases the cancer is advanced when first seen and little of therapeutic value can be attempted.

Rarely, cancer of the liver involves only one lobe and this can be excised surgically.

Nasal cancer is also nearly always fatal, but surgery and radiotherapy can be of value in early cases. Primary lung cancer is rare in dogs compared with man, as dogs are non-smokers. If only one lobe of the lung is affected, surgery can be attempted, but usually the cancer is more widespread.

When cancer of the kidney involves only one kidney and has not spread to other organs, the affected kidney can be removed surgically. Cancer of the bladder if diagnosed early can be treated surgically, but most cases are advanced when first diagnosed. Palliative therapy with anti-cancer drugs may prolong life without toxicity in some cases.

Testicular tumours, of which there are three main types, are more common in undescended testicles than when testicles are in the scrotum. One type of tumour produces oestrogens (female hormones) which affect the appearance of the dog, i.e., loss of hair, enlarged nipples, pendulous abdomen and decrease in the size of the other testicle. Following castration these changes, if not too advanced, can be partially reversed, especially hair loss. A small percentage of these hormone-producing tumours are malignant and spread to other sites.

There are many different types of tumour of the ovary; some can be removed successfully surgically and others are more malignant and metastasise widely. Unlike the position in women, where cervical carcinoma is relatively common, uterine cancer in the bitch is rare. More common are vaginal tumours, some of which can be successfully treated surgically.

Tumours of the adrenal gland can produce hair loss and changes in the appearance of the dog. Benign tumours, if unilateral, can be treated surgically. If bilateral, therapy is sometimes successful using a drug. Malignant tumours can spread widely around the body. A similar position is found with tumours of the thyroid gland; some benign tumours can be excised surgically or benefit can be obtained by giving drugs. Malignant tumours usually rapidly metastasise and euthanasia may be the only course open.

29

CANINE DENTISTRY

Dentistry in man has a long history, almost as long as civilisation itself. Techniques have been performed and refined over many generations. Dental problems in dogs have also been recognised for a long time, but it is only relatively recently that specific methods of prevention and repair of canine dental disorders have been developed. Dogs need teeth to cut, chew, tear, hold, carry and to groom themselves properly. Without teeth the gums harden and although the dog can manage to eat chopped-up food adequately, the tongue usually hangs out of the mouth so that it dries and is often damaged. Many techniques current in human dentistry can, with a little modification, be used on our pets, but it is important to remember that a dog's behaviour is very different from ours. In addition, canine teeth have to withstand enormous forces compared with those of man (1,200 lb/sq in. compared with 150 lb/sq in. in man). This obviously makes the use of delicate appliances impractical and can lead to disappointment, not to mention expense, if some of the common dental techniques involving bridges and crowns are used on our pets.

Dogs undoubtedly function more efficiently with a complete set of healthy teeth, and it is the aim of veterinary dentistry to preserve teeth as long as is practicable. This aim can be realised by preventing the build-up of plaque or calculus, just as with us, and involves the training of the dog to accept a daily tooth-brushing routine. Today special brushes and specially flavoured toothpastes containing products to fight bacterial build-up are available for use in dogs. The aim of preserving teeth is helped if the dog receives regular dental check-ups from the veterinary surgeon. If you are lucky enough to find someone who has a special interest in veterinary dentistry, you will find that the question of home care, in other words regular brushing of the dog's teeth, will be increasingly emphasised, particularly in those breeds more prone to periodontal disease.

The materials available to repair dogs' teeth are the same as for ours and the techniques are similar. Canine teeth tend to be much whiter than ours, which makes it difficult to match exactly the colours of the filling materials to the tooth, since these are, at present, only available in 'human' shades. Originally, silver-coloured amalgam was used, but this is used in dogs less commonly; composite, a white-coloured filling material, is often used nowadays. It is placed in a specially prepared undercut hole, where it sets hard. It is held in place by the undercut, which is made so that the entrance is of a smaller diameter than the rest of the hole. In this way, when it has set hard it cannot fall out. Using special solutions this composite can also be stuck to the surface of the tooth to make good defects which are often unsightly, since exposed dentine becomes stained. However, these surface applications are frequently knocked off during a dog's normal chewing activities. Recently, another filling material known as glass ionomer has been developed. This actually bonds to the enamel and the dentine and releases fluoride into the tooth. It is available in silver- or enamel-coloured shades and is a very important development as far as the restoration of defects in dogs' teeth is concerned.

All the techniques used in human dentistry today are available: for example, crowns can be built, but are rarely necessary and usually are made of metal rather than the porcelain of human dental crowns. Orthodontic appliances can also be fitted to correct abnormalities of the bite, known as malocclusions.

Normal functional anatomy of the mouth

A normal adult dog possesses 42 permanent teeth, 20 in the upper jaw and 22 in the lower jaw. The teeth are divided into four main types, according to their function.

There are six *incisors* at the front of each jaw. These small single-rooted teeth are used mainly for the more delicate operations of nibbling that occur when grooming. They are used for cutting, nipping and biting off small pieces of food.

The two *canine teeth* (fangs) in each jaw are situated just lateral to and behind the incisors. They are the largest single-rooted teeth in the mouth and are used for holding and tearing. They also help to keep the tongue in place (see Fig. 199).

There are eight *premolar teeth* in each jaw; they can be single rooted or multi-rooted and are primarily designed for cutting and shearing.

The *molars* at the back of the mouth are the chewing teeth. There are 4 in the upper jaw and 6 in the lower jaw.

The right and left sides of the jaw should be symmetrical, so there is a neat, shortened form for recording the number and type of teeth in each jaw. This is the dental formula:

$$2(I_{\frac{3}{3}}^{} \; C_{\frac{1}{1}}^{} \; P_{\frac{4}{4}}^{} \; M_{\frac{2}{3}}^{}) = 42$$

I = incisors, C = canine, P = premolar, M = molar

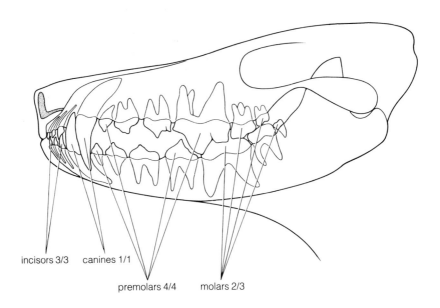

incisors 3/3   canines 1/1

premolars 4/4   molars 2/3

Figure 199   Mature dog's head showing relationships between teeth roots and jaw bone and dental formula

The teeth are arranged to meet in very specific ways as shown in Figure 199. The incisors should meet to form a scissor bite where the upper, central incisors (the two middle teeth) overlap the outside surfaces of the two lower central incisors. The incisal or biting edges of the lower central incisors should just contact the back edge (cingulum) of the upper central incisors. The lower lateral incisor rests on the small outside cusp of the upper intermediate incisor and on the inside cusp of the upper, lateral incisor. The lower canines pass in front of the upper canines and fit neatly in the gap between the upper lateral incisor and the upper canine. The upper canine rests in the gap behind the lower canine, in front of the lower premolar. There should be no contact between the canines and the teeth on either side. The points of the crowns of the premolars sit in the gaps between the premolars in the opposing arcade, giving a pinking shear effect with the lower first premolar nearest the front. The molars (except for the rostral half of the lower first molar) are in occlusion, their grinding surfaces meeting when the mouth is closed.

Head shapes

The shape of the head obviously alters this occlusion quite considerably. There are three basic head shapes:

1. Dolichocephalic: long, narrow muzzle, e.g., Borzoi, Greyhound, Saluki.
2. Mesaticephalic: medium-length muzzle, e.g., German Shepherd Dog, Labrador, Retrievers, Terriers. Three-quarters of all our dogs fall into this category (see Fig. 200).
3. Brachycephalic: short, wide muzzle, e.g., Pekingese, Pug, Shih Tzu, Bulldog, Boxer.

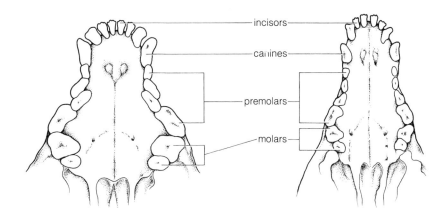

Figure 200 (a) Upper jaw of brachycephalic skull
(b) Upper jaw of mesaticephalic skull

In this last group the lower incisors close in front of the upper incisors, a reverse scissor bite. In extreme cases the lower incisors can be up to 2 inches in front of the upper incisors, e.g., Bulldogs (see Plate 16).

DECIDUOUS TEETH

Dogs, like humans, possess two sets of teeth during their lifetime. First, in puppyhood, is the deciduous or temporary set. These teeth are cut within a few weeks of birth. The incisors and canines are the first to erupt, at about 3–4 weeks, followed by the premolars. Puppies have no temporary molars, so the dental formula for their temporary teeth is:

$$2(I\tfrac{3}{3} \ C\tfrac{1}{1} \ P\tfrac{3}{3}) = 28 \text{ teeth}$$

All the temporary teeth should have erupted by the time the puppy is 12 weeks old (see Plate 17). From this age onwards the roots of the temporary teeth are resorbed, the crowns fall out and the adult, permanent teeth erupt. Incisors erupt at between 3 and 5 months, canines and premolars between 4 and 6 months and molars, which have no temporary counterpart, are cut between 5 and 7 months of age. Thus a 'guestimate' of the age of a puppy can be made, up to 7 months, after which it is a matter of speculation!

THE TEETH AND THEIR SURROUNDING STRUCTURES

The teeth are the hardest structures in the body, but nevertheless they are composed of living tissue. The pulp in the core of each tooth contains the blood vessels and nerves necessary for the growth and repair of the tooth. The outside of the pulp chamber is covered in a fine layer of special cells called odontoblasts, which lay down dentine (see Fig. 201).

Dentine is the chief substance or tissue of the tooth. It surrounds the pulp of the tooth and is covered by enamel on the crown and by cementum on the root of the tooth (Fig. 201). The function of the odontoblast is to produce the dentine. The newly erupted permanent tooth has a very large pulp chamber and a thin dentine wall (see Fig. 202, overleaf). During the first eighteen months odontoblasts lay down a huge amount of dentine, thickening the dentine wall, strengthening the tooth and reducing the size of the pulp chamber.

The *crown* of the tooth is that part which protrudes above the gum and is covered by a layer of enamel.

Enamel is the hardest substance in the body and protects the underlying dentine and the pulp from damage. Near gum level the enamel is shaped with a special bulge, the enamel bulge, to deflect food from the delicate junction of gum and tooth. Without this, during chewing, food would be forced down the tooth and into the gingival crevice, pushing the gum or gingiva further down the tooth. The *gingival crevice* is a shallow pocket up to 4 mm deep which protects the delicate attachment of gingiva to tooth from abrasion and damage. The gingiva is attached to the *cementum* at the *cemento-enamel* junction, the point at which the enamel covering the dentine changes to cementum at the beginning of the root. The *cementum* is the third hard substance of which the tooth is composed. It is a bone-like connective tissue covering the root of the tooth. The *periodontal ligament* is attached to it. This ligament holds the tooth into the *alveolar socket*, allowing the tooth a tiny amount of movement, which acts as a shock absorber.

The largest of the cheek (or premolar and molar) teeth of the dog are known as the carnassials and are immensely strong. They provide a shearing or scissor action so that natural tough food can be efficiently reduced to pieces of a size suitable to swallow. The carnassial teeth in the dog are the lower first molars (2 roots, see Fig. 203, overleaf) and upper fourth premolars (3 roots). It is this tooth, or the adjacent upper first molar, also with 3 roots, that can often be the site of a root abscess. This frequently results in facial swelling and can discharge just below the eye.

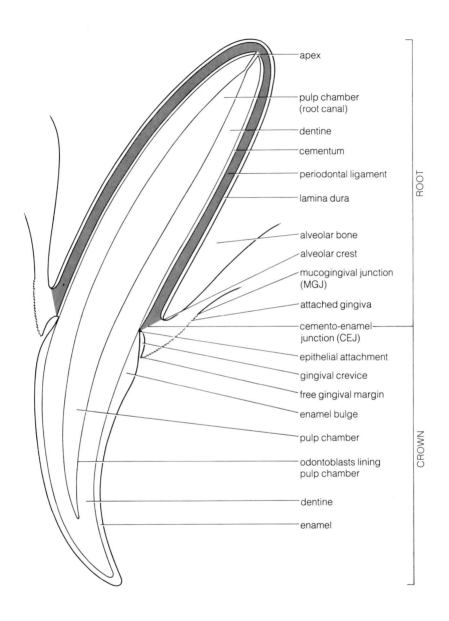

Figure 201 Section of an upper canine of an adult dog

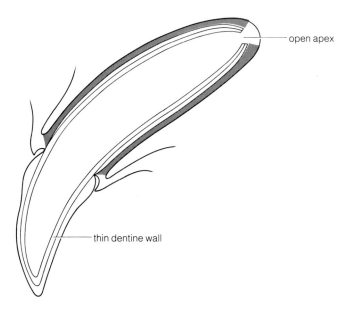

Figure 202   Section of an upper canine of a 6-month-old dog

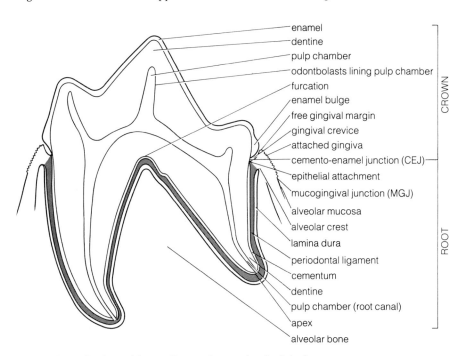

Figure 203   Section of lower first molar tooth of adult dog

The number of roots varies according to the tooth. Incisors, canines and first premolars, together with the second premolar and third molar in the lower jaw, have a single root, while all the rest have 2 roots, except the upper fourth premolar and upper first molar, which have 3 roots. The roots of multi-rooted teeth are slightly divergent, ensuring great strength and stability but making these teeth particularly difficult to extract should the need arise.

Dental disease

CLINICAL SIGNS

The range of signs of dental disease varies greatly from dog to dog as each has a different response to discomfort and pain. Any of the following symptoms may indicate the presence of dental disease:

- Bad breath (halitosis)
- Drooling from the mouth (excess salivation)
- Facial swelling between the nose and the eye, below the eye, under the chin or along the lower jawbone
- Nasal discharge
- Conjunctivitis
- Difficulty with eating
- Chewing on one side
- Refusing biscuits but eating soft food
- Losing food from the mouth whilst eating
- Refusing to play with chews or other toys
- Unwillingness to pick up or carry things
- Gradual change in nature, quieter than normal, not interested in playing or going for walks
- Unable to settle
- More irritable than normal
- Dislike of being patted on the head

Thus the signs can be very varied and many of the changes are so insidious in onset and so non-specific that they often go unnoticed. Hence it is very important for the dog's mouth to be examined frequently by owners and at least once or twice a year by a veterinary surgeon. This is usually carried out at the time of the annual vaccination, when a general health check is always a good idea.

TO EXAMINE YOUR OWN DOG'S MOUTH

Lift the upper lip gently with the mouth closed. This will reveal the teeth and gums. The gums should be glistening, smooth, firm, pink and free from any debris. Some dogs have dark or pigmented areas on the gums, lips, tongue and hard palate, which are quite normal. Diseased gums have a different appearance; they may be dull and rough, soft, red or bleeding. They may have receded, exposing part of the root. They can be swollen, puffy and irregularly shaped. Sometimes gum boils are visible as red or white sores on the gum over the tooth root. The teeth are normally clean, shining white and fixed firmly in position with a smooth unbroken outline. Anything other than this appearance is abnormal. Dogs' teeth and gums behave in essentially the same way as people's. Broken and decayed teeth hurt us and they also hurt our dogs, although they may not show obvious symptoms.

MALOCCLUSIONS

Earlier in the chapter the normal meeting or occlusion of the teeth was described. If the teeth are not in the correct position in the mouth, the abnormal positioning and relationship between the teeth is called a *malocclusion.*

Causes

Malocclusions can be hereditary or acquired. The genetic information dictating the positions of the teeth and the length of the jaw can be passed on from generation to generation. If this information is incorrect, an hereditary, genetic malocclusion will result.

Retained deciduous teeth often interfere with the eruption of the permanent teeth and are *the commonest cause of malocclusions.* The tendency to retain deciduous teeth seems to be passed on from one generation to the next, but its exact mode of inheritance is unknown. It is particularly common in some of the smaller breeds (see Plate 18).

Acquired malocclusions occur when the genetic information is correct but some other factor prevents it from being implemented.

During normal development the upper jaw, or maxilla, and the lower jaw, or mandible, do not grow at exactly the same rates. At some stages one jaw may be somewhat in advance of the other, but provided the genetic information is correct, and no other factors intervene, the end result when growth is completed will be a normal occlusion.

Hereditary malocclusions

Most abnormal occlusive patterns can be classified into two general categories – overshot and undershot.

1. *Overshot or brachygnathic bite*
Some or all of the teeth of the upper jaw are in front of their counterparts in the lower jaw. The upper jaw may be longer than the lower jaw. The upper incisors are some distance in front of their lower counterparts, so there is no physical contact between them.

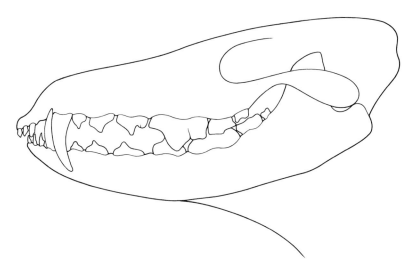

Figure 204 Overshot (brachygnathism)

The severity of the condition varies from a 1 mm gap between upper and lower incisors (with the upper premolars approximately half a tooth width further forward than normal) to a 5 cm (2 in.) gap between upper and lower incisors, with the upper premolars 2–3 teeth too far forward and the upper canines some distance in front of the lower canines (see Fig. 204). In many cases it is difficult to detect minor brachygnathism by looking at the incisors alone – it is always essential to check the alignment of the premolars and the canine teeth.

Other colloquial names for the condition are parrot-mouthed or pig-jawed.

2. Undershot or prognathic bite (see Fig. 205, overleaf)
In this condition the teeth, notably the incisors of the lower jaw, are in front of those of the upper jaw; the lower jaw may be visibly longer than the upper jaw. In other words, there is a long mandible or lower jaw and a short maxilla or upper jaw. The brachycephalic breeds, e.g., the Pug, Boxer, Bulldog and Pekingese, show this as a normal anatomical feature and it is indeed part of the breed standard.

The severity of the condition varies in the same way as brachygnathism and in borderline cases the presence of prognathism can sometimes only be detected on close examination of the premolar and canine teeth.

When discussing these overshot and undershot bites, which are of especial interest to dog breeders, confusion can sometimes arise because

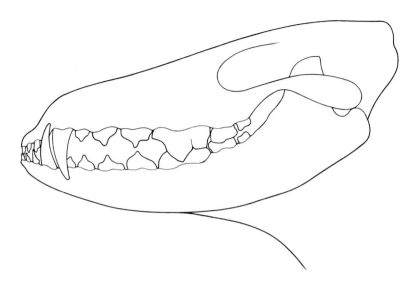

Figure 205   Undershot (prognathism)

the brachycephalic breeds have a prognathic, undershot bite, while it is the longer-headed breeds that are more likely to have an overshot (or brachygnathic) bite. This becomes logical if one thinks of the word meanings. In this context

Brachy . . .   means short
Pro . . .   means long
. . . cephalic   refers to the maxilla and head
. . . gnathic   refers to the mandible length (lower jaw)

So, 'brachycephalic' means short maxilla and head and 'brachygnathic' means short lower jaw (mandible).

3. Displaced canine teeth
This is a very mild form of prognathism. The incisors occlude normally, but the lower canine is slightly too far forward and comes into contact with the upper, lateral incisor (see Plate 19); the lower premolars are also slightly too far forward, most easily seen where the tip of the lower fourth premolar comes into contact with the upper third molar. This underlines the importance of examining the canine and premolar teeth when evaluating the bite.

4. Level bite
This is a mild form of prognathism and is slightly more severe than displaced canine teeth. The tips of the upper incisors meet the tips of the

lower incisors instead of the overlapping scissor relationship. This damages the incisors, which wear down very quickly (see Plate 20).

5. Open bite
When there is a genetic potential for prognathism but the dental interlock of the canines and incisors prevents the lower teeth from moving in front of their upper counterparts, the mandible, still genetically programmed to grow longer than the maxilla, bends downwards and even outwards to accommodate this extra length (see Fig. 206). This creates the open bite, where the tips of the lower premolars are further from those on the maxilla than normal. This may interfere with their function. Sometimes, there is a gap between the upper and lower incisors. This is also known as an open bite and is often seen as part of the wry bite (see below). The open bite involving premolars or incisors can occur with any of the other malocclusions.

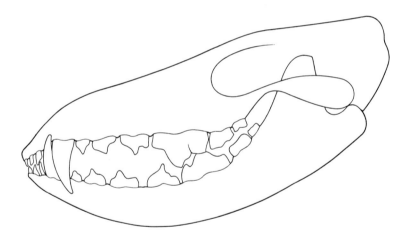

Figure 206   Open bite involving the premolar dentition

6. Wry mouth
In this condition each side of the jaw grows at a different rate. If only the mandible is involved the bite will be prognathic (undershot) and often open as well on the affected side but normal on the unaffected side. If the maxilla is affected the mandible is usually involved as well because of the dental interlock. This alters the development of the whole head, the affected side

being bigger; the midline of the head and bite, viewed with the incisors is deviated. A wry mouth can accompany any of the other malocclusions.

Occasionally these defects may develop as the result of a misplaced temporary tooth interlocking with the opposite arcade rather than being purely due to inheritance. If the mandible and maxilla grow at different rates a misplaced temporary tooth locking the two together at an inappropriate time could force them to retain that particular relationship throughout growth. This may result in the appearance of any of the above defects. If the misplaced deciduous tooth is removed as soon as it is noticed the genetic instructions will be able to dictate the development of the maxilla and mandible. If the genetic information is correct normal occlusion will result. Hence frequent examination of the puppy's mouth and bite is very important. With potential show puppies it is essential; it also helps them to get used to being handled, and prevents them from being mouth-shy when they are exhibited. If in any doubt about the bite of a puppy, seek veterinary advice without delay. Do not forget that they are developing very rapidly.

Other malocclusions

Anterior crossbite. Some of the lower incisors are in front of the upper incisors (commonly the upper central incisors), but all the other teeth are correctly positioned. This is not a true prognathism and is not usually thought to be inherited. It is sometimes associated with retained deciduous incisors. It appears in puppies from 4–7 months of age and concerns the positioning of the incisors rather than the length of the upper and lower jaws.

Malocclusions secondary to retained temporary teeth.
Temporary teeth normally fall out as their permanent counterparts start to erupt. If the temporary teeth are still present, the permanent teeth are forced to erupt next to them. They are then in the wrong place, resulting in a malocclusion. The severity of this depends on which teeth are affected, how the affected teeth are positioned relative to the opposite jaw and how long the retained temporary teeth remain in place. Sometimes the developing permanent teeth are in such a position that they damage the soft tissues of the opposite jaw. This commonly happens when the lower temporary canines are retained (see Plate 21); the permanent lower canines erupt to the inside (medially) of the temporary teeth and frequently grow to impinge upon the hard palate. Each time the dog's mouth is closed, these canines hit the mucous membrane of the hard palate. This soon becomes sore and ulcerated. Eventually, the teeth may puncture the hard palate to make a sinus or hole through it into the nasal passages.

   Apart from causing deviation of the erupting permanent teeth, retained temporary teeth also produce gingivitis (inflammation of the gums) and periodontitis (inflammation of the deeper tissues supporting the teeth) between them and their adjacent permanent teeth, due to the food and debris which becomes trapped between them.

Retained temporary teeth

As the crown of the permanent tooth appears through the gum, the temporary tooth should be loose, its root mostly resorbed, and should soon drop out. If not, resorption has failed to occur and the temporary tooth will not be shed. Then the whole tooth will need careful removal under an anaesthetic by a veterinary surgeon. Retained temporary teeth should be removed as soon as it is apparent they are not going to fall out naturally. This will prevent a vast number of malocclusions. It is not enough simply to break off the crown of the tooth, since it is the presence of the root which forces the erupting permanent tooth into the wrong position. This cannot be too strongly emphasised.

Malocclusions of temporary teeth

If wrongly positioned temporary teeth are causing a problem, for example by becoming embedded in the hard palate, they should be extracted under anaesthetic by a veterinarian. This will prevent further damage to the hard palate and allow the mandible and maxilla to grow to their full genetic potential. This procedure is known as *interceptive orthodontics*.

Other orthodontic procedures can be *corrective*, which is concerned with the reduction or elimination of an existing malocclusion, or *preventative*, which is concerned with the preservation of normal occlusion by preventing a malocclusion from developing.

Malocclusions of permanent teeth

It is possible in certain circumstances for the permanent teeth to be repositioned with braces in a similar fashion to human orthodontics. Veterinary surgeons are often asked to embark upon orthodontic procedures, particularly with potential show stock that are developing signs of overshot (brachygnathic) or undershot (prognathic) bites. From the previous pages it will be clear that hereditary factors may be responsible, and therefore the ethics of such procedures must be carefully considered.

Orthodontic procedures should not be carried out if the malocclusion is hereditary, unless the animal is neutered, since the condition is likely to be passed on to future generations. If the malocclusion is causing pain, or damage to any structures in the mouth, it should be treated either by moving the offending teeth into an acceptable position, removing the offending part of the tooth and treating it endodontically (i.e., by filling or capping it) or removing it entirely.

Prevention

Selective breeding from lines with perfect mouths will eliminate hereditary malocclusions. Unfortunately there are many breeds where this is impossible, so breeding should be restricted to those with minimal problems. *Removal of retained temporary teeth* at the appropriate time helps to prevent them causing malocclusions. Although the exact mode of inheritance of the tendency to retain temporary teeth is not yet fully understood, it would be sensible to avoid breeding from those which exhibit this problem wherever possible. However, in smaller breeds this tendency has become so widespread that it is often difficult to find unaffected animals.

PERIODONTAL DISEASE

This is disease affecting the tissues surrounding the tooth. More teeth are lost as a result of periodontal disease than any other condition of the mouth. The teeth themselves are usually perfectly healthy, but the structures surrounding the teeth, called the periodontium, become diseased and unable to support them. Eighty-five per cent of dogs and cats over 3 years old suffer from periodontitis to some degree; it is the most common and most easily prevented oral disease.

The mouth is naturally an unhygienic environment, containing many bacteria. These come from food and grooming and also from some of our pets' less attractive habits such as investigating rotting carcases and faeces. Some of these bacteria stick to the tooth surface, forming a layer called *plaque* (see Fig. 207). Up to 9–12 months of age, the dog's teeth are usually so smooth that the plaque is wiped off whilst gnawing some tough material. With the passage of time, the surface of the teeth becomes minutely roughened, making it easier for the plaque to adhere. Although this may not be readily visible to the naked eye, it soon becomes apparent if one of the 'human' disclosing solutions is used. These work just as well with dogs' teeth as with ours and are readily available from the local pharmacy. As the plaque accumulates, it becomes mineralised and hardens to form a yellowish-brown layer. This is called *calculus*. Plaque continues to build up on the surface of the calculus, becoming mineralised and thus continuing the process (see Fig. 208). However, it is the plaque bacteria that do the damage, not the calculus. Plaque on its own causes periodontal disease, whereas calculus on its own does not. Calculus is so rough though, it is rare to find calculus without a coating of plaque. From their vantage point on the teeth the plaque bacteria then invade the gums at the gingival crevice. Inflammation of the gums, or gingivitis, then occurs, which is the gum's method of increasing its defences to fight off the bacteria. The blood supply is increased so that more white blood cells, which protect all the

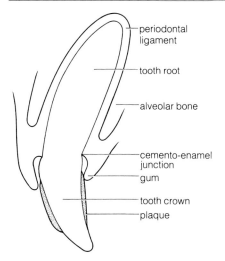

periodontal
ligament

tooth root

alveolar bone

cemento-enamel
junction

gum

tooth crown

plaque

Figure 207 Plaque adheres
to the enamel but is
constantly worn off the tip
of the tooth, accumulating
mostly nearer the gum

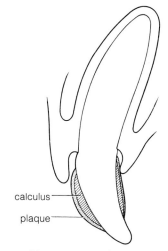

calculus

plaque

Figure 208 Calculus
builds up more on the
surface next to the lips. On
the other surface the tongue
is constantly licking it off
although a thin layer does
accumulate

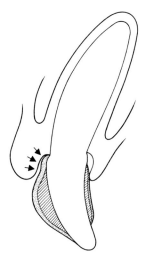

Figure 209 Defence
mechanisms try to fight off
the advancing bacteria, the
gum swells, often bleeds
and is pushed away from
the tooth by the
accumulating calculus and
plaque

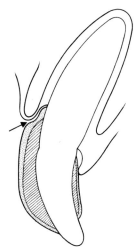

Figure 210 The gums
recede; the bacteria attack
the periodontal ligament as
well as the gums

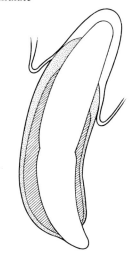

Figure 211 The bacteria
have destroyed much of the
gum, periodontal ligament
and alveolar bone. The
tooth is loose, exudes pus,
and plaque and calculus
accumulate

body systems from infection, are available. The extra blood, however, results in reddening and swelling of the gums, which is clearly visible (see Fig. 209). As the bacteria advance along the tooth, the gums recede (see Fig. 210); the bacteria also change to more aggressive, destructive types known as anaerobes, which can live with little or no oxygen. These further destroy the gum, alveolar bone and periodontal ligament as they work their way down the tooth root (see Fig. 211). Pus exudes from around the tooth as the destruction of the periodontal structures continues. Eventually the supportive tissues are destroyed and the tooth is lost along with most of the invading bacteria. The body defences then overcome the remaining bacteria and slowly the socket is filled. The hole left by the avulsed tooth weakens the jawbone considerably as it is not immediately filled in with new bone but just with fibrous tissue. After 4–6 months, however, new bone will gradually fill the socket.

The tragedy of the situation is that seldom, if ever, are the teeth that are lost anything other than healthy. With early dental attention they could undoubtedly have been saved (see Plate 22).

Complications

Apart from the discomfort of the periodontal disease and the loss of these otherwise healthy teeth, the bacteria on the teeth enter the bloodstream and are carried around the body. All the blood from the body passes through the heart, lungs, kidneys and liver. Bacteria carried in the blood can settle in any of these or other organs and set up a focus of infection which may interfere with their functioning, thus causing numerous serious problems. This is especially important in the older animal. Endocarditis, for example, a serious heart condition, could be directly attributable to lack of dental care.

Treatment

Effective treatment of periodontal disease depends on the total removal of the plaque bacteria and all the calculus not only from the visible crown of the tooth but also from below the gums, where calculus and bacteria are moving down the root. To be done properly this should be performed under anaesthetic by a veterinary surgeon using special hand scalers, curettes and possibly ultrasonic scaling equipment (see Plate 23). Once the crowns, affected roots and gingival crevices have been perfectly cleaned they must be polished to give the tooth its original, absolutely smooth surface. This will make it more difficult for the plaque to adhere to the tooth. Thus, to be done properly, a dog's teeth scaling involves a general anaesthetic and a fairly time-consuming procedure, so it is likely to be more expensive than private dental treatment involving scaling and polishing for us.

If the periodontal disease is advanced, the gingival crevice may have deepened to form a pocket as a result of the bacterial invasion. If this pocket is more than 3–4 mm deep, it is very difficult to keep clean. If the pocket is left, despite being thoroughly cleaned during the scaling and polishing process by the veterinary surgeon, bacteria will soon recolonise it and continue to invade the deeper structures of the tooth. It is therefore necessary to reposition the gum edge further down the tooth to eliminate such a pocket. Then with thorough home care, further progress of periodontal disease can be prevented.

Antibiotics are also often required to help clear up any remaining bacteria. Oral hygiene sprays containing antiseptic and zinc to apply to the gums will help damaged gum tissue to heal.

Although periodontal surgery can be very successful with people, its application can present problems in the dog. If too much of the tooth's supporting structure has been destroyed or, alternatively, if effective home care is not feasible, the badly affected teeth will have to be extracted. Loose incisors can be saved by splinting them to firm teeth after thorough cleaning and with meticulous home care some degree of repair can occur.

From the above it will be realised that treatment at best is only a salvage procedure and prevention obviously is preferable. *This involves home care.*

Daily tooth cleaning is the only way to prevent periodontal disease (see Plate 24).

Gnawing on rawhide chews, tough rubber toys, large pieces of raw vegetable or barely cooked tough meat and chunky, hard, dry food helps, but is no substitute for brushing the teeth with a soft but firm toothbrush and a specially formulated dog toothpaste.

Human toothpaste is not suitable because it froths. It frightens most dogs, lacks the appealing taste of specially formulated dog toothpaste and should not be swallowed in excess. On the market today there are dog toothpastes containing agents which kill the bacteria in plaque. These are available through veterinary surgeons. Because the market is much smaller than that for human toothpaste the cost is considerably higher.

How do you brush a dog's teeth?

The easiest approach is with the dog sitting down. Approach from the side and gently lift the upper lip. The teeth are then brushed with a circular motion, which massages the gums as well as cleaning the teeth. Finally a downward stroke is used to brush the debris away from the gums. Since teeth-cleaning procedures are best started at 6–9 months of age, before the inflammatory processes have begun, and as it needs to be performed daily, it needs to be an enjoyable event. At first only one or two teeth should be brushed at a time, then, as the dog grows accustomed to the new routine, more teeth can be tackled. When the outsides of all the teeth can be brushed with ease, the inner aspects may be added to the routine, although this is less important as the tongue rubbing on the teeth helps to keep them clean and reduce the amount of plaque that is laid down.

More abrasive pastes are available which help to remove any minor deposits from the crowns of the teeth, but these cannot reach the calculus and plaque below the gum margin. After professional scaling and polishing has been carried out, daily brushing with special toothpaste will help to prevent the recurrence of periodontal disease by removing any plaque deposits.

EPULIS

This is the commonest growth in the dog's mouth and is usually benign (non-cancerous). It is an excessive growth of gum tissue. As the growth enlarges it can change shape and become cauliflower-like (see Plate 25). These tumours often grow from the gum line up the side of the tooth. Bacteria and debris, trapped between the epulis and the tooth, invade the normal gum, thus causing periodontal disease. Epulides are particularly common in Boxers, but any breed of dog can be affected.

Treatment

The growth should be removed under anaesthetic by a veterinarian and normal gum anatomy restored. Any periodontal disease must be treated as previously described. Unfortunately these growths do tend to recur and should be removed when pockets deeper than 4–6 mm are formed.

Complications

Not every growth in a mouth is an epulis. It is important that the growth is properly identified and treatment pertinent to each particular tumour carefully followed. Veterinary advice should be sought if you are at all concerned about any unusual gum formation in your dog's mouth.

CARIES

Caries is the decay or demineralisation of the enamel and dentine in the crown of the tooth, or the dentine of the root. It is less common in the dog than in man, but still affects over 10 per cent of all dogs. It is visible particularly on the biting surfaces of the molars and is easily seen when the dog yawns (see Plate 26). It can also be detected on any exposed root surfaces and often occurs at the gum margin. At first, the decay appears as a dull, white, powdery looking area which gradually becomes yellow, then brown and finally black as the lesion advances. Sometimes all that is visible is a small black dot on the surface of a tooth, but hiding underneath may be a much larger cavity of decayed dentine. Eventually the decay will penetrate the pulp and a painful tooth root abscess can result. The tooth will gradually disintegrate and will be lost.

Symptoms, apart from those visible, may include a reluctance to eat and jaw chattering, but usually there are few specific symptoms. The dog's premature ageing and unwillingness to play often disappear once the toothache is treated.

Cause

Lack of oral hygiene and the consumption of excessive sugar in the diet contribute to dental decay in the dog as in man. Defects in the formation of enamel during development of the teeth may leave areas of exposed dentine which are more susceptible to decay. This enamel deficiency is called enamel hypoplasia and may be the result of:

1. Illness or damage during the tooth's development, commonly producing a band of exposed dentine round one or more teeth. In the days when distemper was rife this was a very common finding. Affected teeth were often called 'distemper teeth', indicating that the puppy had had a fever and illness whilst the teeth were developing
2. A developmental anomaly, where the enamel did not form a complete covering over the dentine, resulting in a small defect sometimes found on the biting surfaces of the molars and premolars.

Complications

If the caries lesion is not treated early in its course, and enters the pulp chamber (root canal), root canal therapy (see later) is required if the tooth is to be saved; otherwise it will have to be extracted.

Treatment

The sooner a caries lesion is treated the better. As the cavity encroaches upon the pulp chamber so it becomes more painful and difficult to treat. The decayed dentine is drilled out under general anaesthesia. If the cavity has reached the pulp chamber the pulp must be protected (capped) or removed, depending on its state of health. Small undercuts are made in the dentine to retain the filling. Once it is set, the surface is carved to follow the contours of the tooth, then polished to make it perfectly smooth. Some filling material such as the glass ionomers release fluoride, which helps to strengthen the dentine and prevent further spread of the lesion, but it is not strong enough to be used alone on the biting (occlusal) surfaces of teeth. It should be covered with composite or amalgam to provide a strong biting surface.

Prevention

Examination of the teeth for signs of early decay is mandatory. This can be carried out easily by owners who have trained their dogs to allow dental inspection. Early recognition allows early treatment and it is imperative that any exposed dentine should be treated, preferably before it begins to decay. If in doubt about any marks on your dog's teeth, do consult your veterinarian in the first instance.

Home care on a daily basis, involving brushing of all the surfaces of the teeth with a specially formulated dog toothpaste together with the avoidance of sugary foods, will help to prevent tooth decay.

PULP NECROSIS AND ROOT CANAL TREATMENT

The death of the pulp (pulp necrosis) spells the death of the tooth. A tooth root abscess (apical abscess) will result which can be very painful. If the tooth is to be saved, root canal therapy is necessary just as in man. In the dog, the canine and the upper fourth premolar (carnassial) teeth are the most commonly affected.

Causes

Pulp will die as the result of:

1. Infection. Disease can enter the pulp via the bloodstream if the dog is suffering a severe, generalised infection. More commonly, the infection is the result of exposure of the pulp by an extensive caries lesion or a fracture.
2. The blood vessels to the pulp can be damaged as they enter the tooth at the apex. A hard blow to a tooth can move it enough to damage the apical blood vessels without actually breaking the tooth.
3. Excessive heat can damage the pulp and result in its death. This is rare, but can occur, for example, when a puppy chews through an electric cable and survives.

Symptoms

Apart from possible toothache, which in its early stages is often undetectable, there will be no obvious evidence that the pulp is dying until weeks or even months later. The tooth then begins to change colour. It normally turns pinkish grey, reflecting the colour of the degenerated blood in the fine tubules of the dentine (see Plate 27). This should not be confused with oxytetracycline staining (see below). If the tooth has been broken, the pulp will be visible at the fracture site, if it is exposed. At first it will be red-pink; as it deteriorates, it becomes black.

Treatment

Treatment is a little complicated if it is to be successful and the tooth saved. Under general anaesthesia the tooth is first X-rayed to ensure there are no hidden complications. If there is not already a convenient hole in the tooth from a fracture, an access hole is drilled into the pulp chamber, the dead and dying pulp is removed from the root canal (pulp chamber), using special veterinary instruments similar to, but larger than, those used in human work. The wall of the canal is then filed clean. This has to be done meticulously, starting with tiny files and working up to the largest file necessary to bring out clean filings. The canal is then disinfected, dried thoroughly and filled with a cement, often zinc oxide and eugenol, as with human dentistry. This is compressed into the canal using gutta percha points, which are long fine conical rolls of a special type of rubber, and instruments, called pluggers and condensors. Small undercuts are made in the dentine and the access hole is filled. Any rough or sharp edges are smoothed off, and the tooth is polished. The pinkish grey discoloration is very difficult to treat. Treatment follows the same lines as that for tetracycline staining described later in this chapter.

Complications

Necrotic pulp is very susceptible to infection as it has no defence mechanism. The infection spreads throughout the pulp, through the apex of the tooth and invades the alveolar bone, forming an apical abscess. This is visible on an X-ray as a halo around the root tip. Eventually, the infection works its way through the bone and appears under the skin as a swelling or on the gum as a red gum boil, a little distance from the root tip. This bursts, releasing pus and serum, which will continue to discharge for as long as the infected pulp exists.

Pulp necrosis is very serious in young dogs. When the pulp is dead no more dentine is produced, so the dentine wall remains thin. Thus it is weak and the tooth is vulnerable to fractures.

Prevention

Avoid the causes where possible by providing dogs with tough rubber toys to chew, *not bones*, which are a common cause of tooth fracture and apical damage.

Fighting, collisions with cars, walls and other dogs, and catching stones are also to be avoided.

Early treatment of any suspected lesion should prevent its progression to an abscess or a discharging sinus, which often leads to loss of the tooth.

BROKEN TEETH

Approximately 50 per cent of dogs break one or more teeth at some time in their lives. Sometimes a dog can break the tip of a tooth without exposing the pulp, but more often than not the fracture does involve the pulp chamber. Being composed mainly of small blood vessels, the damaged pulp usually bleeds, but this soon stops (see Plate 28). As the pulp rapidly becomes infected, treatment should be sought as soon as possible.

Causes

Chewing bones is mistakenly thought to be good for dogs' teeth and often results in slab fractures of the upper fourth premolar (see Plate 29). A slab of enamel and dentine is broken off the lateral side of the tooth, usually extending from the tip of the tooth down sometimes below the gum margin and often involving the pulp.

The canine teeth are commonly fractured in head-on collisions with other dogs, cars, walls or during fighting. However, a common cause is the diabolical pastime of catching stones. *Never, ever throw stones* for your dog.

It is sometimes necessary to reduce the height of the canine teeth, for example if a tooth has erupted incorrectly and impinges upon a structure it should miss. Sometimes owners of working dogs request that the length of the canines be reduced if they are thought to be damaging their charges with over-vigorous use of their teeth. The procedure is similar to that used for dealing with freshly broken teeth, which is described below.

Treatment

The teeth must first be X-rayed under general anaesthesia, but provided the pulp is fresh and healthy and there are no complications, pulp capping can be carried out. This is a sterile procedure carried out under general anaesthesia and full aseptic conditions. The tooth and mouth are cleaned thoroughly and if the canine teeth are intact but are to be reduced in height the required length of tooth is cut off with a dental drill. Using special sterile instruments the top 8 mm (½ in.) of pulp is removed. Bleeding is controlled and calcium hydroxide gently packed on top of the pulp to stimulate it to produce reparative secondary dentine. Small undercuts are made, cavity liners are placed and the hole is then filled in the usual way and antibiotics administered.

This procedure, although complicated, is of particular importance in young dogs up to 2 years of age. It keeps the tooth alive, allowing the pulp to continue producing dentine to thicken and strengthen the tooth wall.

If the tooth is broken below gum level the root can be saved with root canal treatment. It is possible but unwise to put a post into the treated root and attach a small crown. Due to the forces exerted within the dog's mouth, it would be injudicious to build the crown to the same height as the original tooth. The chances are it would soon be broken and damage the remaining root too.

Why should one treat the root and not remove it? Removing the tooth root will initially weaken the jaw as the socket does not fill with bone for 3–6 months. This will make the jaw more likely to fracture until then. Extraction of dogs' teeth is more difficult than in man as the roots are much larger. Hence it is traumatic for the dog and may be complicated by jaw fracture, oro-nasal fistula formation and post-operative pain and infection (see Extraction on page 511).

Complications

If the tooth is not treated within 24 hours of the injury, infection is likely to become established in the pulp. This leads to pulp necrosis and the complications associated with it. In young dogs it is very serious. The dead pulp does not produce dentine, so gradual thickening of the dentine walls ceases, rendering the thin wall weak and susceptible to further fractures. This relative weakness is also a problem even if full root canal treatment has been carried out in a dog less than 2 years old.

Prevention

It will be obvious from the above that tooth-breaking activities should be avoided wherever possible! Stones should never be thrown for dogs to catch; bones should not be given to dogs, particularly young dogs, because the dentine wall is so fragile and thin.

WEARING DOWN OF TEETH (TOOTH ATTRITION)

Normally a dog's teeth only wear down slightly with the normal habits of feeding, grooming and lifestyle. Some dogs develop habits such as stone chewing, brick carrying and excessive grooming. This latter may possibly be secondary to flea infestation. The result is to wear the teeth down abnormally fast, a process known as *attrition*. As the enamel and dentine is worn away, the pulp rapidly lays down reparative dentine to protect itself from the encroaching irritant. This process is continuous and the reparative dentine is visible as a brown mark in the middle of the wearing tooth surface. No treatment is necessary unless the rate of wear exceeds the rate of repair and the pulp is exposed. Treatment is then the same as for broken teeth.

THE TETRACYCLINES

These very useful broad-spectrum antibiotics are now known to cause discoloration of developing teeth when administered to dogs of less than 6–8 months old. All the teeth that were developing at the time the drug was given will become brown, yellow-orange or grey. These teeth are not weakened or damaged in any way; they are only discoloured, so no treatment is required except for aesthetic reasons.

Treatment

Complicated bleaching techniques may remove these discolorations. Affected teeth are more successfully coated with enamel-coloured resin to cover the discoloration. In either case general anaesthesia is required and the treatment is not simple.

REBUILDING OF CROWNS

Rarely is it necessary to build up the crown of a dog's tooth to its original height. Dogs can manage very well with short crowns. Only for aesthetic reasons and for some working dogs, building a crown may be desired. The forces imposed on dogs' teeth are far greater than on human teeth as the jaws and jaw muscles are so much stronger. A human tooth has to withstand forces of approximately 150 lb/sq in., whereas a dog's tooth is subjected to up to 1,200 lb/sq in. It is for this reason that rebuilding crowns rarely succeeds for any length of time. The playful nature of the dog also endangers any false crowns, which frequently disintegrate whilst chewing fences, fighting or just playing. Hence it is not recommended to have a crown fitted to a broken tooth, as it is unlikely to last, and is usually of no benefit to the dog.

Techniques

Techniques vary according to the tooth involved. Incisors can be rebuilt up to almost their normal height. Small holes are drilled in the remaining part of the tooth or root to accept tiny metal pegs, pins or posts, having performed root canal treatment if the pulp is involved. The crown is then rebuilt on the pins and posts using composite or dental acrylic. If a porcelain-bonded metal or a metal crown is to be fitted, an impression is taken after the posts have been placed and sent to a dental laboratory, which will make the crown according to the impression. This is then cemented in place.

The canine teeth are of course much larger and hence subjected to greater leverage forces. Porcelain-bonded metal crowns often chip, so metal crowns are preferred. Root canal treatment is performed when necessary, and the tooth prepared for the crown. An impression is taken from which the dental laboratory makes the crown. This is then cemented into place.

Premolars and molars are more difficult. It is not recommended that these are built up higher than the level of the remaining tooth structure since they are likely to disintegrate with a dog's gnawing activities. However, it is essential that the root canal is treated if it is involved.

EXTRACTION

If teeth are so badly diseased or decayed that they cannot be saved, they will have to be extracted. Extracting dogs' teeth is more difficult and traumatic than extracting humans' teeth, because the roots of dogs' teeth are much longer and more firmly attached. In man, normal teeth can be removed by twisting and pulling each tooth with dental forceps. This is not true of dogs' teeth. Sharp-ended fine instruments (elevators) are worked in between the alveolar bone and the tooth root, breaking and tearing the periodontal ligament and, inevitably, breaking some of the surrounding alveolar bone. Eventually, when the whole periodontal ligament is destroyed, the small single-rooted tooth will come out. If the tooth is pulled using dental forceps the root will usually fracture, leaving part of it behind in the socket. Removal of the broken fragment is very difficult but must be achieved to prevent infection and suppuration.

For larger teeth and multi-rooted teeth, extraction is even more difficult. Multi-rooted teeth, i.e., premolars and molars, are cut into single-rooted segments, using a dental drill. The junction of the roots must first be located, then the crown cut through in a straight line to this junction (called the furcation, see Fig. 203). Each root is then elevated individually, as described above for small single-rooted teeth.

The canine teeth are probably the most difficult to extract. The root extends a very long way into the jaw bone. In the lower jaw, the tooth's tip is very close to the edge of the jaw bone. In the upper jaw, the canine's root is adjacent to the nasal cavity, separated from it only by a very thin plate of bone.

Extraction of these teeth requires great care and patience. To avoid penetrating the nasal cavity the tooth must not be tilted during extraction and the elevator must be used very precisely. It is usual to incise the gum with a scalpel and lift it from the bone over the tooth root. The bone visible over the root is then drilled away. The fine elevator is carefully worked through the periodontal ligament between the root and the remaining bone, being careful not to penetrate the nasal passage when extracting upper canines. Thus loosened, the tooth is lifted off. The gum is then sutured back into place, closing the large empty socket.

From Fig. 199 it can be seen that the roots of dogs' teeth are very large. Once extracted the empty socket weakens the jaw. It takes many months for the socket to fill with bone and regain some of its former strength.

From the above it will be obvious that dental problems can occur in dogs just as they do with us. Unfortunately dogs cannot tell us how much discomfort these problems cause, but specialist treatment is now available. Dental techniques are just as unpleasant to the dog as they are to us, and since explanations are impossible, general anaesthesia is essential. This presents additional cost to the specialised and often time-consuming techniques that have been described. Nevertheless, these techniques can be successfully applied and present a positive alternative to the inevitable extraction.

Today there are a few practices specialising in the dental techniques described. If your veterinary surgeon has not specialised in this particular field, you are likely to be referred to one that has. This may mean travelling some distance, but it is well worth the journey to save your dog suffering toothache.

30
RUPTURES AND HERNIAS

'I am afraid Zak has ruptured the cruciate ligament in his knee joint, that is why he is lame and in pain.'

'Poor Polly has an inguinal hernia, that's what the swelling is between her back legs, she will have to have an operation.'

'As a result of the road traffic accident Rambo has suffered a severe ventral rupture. We will have to operate immediately.'

These are typical of comments heard frequently in veterinary consulting rooms and they must be confusing in the extreme to many dog owners. Throughout this book there has been reference to various types of ruptures and hernias and it was felt that a chapter on these disruptions and their consequences might help unravel some of the complexities.

Confusion has arisen since, by common usage, ruptures and hernias have become synonymous terms whereas strictly they are not. A rupture describes tearing or disruption of tissue. Thus the ruptured ligament mentioned above is a torn ligament. A hernia on the other hand describes the abnormal protrusion of part of an organ or tissue through the structures normally containing it. The above mentioned inguinal hernia describes the protrusion of some of the abdominal contents – fat, loops of intestine or occasionally uterus in the bitch – through the abdominal wall to form a visible swelling in the groin. Discussion of the ventral rupture will make the situation clearer. The veterinary surgeon has realised that, as a result of the road traffic accident, the abdominal muscles which help to contain Rambo's abdominal contents have been torn and therefore the abdominal contents are able to prolapse and lie just below the skin (subcutaneously). Thus a ventral rupture is in this case a ventral hernia. However, in the case of ruptures involving tissues other than those associated with the abdomen the rupture may not involve herniation. For example, a ruptured or torn bladder, a not uncommon sequel to a road traffic accident, is not usually associated with herniation of the bladder since again this would involve rupture of the abdominal wall.

Hernias may be reducible or irreducible.

If irreducible they are incarcerated: in other words, the herniated contents cannot be returned to their normal position.

Reducible hernias on the other hand are responsible for those abdominal swellings, which disappear. Inguinal hernias are frequently reducible and on coming to the vet the swelling in the groin which had been so worrying has miraculously gone. However, the veterinary surgeon will soon be able to tell whether there is a rupture in the abdominal wall through which the bowel contents are herniating so there is no need for embarrassment even if the swelling has disappeared. It is worth remembering that not all abdominal hernias follow a rupture. In the case of inguinal hernias sometimes the abdominal contents will pass down the natural inguinal canal which just happens to be sufficiently large to allow the abdominal contents to escape. In this case there is strictly no rupture involved.

Thus we can have ruptures without hernias and hernias without ruptures.

Hernias are classified according to their anatomical position and a few of the more common ones affecting the dog will be described. The majority of these also involve ruptures, but ruptures that do not involve herniation will be described subsequently.

Diaphragmatic Hernia

In this condition part of the abdominal contents (usually the liver and stomach) pass into the chest cavity. Although occasionally this can be congenital, due to improper closure of the diaphragm separating the chest from the abdominal cavity, by far the greatest number of cases of diaphragmatic hernia follow diaphragmatic rupture as the result of trauma such as a road traffic accident or a fall.

The signs of herniation which include respiratory distress, cyanosis (blue colour of the mucous membranes) and shock may not be immediately evident following the rupture of the diaphragm since it may take some days for the abdominal contents to move forward and initiate the production of pleural fluid and increased intrathoracic pressure, which results in the signs of discomfort and difficulty in breathing. One of the signs often described is of an 'empty abdomen' on palpation, because the abdominal contents have moved into the chest where they cannot be easily palpated, but I have always found this a particularly unreliable sign.

A relatively rare type of diaphragmatic hernia is the pericardio-diaphragmatic hernia or peritonopericardial hernia as it is sometimes called. This is a type that is not associated with concomitant diaphragmatic rupture but is congenital (has been present from birth) and is due to incomplete formation of the diaphragm in such a way that it permits the abdominal cavity to communicate directly with the pericardial sac surrounding the heart. Signs depend entirely on the type of abdominal contents which move forward to occupy a position in the pericardial sac adjacent to the heart. In some cases signs may be entirely absent. However, the condition is usually associated with digestive upsets, difficulty in breathing and, on occasions, heart failure.

Femoral Hernia

This is very rare but is reported to occur sometimes in performing dogs which have been trained to walk on their hind legs. It is always acquired and it is considered that the vertical position of the body imposes an unusual strain on the muscles at the fold of the thigh. The femoral canal is the tubular passage that carries nerves and blood vessels to the hind leg and a femoral hernia classically contains a loop of bowel.

Hiatus Hernia

This is much rarer in the dog than it is in man. It strictly describes the protrusion of one of the abdominal structures through one of the natural openings or hiatuses in the diaphragm. These natural openings allow the vena cava, aorta and oesophagus to cross from the thorax to the abdomen and are all situated in the upper (dorsal) part of the diaphragm which in the dog is particularly muscular. However, cases have been reported of herniation of part of the stomach through the oesophageal hiatus.

Incisional Hernia

This is the term used to describe the swellings that sometimes appear following an operation when there has been breakdown of the wound internally although the skin has healed. An incisional hernia can be due to several factors, but basically is the result of improper healing or excessive strain on the wound. This may be caused by undue muscular effort on the part of the dog, obesity or jumping from a height which creates undue pressure on the weakened area. Frequently incisional hernias are referred to as wound breakdowns.

Inguinal Hernia

In the dog this is more common that a femoral hernia although the site is similar. The first sign noticed is a swelling of varying size in the groin. The hernia may be the result of rupture of the abdominal muscles at a weak point in the groin or, as is more usual, passage of the abdominal contents through the inguinal canal. This canal is an oblique passage in the ventral abdominal wall and carries the round ligament of the uterus in the female or the spermatic cord in the male. Most commonly a loop of bowel, omental fat or occasionally a gravid uterus is found in the hernia. In the male the herniated contents will sometimes descend into the scrotum when it is known as a scrotal hernia. (See Fig. 212 and Fig. 213, overleaf.)

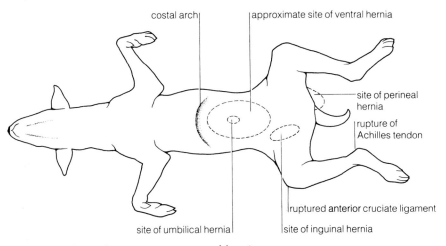

costal arch

approximate site of ventral hernia

site of perineal hernia

rupture of Achilles tendon

ruptured anterior cruciate ligament

site of umbilical hernia

site of inguinal hernia

Figure 212   Sites of common ruptures and hernias

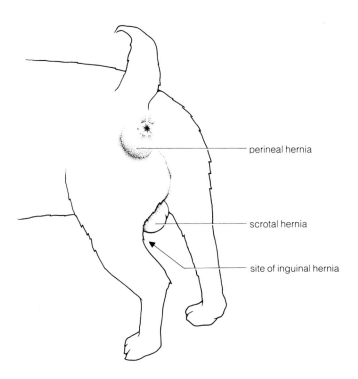

perineal hernia

scrotal hernia

site of inguinal hernia

Figure 213   Diagrammatic representation of perineal hernia also showing sites of inguinal and scrotal hernias

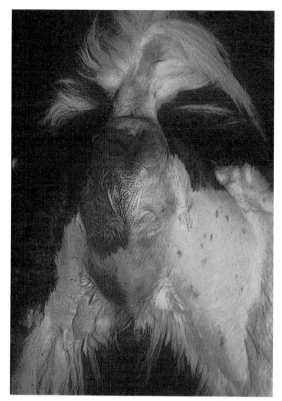

Figure 214 An 8-year-old male mongrel with a
double perineal hernia with right side haematoma

Perineal Hernia

The region surrounding the anus and bounded by the tail and the pelvis is
known as the perineum. Beneath the skin there is a muscular diaphragm,
a defect in which can allow deviation of the rectum and protrusion of
pelvic and sometimes abdominal contents including the bladder.

Many factors have been incriminated in the aetiology. Although the
condition can occur in bitches, it has long been recognized as a disease of
older uncastrated male dogs. The peak age incidence is approximately 8
years. Straining, diarrhoea, congenital weakness, hormonal imbalance
have all been implicated. Signs include swelling on one or both sides of the
anus with constant straining. (See Fig. 212 and Fig. 213.)

Strangulated Hernia

A simple (reducible) hernia, particularly when involving a loop of bowel,
can become strangulated. The hernia becomes tightly constricted. As any
hernia progresses through its weakened retaining wall the opening in the

wall tends to close behind it, thus forming a narrow neck. If the constriction is great enough the blood supply is cut off and the hernia will quickly swell and become strangulated. It is vital that blood supply is quickly restored to the organ otherwise necrosis and gangrene can result which can lead to the death of the dog. It is for this reason that veterinary surgeons will frequently advice surgical correction of even very small, simple hernias solely as a preventative measure.

Umbilical Hernia

This is the classical 'little rupture of the belly button'. It is a protrusion of the abdominal contents through the abdominal wall at the umbilicus. The opening in the abdominal wall is natural but this should close at birth. Many defects do close with time. In the puppy it is only a persistent or irreducible umbilical hernia that will need surgical intervention. Do not be alarmed if your veterinary surgeon advises 'masterly inactivity' for a little while; he is merely waiting to see if the condition will be self-correcting.

The condition appears to be familial in some breeds. Those showing a higher risk of umbilical problems include the Airedale, Basenji, Pekingese, Pointer and Weimeraner.

Cutting the umbilical cord too close to the body wall by the bitch, breeder or veterinary surgeon has been implicated in some cases. This is more likely to result in evisceration of abdominal contents than in the formation of a hernia, however.

Umbilical hernias are potentially serious if irreducible since strangulation can occur or if a loop of bowel is involved, obstruction of the bowel may result. (See Fig. 212.)

Ventral Abdominal Hernia

This has already been mentioned. It is worthwhile remembering that by definition it is 'an interruption in the continuity of the abdominal wall at any point other than the umbilicus or inguinal ring'. In addition to the ventral abdominal muscles 'ventral' hernias can also occur laterally and can be found in the flank close to the pelvis. This has been attributed to the elasticity of the tissue in this area compared to the midline which is highly fibrous (*linea alba*), or the anterior paracostal area where the muscle is thicker and stronger. Usually ventral hernias are the result of trauma, often a road traffic accident, but fights can result in the condition. Occasionally weakness or maldevelopment of the abdominal muscle will predispose. (See Fig. 212.)

Treatment of hernias

With ourselves many hernias are treated by palliative measures, trusses, bandages etc. These are of no use whatsoever in the dog. In young animals it is common practice to leave simple hernias alone, often the animal will 'grow round' the hernia and it will disappear. Failing this, surgery is advised, irrespective of the type of hernia. Even complicated diaphragmatic hernias now carry a good chance of recovery due to modern surgical methods and anaesthesia.

The operation for strangulated hernia is urgent and obviously carries a much poorer prognosis, particularly if gangrene has set in. Today with modern antibiotics and other drugs to combat shock even these previously poor risk cases are tackled with more confidence and success.

RUPTURES

Rupture of the Heart

This condition is not common but can occur following certain types of heart disease. Small breeds of dogs in particular are affected.

Rupture of Abdominal Organs

Rupture of the alimentary canal tract can occur as the result of tumours, dilation and torsion (in the case of the stomach), foreign bodies etc. If diagnosed sufficiently quickly prompt surgery and resection of part of the bowel can be successful.

Ruptured Bladder

The urinary bladder can rupture as the result of obstruction, usually due to calculi (stones) although it can follow trauma. Again prompt surgery is essential.

Similar causes can result in rupture of the urethra.

Rupture of the Liver

Rupture of the liver, spleen and kidney can also occur either spontaneously (usually as the result of tumour formation) or as the result of trauma.

Abdominal pain and sudden collapse are the cardinal signs. The dog is invariably very shocked and requires very prompt and aggressive treatment. Even then the chances of recovery are limited.

RUPTURES OF LIGAMENTS, MUSCLES AND TENDONS

Ligaments

In the dog the ligaments most commonly ruptured are the anterior cruciate ligament in the knee and the round ligament in the hip joint.

The anterior cruciate ligament serves to stabilise the stifle (knee) and tearing and stretching of its fibres can be gradual, resulting in chronic lameness, or sudden, as the result of uncoordinated movement such as occurs if the dog slips when moving at speed. Without surgery the animal is unlikely to regain a normal gait but sophisticated surgical techniques now available are extremely effective in restoring normal function in a relatively short time. Many dogs having undergone successful joint surgery are able to compete both in obedience and working trials as well as shows for beauty.

Rupture of the round ligament of the hip is invariably associated with dislocation of the joint. Modern surgical techniques aimed at restoring the integrity of the joint are remarkably successful.

Muscles

An example of rupture of a muscle is that of the gracilis muscle in the racing greyhound. This is a small muscle which occupies the medial surface of the thigh. Rupture causes lameness and inability to extend the stifle and there is usually an obvious swelling on the medial surface of the thigh. Treatment involving careful suturing coupled with prolonged rest often results in restoration of function. (See Chapter 19, The Locomotor System.)

Tendons

The Achilles tendon is the common tendon of the gastrocnemius, superficial digital flexor, semitendinosis and biceps femoris muscles. Partial or complete rupture occurs as the result of trauma or lacerations. Ruptures usually occur at the point of insertion into the calcaneus (point of the hock) and often are associated with an avulsion fracture. The signs are characteristic since the hock is 'dropped' and the dog is no longer able to stand or walk on the toes of the affected limb. The plantar or posterior surface of the metatarsus may touch the ground and the ruptured ends of the tendon can usually be palpated through the skin. The condition does not usually appear acutely painful. Treatment is surgical.

By definition some hernias are also classified as prolapses – but just as with ruptures all prolapses are certainly not hernias. Thus a prolapsed intervertebral disc can be rightly described as a herniated disc, whereas a prolapsed rectum is certainly not a hernia. Beware!

Miscellaneous

31

KENNELS AND KENNEL MANAGEMENT

It is a lucky dog that does not have to be kenelled at sometime during its life and it is for this reason that this chapter has been written.

The family holiday is probably the main reason for kennelling Rover. Please do not be tempted to take him with you even if you are only popping across the Channel for the weekend in your new boat. If you do, you are liable to be faced with six months quarantine for Rover on his return due to the strict enforcement of quarantine laws in the UK, laws which are unlikely to be lifted despite further harmonisation within the EEC in 1992.

Whatever you do, do not be tempted to try to smuggle him back.

Dogs also have to be kennelled for other reasons. Have you ever wondered what happens when the veterinary surgeon says he is going to keep Rover in or where he is put when he is recovering from an operation (Fig. 215)? There are also animals that, for a variety of reasons, have to be accommodated, partially if not entirely, in kennels within the home environment.

Thus, all told, there are many reasons why you need to know about kennels.

Numerically speaking, commercial boarding kennels are the largest group, but quarantine kennels are more stringently governed by legislation with regard to construction and management. They have therefore, over the years, become regarded as the pattern from which other commercial kennels have evolved.

All kennels have broadly the same requirements. They must cater for the needs of the dogs and the personnel looking after them. The dog's needs are relatively simple. Warm, comfortable accommodation with adequate ventilation and sanitary facilities are the requirements of the inmate. The personnel looking after both the kennels and inmates require kennels that are escape proof, easily maintained and cleaned and that have adequate drainage and lighting. Other requirements are added for special purposes. Dogs in quarantine have to spend six months in the same kennel and

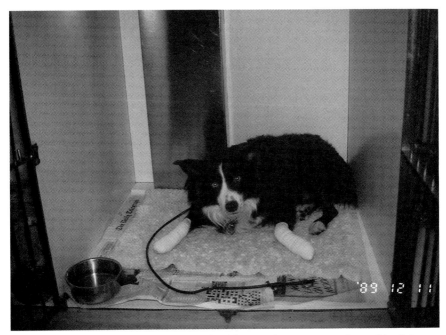

Figure 215   What happens to Rover when the veterinary surgeon keeps him in?

therefore need more space than is required for a fortnight 'holiday' let. At the other end of the scale, Rover staying overnight at the local veterinary hospital will probably have hardly any space at all but even so may actively discourage disturbance by his caring veterinary nurse, anxious that he has his regular 'comfort breaks'. The fact that he is provided with a thermostatically controlled heat pad in his little cell will no doubt be much appreciated during recovery from the effects of his general anaesthetic but that same heat pad, provided for a fortnight holiday boarder would be totally ignored, if not actively vandalised! These are just some examples of different needs for different circumstances.

QUARANTINE KENNELS

Quarantine kennels in the United Kingdom are designed and maintained for the sole purpose of keeping imported dogs out of contact with other animals for the statutory six months quarantine period. Although considered by many to be draconian, the quarantine regulations are designed to keep the British Isles rabies free. It must be realised that it only needs a rabid animal to attack some of our native wildlife, particularly foxes, for the disease to become rapidly endemic in this country.

One of the signs of the disease is a dramatic change in the dog's temperament. Thus, the quiet comfort-loving Collie suddenly goes on the rampage, gets the wanderlust and starts attacking everything in sight. One of the problems of the disease is that the incubation period is long and variable. This is the period between the dog becoming infected, usually from the bite of another animal, and the time that obvious signs of the disease begin to show. It is for this reason that quarantine has been set at six months. In some cases even this may not be long enough.

Quarantine kennels are under the daily inspection of a veterinary surgeon appointed by the Ministry of Agriculture, Fisheries and Food and it is to this veterinary surgeon that the licence is granted, not to the owner of the kennels. Every eventuality is covered in the regulations governing both the construction and the maintenance of quarantine kennels. The kennels must be constructed so that nose and paw contact between animals that are strangers to one another is impossible. Escape must also be prevented and for this reason entry to any kennel unit is through a 'lock' or 'trap' with inwardly opening doors, the first of which must be closed before the inner door is opened (Fig. 216). All doors must be fitted with locks and the doors must be self-closing.

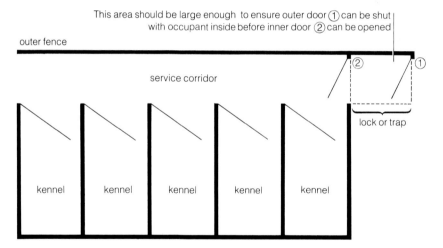

Figure 216 All access doors to quarantine kennels must have a lock or trap system to ensure security and prevent escape

Dogs from the same home can share a kennel with up to a maximum of three animals, but this is strictly at the discretion of the veterinary surgeon in charge. Separate accommodation must always be on hand in case it is required.

The minimum size of each kennel is specified and a rough guide to minimum area is that the width of each unit must be at least one and a half times the length of the dog and the length of each unit twice the length of the dog. Each kennel must open on to an individual run.

Minimum sizes of units

Small dogs to 25 lbs in weight (11.3 kg) must have a minimum internal compartment of 12 square feet (1.1 sq m). The width and the length must not be less than 3 feet. **Medium dogs**, which are classified as weighing up to 65 lb (30 kg) must have a minimum of 16 sq ft (1.5 sq m) and a width and length of not less than 4 sq ft (1.2 m). **Large dogs**, over 65 lb (30 kg) have a minimum of 16 sq feet of internal accommodation (1.5 sq m) and the width and length must not be less than 4 sq ft. Even for small dogs the height must not be less than 6 feet (1.8 metres). In other words, two tier units are not allowed. The partitions have to be solid between the internal compartments and extend up to 6 ft (1.8 m) or to the roof.

The size of runs is similarly controlled. **Small dogs** must have a minimum of 40 sq ft (3.7 sq m) **medium dogs** 60 sq ft (5.5 sq m) and **large dogs** 80 sq ft (7.5 sq m). The partitions between runs must be solid: up to 18″ (45 cm) for small and medium dogs and 2 ft (61 cm) for large dogs. If the rest of the partition is wire, it must be double with a gap that ensures there can be no paw or nose contact. For reasons of hygiene no grass exercise areas are allowed. As stated, the entrance to a block of kennels must have a 'trap' or 'lock' system with self-closing double doors opening inwards. All doors, including those of individual kennels, must be fitted with a lock and key.

Staff must be aware of the dangers of rabies to themselves and the implications should the disease become established in the United Kingdom. Basic hygiene and methods of preventing cross infection between animals in the kennels have to be understood.

Quarantine kennels have to be run as a totally separate unit and cannot form part of either a boarding or hospital kennels. Animals have to be vaccinated against rabies on entry to the kennels and clear identification must be evident at all times while the animal is in residence. [Surely yet another reason for a permanent identification system. Editor]

There are further regulations on cleanliness and disposal of waste material. Visitors may visit their own animal, but for the first 14 days after arrival and administration of rabies vaccine, the animal cannot have visitors except under very special circumstances.

Even the method of transport of the animal from the port of entry to the quarantine facility is controlled and must be by authorised carriers.

The regulations are designed solely to prevent rabies becoming established in this country. It behoves all of us to observe them and to ensure that they are not broken, because once rabies is established in our native population of foxes it would be very difficult to eradicate the disease.

BOARDING KENNELS

These are numerically by far the largest group of kennels found in Britain. A glance through any *Yellow Pages* will demonstrate that boarding kennels are to be found in all parts of the country. Their operation is governed by legislation under the Animal Boarding Establishments Act 1963. Under this Act it is forbidden to keep a boarding establishment for animals except under the authority of licence granted by a local authority. A boarding establishment is defined as 'any premises which provides accommodation for animals for return'. There are certain exceptions to this, particularly if the kennels are ancillary to the main business. Veterinary surgeons' practices or hospital kennels are not covered by the Act. Training kennels for Police dogs, Guide dogs or those for Obedience training are exempt as are Greyhound kennels and Hunt kennels. Kennels at airports and hotels are also exempt. Breeding kennels with more than two bitches are covered by the Breeding of Dogs Act 1973.

The legislation was designed to improve the standard of commercial kennels. Unfortunately the standards as set by the Act are imprecise and are open to varied interpretation by the inspecting officer of the local authority, who does not have to be a veterinary surgeon.

The Act states that 'animals must be kept in accommodation that is adequate in construction and size.' Some local authorities will interpret this to allow wooden kennels – others will not. The Act states that adequate exercise facilities 'should be provided' and unlike quarantine regulations, this does not include individual runs for each kennel unit. Grass exercise paddocks are allowed by some authorities. The Act states that 'sleeping compartments must be kept at an adequate temperature'. The interpretation of 'adequate' is also open to variation. Animals must be 'adequately supplied with food, drink and bedding' but there have been, on occasion, considerable differences in the interpretation of these provisions by the kennel's veterinary surgeon and the inspecting officer from the local authority.

Another condition of the Act states that 'While animals are boarded at the establishment there must always be someone resident at the premises and all animals must be visited at suitable intervals'. Obviously lock-up premises with the nearest responsible person out of sight and sound are disallowed but boarding kennels established in country areas are a different matter. Often these will utilise farm buildings or stables which are some distance from the main house. Nevertheless the occupant of the house is, within the meaning of the Act, living on the premises.

Thus, the caring owner cannot place too much reliance on licence by the local authority as a guarantee of quality in commercial kennels.

How then can one assess a boarding kennels? What are the criteria that one should look for when selecting a suitable kennels?

Firstly it is imperative that you do not leave the selection of the kennels until the last moment. If you do, your choice will be severely restricted and you may have to opt for sub-standard accommodation even though it is a licensed kennels.

It is worthwhile inspecting the kennels but choose the time carefully. It is unreasonable to expect to be shown round any kennels in the middle of a busy boarding season when the staff are working flat-out from dawn to dusk. With the exception of Christmas, Easter and Bank Holidays, most kennels are relatively quiet from October to June. Even if you have no firm holiday dates it is advisable to contact the kennels of your choice during this period to find out more about prices, accommodation, and services.

How do you select the kennels of your choice?

Yellow Pages is always a good starting point. Your veterinary surgeon should also be able to help with the name and address of reputable local accommodation. Direct recommendation from other dog owners is also worth following up.

Having listed a few names and addresses, what is the next step?

Ring the kennels and ask for details of their fees and services. Do they have a brochure and could you have a copy? From the brochure you can learn a lot. Is a specific deposit required and if so, under what conditions is the deposit returnable? Are inoculations required and evidence that they have been carried out? Are regular boosters mandatory? Are details of food preferences requested and contact addresses and telephone numbers in the event of an emergency?

The casual friendly kennel that sounds heaven-sent in the last-minute crisis: 'Oh yes, we've got room, drop him in when you're passing', should be avoided at all costs. Nice though the management undoubtedly are, and delightful to poor, bewildered Bertie, abandoned while his family fly off to the sun, these same casual folk may be totally incapable of responding to an unexpected emergency. They are unlikely to have taken any contact telephone numbers and will not have any means of contacting you should any mishap occur. They would, of course, be genuinely very distressed should anything go wrong.

Far better is the business-like approach: 'If we have to contact you in an emergency, can we have an address and 'phone number, either of yourselves abroad or your appointed representative.

'What are Bertie's food preferences? We try as far as possible to ensure that dogs in our care are happy and contented and if Bertie is disinclined to eat our brand of dog food, we'll try his.'

Then comes the question of the deposit. Reputable kennels have made a tremendous investment and their period of return is concentrated into a relatively short season. Owners who book at peak times and then do not turn up cause considerable waste of revenue since at good kennels accommodation is always at a premium during the boarding season. Therefore, do not be upset if a fairly hefty deposit is requested and a note to the effect that this is only returnable in special circumstances.

Before making a commitment to board Bertie, ask to see the kennels if at all possible. It is courteous to make an appointment. Do not think this gives the kennel management time to prepare for your visit. If they are a successful boarding establishment, they are far too busy to contemplate such action. When you do go to look round, prepare a check list of questions that you can put to the kennel personel to cover important points. A suggested list is as follows:

1. Do you insist upon a current vaccination certificate being produced?

2. What will happen if Bertie is ill while in your care?

3. Are you covered by pet health kennel insurance? Today many kennels are insured with leading pet health insurance companies which ensures that any necessary veterinary attention is carried out without delay. The owner does not then come back to face unexpected and sometimes quite large veterinary bills.

4. Ask about exercise during boarding. Are dogs taken for walks on leads? This is not a good idea. The provision of proper runs is a sign of a better kennels.

5. Ask about lost animals. Have the kennels ever experienced this? What is the procedure in such cases? Although escape from a boarding kennels is relatively rare it does occur and can occur even in the best run establishment. It is worthwhile knowing how the management would tackle the problem. The vague, 'Oh, I don't know, it's never happened here' is really not good enough.

6. Ask about feeding and whether food preferences are taken into account.

7. Another question which invariably invokes an interesting response concerns 'doubling-up.' 'Doubling-up' is a practice carried out by many kennels where two dogs, usually of the same sex will be put together if one appears to be pining. As a veterinary surgeon I can only deprecate this procedure. I think it is dangerous and can lead to fights and injury since the animals cannot be kept under surveillance 24 hours a day for the whole of the boarding period. At the same time, I can appreciate the reasons for the practice: dogs are social animals and some do miss their owners and pine if they are in the solitude of a kennel on their own, irrespective of how caring the staff appear to be.

Another reason for 'doubling up' is the problem of weekends. Invariably people want to bring their animals on a Friday or Saturday and collect, on either Sunday or Monday. At weekends in the middle of the season kennels will sometimes have more animals on the premises than is theoretically allowed by the boarding licence, which clearly states the number of dogs that can be accommodated. This is always a difficult problem even in the best run kennels and some overcome it by 'doubling-up'. Sometimes it is unavoidable since flights and estimated times of arrival are subject to delay. I much prefer the system of temporary kennelling or 'overflow' accommodation into which dogs can be housed for just 24 to 48 hours in an emergency.

8. One final question to ask is whether the kennels will allow you to place Bertie in the accommodation that he is going to occupy. Much can be inferred from the reply. If you are told frankly that due to constraints of time and staff you cannot put Bertie in his kennel that is acceptable. If there is prevarication and excuses, be a little careful for it well may be that Bertie has an accommodation earmarked for him which bears no resemblance to the sort of kennel you were originally shown.

During your visit note any parts of the premises that appear to be 'out of bounds'. Are there kennels of differing standards and you are only being shown the best ones? Do some of the units appear to be without runs or adjacent exercise compounds?

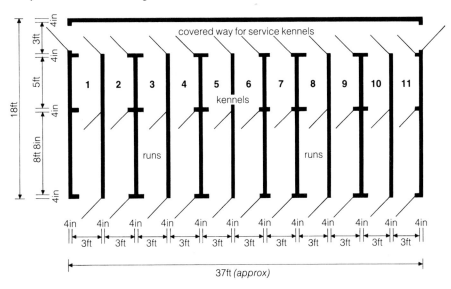

Figure 217 Commercial kennels vary widely in size and type. This plan is typical of the layout of a modern kennel and run system

What about the size and type of kennels (Fig. 217)? Commercial boarding kennels, unlike quarantine kennels, do not have to conform to stringent construction regulations and thus can vary widely in size and type. Some can be individual chalets in a paddock, or indoor units each opening on to a service corridor and with individual runs. In some kennels

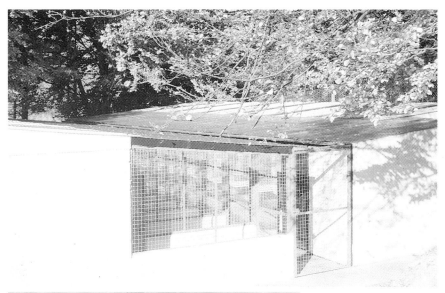

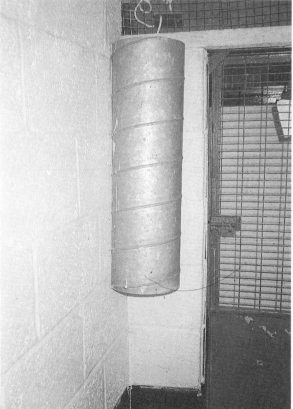

Figure 218　(Above) In some kennels even the exercise runs are covered

Figure 219　(Left) Individual overhead heating must be suitably protected from damage by the occupants

even the exercise areas are covered so that animals do not get wet during rainy weather (Fig. 218). Individual exercise runs attached to each sleeping unit after the fashion of quarantine kennels are common, but so are communal exercise compounds of concrete or in some cases of grass. Although the latter look much nicer they are difficult to keep clean and can become extremely muddy in winter, despite the fact that the Boarding Establishment Act insists upon a paved area around the edge and at the gateway to the compound.

Heating, ventilation and lighting all vary. Some kennels have background heating in the form of central heating, electric convectors etc. while others have individual heating in each kennel. This can be in the form of underfloor heating in part of the sleeping area or suitably shielded and protected infrared overhead heating (Fig. 219).

The sizes of individual kennels and runs vary tremendously. The basic quarantine reequirement previously mentioned of a width of one and a half times the dog and a length of at least twice the dog's length is a useful yardstick by which to judge the accommodation. Remember that most dogs like relatively cosy sleeping quarters so provided the run accommodation is adequate, do not be too dismayed if these appear small. Check the drainage and the state of the concrete or other material used for flooring and walls. Does it look clean? Is it hygienic? Remember that dogs are great destroyers of kennels and wear and tear during any boarding season is tremendous. Is maintenance being carried out and if so, to what standard?

Check the feeding bowls, and the provisions for cleaning and sterilising them. Are they in reasonable condition or are they very battered and tatty looking?

Figure 220 Small breeds from centrally heated homes need relatively more bedding than larger, more active dogs

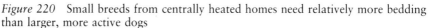
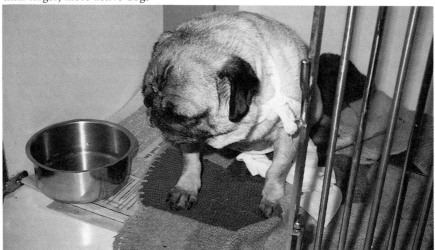

What sort of bedding is being used? This of course depends on the season. In the height of summer many dogs will eschew if not actually chew any form of bedding provided. In summer I would not be concerned if there was little bedding in evidence provided the bed area was raised above the level of the rest of the internal accommodation. In the colder months of the year heating and bedding depends very much upon the breed and lifestyle of the animal. Obviously the all outdoor, hunting, shooting, fishing work-dog is less likely to appreciate a heated kennel and the provision of lots of synthetic acrylic bedding than Penelope the pampered Pug, visiting kennels for the first time from the relative luxury of her penthouse flat (Fig. 220).

One final question in the selection of a boarding kennels is the size of the enterprise. Small units are usually under the direct supervision of the owner who frequently runs the kennels without any external help. This has much to commend it and these kennels usually have an established clientele and are frequently unable to accommodate much 'new business'. The larger kennels, on the other hand, if sensibly run, are organised on the same broad lines as the small owner-run concern. Each unit or block of kennels is usually under the supervision of one member of staff and in consequence the same rapport can be built up between the animals and those looking after them. The larger kennels, like the larger veterinary practices, are also at an advantage in that staff are more likely to be available at anti-social hours. Should Bertie develop a problem at 10 o'clock at night it is less likely to go unnoticed. However, it must be emphasised that boarding kennels are not hospital kennels. They should not be expected to offer a 24 hour-round-the-clock service with staff.

BREEDING KENNELS

Those who keep a bitch or two and breed the occasional litter will seriously consider the provision of kennel accommodation when the bitch is rearing a litter. It should be remembered that under the terms of the Breeding of Dogs Act it is necessary to obtain a licence if three or more boarding bitches are kept. The conditions of this Act are very similar to those of the Boarding Establishments Act in that dogs have to be kept in accommodation 'suitable as regards construction, size of quarters, number of occupants, exercise facilities, temperature, lighting, ventilation and cleanliness' and dogs must be 'adequately supplied with food, drink and bedding material and appropriately exercised'. Emergency situations such as fire have to be catered for and reasonable precautions taken for the prevention and control of the spread of disease among the kennel occupants. Again, this is similar to the Boarding Establishments Act.

Breeders are often divided into 'indoor' or 'outdoor' breeders although there are establishments which are a combination of both.

Indoor breeders

The majority of breeders maintain their stock almost entirely within their own private dwelling house. The animals are often kept for long periods of time in cages within the house, perhaps in the spare bedroom. This is unfortunately the life to which many terriers, toys and other small breeds are condemned when part of a breeding establishment. As far as inspection is concerned the cages must be of sufficient size for the dog to stand up and turn round comfortably and if necessary, to defecate away from the sleeping area. Rather like hospital kennels (which will be discussed later in the chapter), these cages should be considered primarily as sleeping areas and it is essential that the occupants are exercised regularly enough for those areas to remain unsoiled.

These indoor breeding establishments are, of necessity, labour intensive if the animals are going to be kept in tip-top condition and exercised properly. Regrettably many establishments fall short of these criteria despite the fact that the main provisions of the Breeding of Dogs Act are fulfilled. Obviously the cages have to be fairly easy to clean but since there is not the turnover of occupancy that occurs either in boarding kennels or in hospital/practice kennels, the standard of construction of the cages does not have to be of such high quality. Painted hardboard, if well maintained is entirely satisfactory. Inspection of indoor breeding kennels is bound to be somewhat subjective. It is really based on the opinion of the Inspector in reply to questions such as, 'What exercise is given and how often?' 'How often are the animals fed and let out?' 'How many litters are bred annually?'

The larger the concern the greater the risk of disease unless scrupulous hygiene is observed. Under these circumstances kennels or cages of a more impervious and permanent nature may be demanded and this can cause controversy between the breeder and the licencing authority.

Probably one of the most controversial questions put to the owners of these indoor breeding establishments is 'Where do you whelp a litter?' It is a time-honoured tradition among many breeders (not only those of the smaller breeds who practice the 'indoor system') to use a spare bedroom or little-used room in the house as a whelping area. There is certainly nothing wrong with this provided reasonable standards of hygiene are maintained, including the provision of impermeable floor coverings which can be adequately scrubbed and disinfected.

Inspectors perhaps not well versed in breeding matters are often concerned at the frequent lack of adequate bedding in breeding kennels. In full coated breeds, particularly in summer time, this is probably of little consequence but thin skinned, short haired dogs do find comfort in a

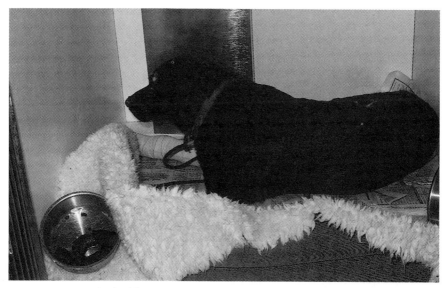

Figure 221 Acrylic bedding is ideal. It is easily laundered and virtually indestructible

reasonable amount of adequate bedding, be it blankets, newspapers or straw. Similarly, large boned breeds who are denied bedding are likely to develop pressure sores on elbows and hocks. From a hygiene point of view the new generation acrylic bedding materials are ideal since they can be laundered easily and are virtually indestructible (Fig. 221). However, traditional bedding such as hay and straw or blankets has been used for generations and should not be discouraged if adequately maintained.

Outdoor breeders

Breeders of larger dogs often keep their stock in accommodation consisting of out-buildings of one sort or another. These are often sheds and do not form part of the dwelling house. Sometimes converted stables or other farm buildings are used. These often cause problems for inspectors particularly in respect of heating and ventilation. It is expected that excreta and soiled material should be removed at least twice a day from the living areas and at least once a day from exercise areas in outdoor kennels. Exercise facilities must be provided as should facilities for the hygienic disposal of waste materials. This may be in the form of on-site incineration or collection by the local authority. The larger breeding establishments obviously have to make provisions for food preparation and storage in just the same way as provision has to be made under the Boarding Establishments Act. Depending upon the size of the undertaking isolation facilities should be available in order to minimise the spread of any infectious or contagious disease.

Anyone considering establishing outdoor kennels for breeding dogs should consider investing in purpose built units rather than endeavouring to convert existing sheds and buildings. Many precast kennel buildings are available today from specialist manufacturers who regularly advertise in the two weekly dog papers, *Our Dogs* and *Dog World*, as well as other specialist publications such as *Kennel and Cattery Management*. These can be ordered from your newsagent.

VETERINARY KENNELS

Pet owners are often worried when the veterinary surgeon decides to hospitalise the family dog for any purpose. Few people unfortunately, have the opportunity of seeing the type of accommodation provided, often solely due to lack of time. Veterinary premises are exempt from the terms of the Boarding Establishments Act unless boarding commercially. Veterinary accommodation is short stay and the kennels are designed to fulfil special purposes. They should be easily cleaned and maintained since they have a high turnover of occupancy (Fig. 222). In consequence many of these kennels today are made of plastic, glass fibre or stainless steel and involve high capital outlay.

Veterinary hospitals

The protected title, Veterinary Hospital, is only granted by the Royal College of Veterinary Surgeons to certain practices in Britain fulfilling stringent conditions. Among these conditions are suitable kennel accommodation and sanitary areas on site. Readers can rest assured that when

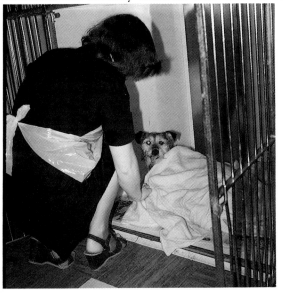

Figure 222 Veterinary kennels should be easily cleaned and maintained

the much loved dog is kept in veterinary premises, care is of a high standard. It is usually provided by skilled veterinary nurses who are well aware of the sick animals' needs to attend to the calls of nature and so regular visits to the 'sanitary area' are an established part of the routine.

Practice boarding kennels are not allowed under the provisions for veterinary hospitals. Veterinary practices, which are not veterinary hospitals and are running boarding kennels are subject to licence by the local authority in the normal way.

Home kennels

Finally, let us discuss 'home kennels'. These do not come under any legislation although those who keep a bitch or two and breed the occasional litter may wish to consider the provision of kennel accommodation even though they do not come under the provisions of either the Breeding or Boarding of Dogs legislation.

There are also other reasons for providing kennels. There is certainly no harm in housing the destructive dog in a kennel if it has to be left unattended. If dogs of both sexes are kept there is a need to kennel a bitch when in season to avoid the unplanned mating and subsequent pregnancy. Boarding the bitch for approximately three weeks twice a year can prove expensive and on site facilities will reduce strain on the budget as well as stress on the animal!

Types of kennels

The type of kennel required depends on the breed of dog and the amount of time kennelled. If your animals have to be left for lengthy periods each day there must be adequate room for the dog or dogs to move about, to lie down at full length and to stand up without touching the roof. The dimensions laid down by the quarantine regulations, i.e., a width of kennel of one and a half times the length of the animal and depth of kennel twice the length of the dog with a minimum height of approximately 6 ft is a good guide. A run or sanitary area should be provided in order that the dogs can go somewhere to relieve themselves. In an adequately fenced secure garden, outside kennels may not need a separate run. However if you do provide a run this should be long enough and wide enough for the dog to move around comfortably. Its size obviously depends on the amount of exercise the dog receives. Even if your dogs live together in complete harmony in your presence it is better to arrange kennelling so that they can be separated when necessary. Get them used to this separation at an early stage. Fights in the owner's absence do occur and are best avoided.

Purpose-built prefabricated kennels for both inside and outside use are available in a wide variety of materials from specialist manufacturers. The simplest and cosiest kennel is constructed of wood and for home use this is very satisfactory. However, kennels of precast concrete, metal and plastic materials avoid the fire risk of wooden buildings.

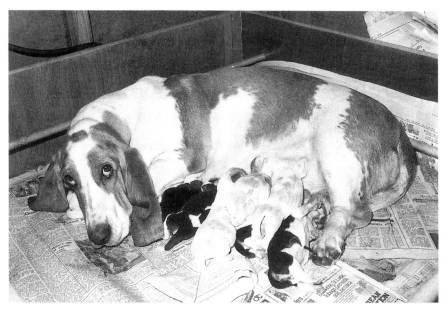

Figure 223   Newspapers are cheap, bacteriostatic and easily disposed

Whatever type of kennel you decide upon your dog should have a draught-free sleeping area. This is usually a raised bed some inches off the ground.

Bedding

Bedding ranges from newspapers or blankets to the modern acrylic fur fabric materials. Hay and straw is not recommended since they can cause skin problems and harbour skin parasites. Newspapers are cheap, bacteriostatic and easily disposed (Fig. 223). Wood shavings and sawdust can be used but do tend to work into the coat, ear and eyes and are generally not recommended although many people use these substances for puppies. The type of bedding you select will depend on the breed and size of dog. Small dogs will be happy in fibreglass beds with a blanket or acrylic fur. Old mattresses covered with strong polythene and a blanket are ideal for many of the larger and giant breeds and prevent the development of bedsores and calluses to which these dogs are prone when forced to lie on hard surfaces.

Heating

If you own a full coated breed and want to show, an unheated outdoor kennel will work wonders on the coat! The same however could not be said for the Chihuahua or other small, short-coated animal only kennelled occasionally either in your own 'house kennels' or in a commercial boarding establishment. Thus heating is dependent upon the breed, circumstances, time of year and length of time kennelled. Many commercial kennels have individually switched infrared heaters for each kennel. During the winter months when boarding kennels are often far from full, only those actually occupied are heated. Infrared heaters can also be used in the home kennel which is used occasionally. Depending on the area to be heated, small inexpensive fan heaters intended for use in greenhouses are often effective but should be placed out of the reach of the dog.

Any form of electrical heating should be installed professionally with suitable contact breakers in the circuit. Then, if the dog chews through the cable electrocution is avoided.

Lighting should be provided for all outdoor kennels especially if they are to be used in the winter months. As well as lights in the kennel, outdoor lights for paths and run make winter kennelling less hazardous.

Many readers may consider cleaning of less importance in the case of home kennels than in the commercial situation. However, if you show dogs you can bring home someone else's infection. Even if you only take your dogs out locally, they are still liable to pick up whatever is 'doing the rounds' in the neighbourhood. Therefore sensible kennel hygiene is essential. Kennels should first be swept and then washed with a scrubbing brush or broom and a bleach solution made up at the rate of 2–3 oz. of household bleach per gallon of water. This will protect your dogs against the most common infections. If a particular infection is suspected your veterinary surgeon will be able to provide you with effective viricidal and bacteriocidal disinfectants. Remember that most bacteria and viruses thrive in warm damp conditions and so it is essential to dry the kennel accommodation as much as possible before returning the occupants.

Noise

Do consider·your neighbours when establishing an outdoor kennel. Not everyone is tolerant of dogs and if your pets are protective of their environment they may be more noisy when you are absent than you realise. Train them to their kennel in easy stages: at first kennel them when you are around and then for increasingly longer periods when you are out. Dogs vary in their behaviour; some are noisy when in the company of others, some are lonely when alone and as a result become vocal. There is no way you can predict the reaction of an individual animal. It can only be assessed by trial and error. Therefore it is important that you acclimatise the animal gradually and note the response.

Planning consent

Planning permission is not normally required for small outdoor kennels but checking with your local authority and your neighbours is time well spent. If you do have problems, be it in respect of planning, construction, or noise, consider 'indoor kennels' in a garage, other outbuilding or spare room in the house. This type of kennel can be quite simple in construction provided the animal is not to be confined there permanently. Conservatories are often considered for this purpose but do remember that they can become extremely hot in summer, and are cold in winter. You can combat low temperatures with extra bedding and supplementary heating, but cooling the over-heated conservatory in summer time is altogether a more difficult problem.

Exercise Areas

Grass exercise areas have not been recommended in other kennel situations mainly on hygienic grounds but for the 'home kennel' a grassed exercise area, often the whole or part of the lawn can be used. As with the recommendations for boarding kennels it is worth considering paving the entrance to the sleeping area and areas of greatest activity, i.e., near any gates since these are the areas that become extremely muddy in winter.

32

HOW TO SHOW YOUR DOG

In Chapter 1, when discussing the pleasures and responsibilities of dog owning the point was made that life with a dog is a time- and energy-consuming business. If you decide that you would like to go one step further and not only own a dog but actually exhibit it, you will find that dog showing is a delightful hobby, but it does take up a lot of time.

Your companion does not have to have a pedigree in order to compete. Many local shows have 'fun' classes for the family pet and fun they are too, particularly on a sunny, summer afternoon. In addition, there are the worlds of obedience and agility, excellence in which does not depend on beauty but on ability.

Depending on your type of dog, working trials and field trials may be your pastime and there are many with working dogs or gundogs who regularly show them but have never entered a beauty class in their life, although as pedigree dogs registered at the Kennel Club they are entirely eligible to do so.

However, most people, when thinking of dog shows, are thinking of beauty shows, pedigree dogs competing against one another in order to be judged the most perfect specimen. In consequence this chapter will be concentrated on the beauty side and will not try to cover all the other fascinating ways in which you can take part, pitting 'Fred' against the rest. The worlds of obedience, agility, working trials and field trials will thus have to wait until another day.

The typical show all seems pretty straightforward at first. You enter your dog in the show, take him along, stand him in the ring with a whole lot of other dogs and a judge decides which is the best. That essentially is a dog show, but like any other sport or hobby there is a great deal more to it.

The Kennel Club is the official body that controls very nearly all the dog shows that are held in Britain. This official body registers dogs, checks their breeding against carefully kept records, makes the rules and licenses the shows. Once a dog is registered at the Kennel Club the owner has to sign to the effect that he or she will abide by the rules and regulations. If ownership of the animal is transferred the new owner has to sign a similar form.

Once registered a dog may not be exhibited at a show that is not licensed by the Kennel Club. An owner can be disqualified for exhibiting his dog in an unlicensed show, so it is very necessary to check that a show is licensed. This is always stated in the show schedule, published long before the event takes place, and which also contains the closing date by which entries must be received.

What happens if you own a dog without a pedigree and still want to show him? There are certain shows, which are known as Exemption Shows, at which this will be possible. The Kennel Club have allowed the organisers to have exemption from its normal regulations and thus both registered and unregistered dogs may enter. These shows are usually run by local fund-raising groups in aid of charity. There are customarily four classes for pedigree dogs with a judge who has experience judging at licensed shows. There are also a whole lot of fun classes, where pedigree and mongrel alike compete against one another. These are the shows with the classes for the dog 'with the waggiest tail'; 'the dog the judge would most like to take home'; 'the dog with the most appealing eyes'. These are fun shows, but do not run away with the idea that competition is non-existent. Many a well-established breeder uses the exemption show to introduce a young hopeful to the wide, wide world of dog shows.

Similarly many of us brought up with dogs are thrown into the rough and tumble, the highs and the lows of the show game, by being taken along to the local exemption show with one of the winning dogs in the kennel who will undoubtedly show the novice handler how it was all done. I have known owners of mongrels travel to exemption shows every weekend, covering hundreds of miles by bus and train just because they love winning another rosette and 'Susie seems to enjoy it as much as they do'. Frankly this is no bad way to become introduced to the show scene. If you want to show your dog, pop him in the next local exemption show. There are always masses of them up and down the country, especially in the summer months, and entry could not be easier. Unlike other Kennel Club shows entries are usually taken on the ground before the event starts, so there is no problem of getting schedules and missing closing dates, etc. Your pride and joy will then have the opportunity of meeting all the extraordinary shapes and sizes in which dogs appear. If you are unclear which classes you are eligible for, the Show Secretary or any of the organisers are usually only too happy to help. Do not worry that you have had no lessons in ringcraft, the atmosphere is all very friendly and relaxed and you will soon receive good advice if you happen to do it all wrong, like getting between the judge and the dog when the last critical placing is being made. Do not worry if you see other exhibitors placing their charges in accepted, if

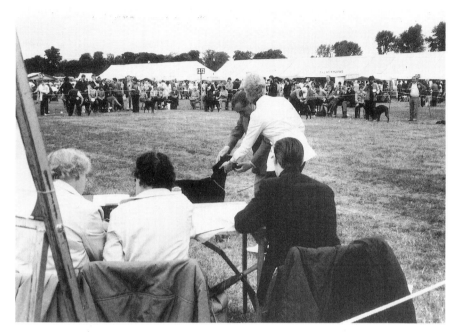

Figure 224 Showing a dog seems straightforward at first. You take him along and a judge decides which dog is best

perhaps exaggerated, poses, you are there to get the feel of the show. I can guarantee you will learn a tremendous amount if you are interested in dog shows, whether you are rejected with the also-rans or find that your pride and joy is as well thought of by the judge as by yourself and actually is placed. Remember that you are there for the experience and so is your dog. I think it is also vitally important to remember that because you did well this week, next week with the same dog at a different show you may get thrown out 'with the rubbish'. That is all part of the show game and happens from the level of exemption show right the way through to the championship show.

The moment that winning begins to matter too much all the fun goes out though the window. Of course we all like to win, but when it gets too serious for you to take losing with good grace, that is when, in my mind, it ceases to be a hobby and becomes a cut-throat business. The chap on the other end of the lead is your mate, your friend for life. Once he becomes a status symbol, a success rating, a £ sign in the stud stakes, it is time to take a deep breath and seriously examine your motives. I am sorry to appear to moralise, but the difference between getting a kick out of a hobby and being hooked on winning at all costs is all too often the sad tale that any veterinary surgeon will tell of another bitch past her breeding age being 'found a good home', another geriatric stud dog being left out in a boring kennel run, not uncared for exactly, but perhaps a little neglected since he is past the bright lights of the big time.

However, I digress; let us return to the bottom rungs of the show ladder. Apart from the exemption shows already described, all the other types of shows are usually run by an official dog club or canine society. These fall into two main groups. There are breed clubs which concern themselves entirely with one breed or the recognised varieties of one breed. There are also the 'all breed' clubs, which are based in one area of the country and cater for everything from Afghans to Anatolian Shepherds, from Weimeraners to Welsh Corgis. If your dog happens to be a Sussex Spaniel it is logical to contact the secretary of the Sussex Spaniel Association and become a member. If you also live in Kettering, your obvious port of call is the Kettering and District Canine Society. The breed club will put you in contact with all the other people who are interested in your favourite breed. The area club will tell you what sort of canine activity is available in the area where you live. Clubs, like dogs, are registered with the Kennel Club. This allows them, among other things, to organise licensed dog shows for which, yes, you are right, licensed dogs may be entered.

The number of registered clubs is quite staggering. There are more than 600 clubs dealing with individual breeds. Some breeds have a single club looking after their interests, while others have several. In the 1989 Kennel Club year book German Shepherds (Alsatians) list no fewer than 49 separate clubs covering the country from Devon to Aberdeen, from North Wales to Kent. There are just as many general societies and, in addition, there are more than 400 dog training clubs as well as more than 50 which concentrate purely on teaching people how to handle their dogs in the show ring. Special ringcraft classes are the next step for you if you have been really bitten by the show bug. These are usually evening classes and serve two very useful purposes. Novice handlers learn the art of showmanship; they get to know the ropes and learn the jargon. Like any other hobby the show game has a jargon all its own. In addition the novice pooch is able to experience the simulated excitement of the show ring and learn how to behave with decorum. Do not be embarrassed to go to ringcraft classes, particularly if your love is one of the more macho breeds. There you will be surprised how many experienced handlers you will meet who are bringing out new dogs. Also, if you happen to have a macho extrovert the experience will be particularly good for both of you and could save embarrassment in the show ring.

The Kennel Club, 1-5 Clarges Street, Piccadilly, London W1Y 8AB, telephone 071-493-6651, publishes a year book which costs non-members £3.50 including postage. This is something of a bargain because it also lists all the rules and regulations governing the whole dog scene, from shows to field trials, from agility to the stud book. The committees who run these breed clubs are tireless in their endeavours to set up programmes of helpful education for members, be they novice or expert. You will meet your fellow enthusiasts at all sorts of get-togethers and if you want to learn, you will.

Initially you do not have to participate any more than by listening and watching. One word of warning however, do not let yourself become seduced by factions which appear in any hobby. In other words, do not take too much notice of the apparent expert who damns all the progeny of one kennel while telling you that another kennel is far superior to the rest. Particular kennels will have their periods when everything seems to be coming up roses. Every dog coming out with their affix, or kennel name, appears to do no wrong in the show ring. Five years later it will be somebody else's turn for the limelight. All of us in dogs know that we all have our highs and our lows. On the whole continued success comes to those with the best dogs.

However, let us return once more to showing. You have now been to one or two exemption shows and you have enjoyed the experience. Therefore you became a member of your breed club and have, let us say, become a member of the local canine society. Is your dog actually registered in your name at the Kennel Club? If so you can enter him for competition at officially licensed shows. If he is not registered or has not been transferred from the previous owner (often the breeder's name) you should apply to the Kennel Club for a registration form or if necessary a transfer form. On payment of the appropriate fee the necessary registration will be effected.

Basically 'beauty' shows can be of two sorts, members-only affairs or open to all.

Shows limited to members of the show society from the simplest upwards are:

Primary Shows: These are small shows with not more than eight separate classes.

Sanction Shows: These 'member' shows restrict the number and standard of classes and can be single-breed sanction shows or schedule more than one breed.

Limited Shows: These are restricted to members of the organising society or to a particular area of residence. This is usually within a certain radius of the show or the location of the organising Society.

All 'members only' shows have an additional restriction in that they do not allow dogs which have won a challenge certificate or any award which counts towards the title of champion to compete.

Challenge Certificates are awarded at Championship shows, which are one of the two types of open show which are open to all registered dogs, irrespective of whether the owner is a member of the particular organising canine society. A challenge certificate is the top prize awarded for each sex in a breed and any dog or bitch which wins three challenge certificates under three *different* judges is entitled to be granted the status of champion, provided at least one of the challenge certificates was won after the dog or bitch had reached the age of 12 months.

The other type of open show is known as an 'open' show and is again open to any registered dog without any restrictions at all.

Challenge certificates, referred to as CCs in conversation and affectionately known as 'tickets' by the cognoscenti, are prestigious awards. The judges have to be passed by the Kennel Club to award them. It is entirely within the judge's discretion. at any show whether or not a challenge certificate is awarded. If it is considered that none of the entries is worthy of the title of champion, the award can and often is withheld.

Open and championship shows may be for only one breed or for a number of breeds. Some shows are so large that they run for up to four consecutive days. The most famous example is Crufts, which is the Kennel Club's own championship show.

The Kennel Club publishes an informative booklet, *The Beginner's Guide to the Kennel Club and Dog Shows*, which covers much of the ground of this chapter. If you are really interested in showing your dog and have not done so in the past, it is well worth sending for a copy.

Let us suppose that you have decided to try your luck at your breed club open show. What do you have to do? It may well be that the secretary of the club has already sent you, as a member, a schedule for the next show. If not, write and ask for one. This schedule gives the date and venue of the show, together with a list of judges and also the closing date by which entries must be received is also stated. It will also tell you which classes have been scheduled and give definitions of those classes.

Shows are organised into classes which are divided up in various ways. The definition of the various classes can be complicated and you should read carefully the explanation for each class. Classes can be organised in various ways:

1. According to sex with classes for bitches and dogs.
2. According to age, thus Minor Puppy classes are for dogs aged 6 and not exceeding 9 calendar months on the first day of the show. Puppy Classes are for dogs between 6 and 12 months of age.
3. According to previous wins. *Novice* classes are for dogs that have not won a challenge certificate or three or more first prizes at open or championship shows. *Undergraduate* classes are for dogs that have not won a challenge certificate or three or more first prizes at championship shows.

Thus, not surprisingly, the more successful the dog is the higher up the scale of classes he has to compete.

If you are unable to understand the wording of the schedule, do not be too bothered, even old hands at times have difficulty deciding whether a particular exhibit is eligible for certain classes. Have a word either with the person who bred your dog or with the secretary of the show. Once you get the hang of it you will realise it is not really all that complicated, although it appears very confusing at first.

It is important that once you have decided to exhibit your dog, you do not think his lifestyle has to change. It is all too easy to think that a show dog has to be pampered so that his coat, especially if it is a long one, is in perfect condition all the time. With certain exceptions this is totally untrue, most breeds of dogs can be restored to show trim by thorough bathing and a good grooming. A good deal of nonsense is talked about the removal of natural oil from the coat by bathing. In much the same way that human hair regains its natural oil within a day or two of washing, so does dog hair, if it is healthy. It may be important that dogs such as gundogs, which work regularly and plunge into icy streams as a way of life, should not have shampoos applied to them too regularly, but the occasional bath will certainly do no harm to those gundogs competing in the beauty classes.

Regular grooming is essential, whatever the breed. The techniques for achieving this end vary hugely from breed to breed and coat-type to coat-type. There are books available on every breed and all of them give detailed instructions on proper grooming whether the subject is an Airedale, a Chow Chow or a Poodle.

The truly successful exhibitors are those who can present a dog in the ring at the top of his form, fit and well groomed, in precisely the same way that a racehorse trainer or exhibitor of dairy cows will bring his charges to their peak on the big day.

Unfortunately, with some breeds the accent on coat length has rather become exaggerated; thus the Yorkshire terrier's show coat has been encouraged to become quite ridiculously exaggerated in length to the extent that regularly exhibited dogs are kept in 'crackers', which is the canine equivalent of human pins and curlers. Hair is actually wrapped around pieces of paper, which are in turn secured with rubber bands. These the dog has to wear during normal exercise in order to prevent the exaggerated hair from being broken and frayed.

The beginner can learn a lot by watching the experts. It is important that you do not become intrusive by asking too many questions, particularly just before they are going into the ring. This is a moment of great concentration for both the handler and the dog. Most breeders are only too ready to demonstrate show preparation and presentation and, in fact, many breed clubs arrange weekend meetings where such things are discussed and debated for the benefit of members. In addition, as already mentioned, specific ringcraft classes are available.

Although it sounds strange, in many ways it is often better to start off a show career with a pretty mediocre dog or bitch. It is just as easy to learn the art of presenting a dog with an also-ran as with one of the high fliers. The handler learns with experience, and by the time the new exhibitor has everything correct there will be no question of wasting the potential of a really good dog. This may be hard to appreciate. Surely if a dog is physically well favoured he really ought to win?

Let us make a comparison with a human beauty competition. If the aspirants simply slouched on to the platform with their hair all over the place, their expensive costume grubby and creased and their feet clad in a pair of wellies, would you really expect any of them to win? Presentation is paramount. In the ring, in any class, the judge will be looking for the animal which most closely fits his interpretation of the breed standard. Obviously then, if the dog you are presenting is to find favour with that judge, you need to ensure that he is looking his best.

Arrive at the show in plenty of time before your class is due and give your dog a final grooming and going over. When the class is called, turn up promptly. The first person you will meet in the ring will be the ring steward. His job is generally to assist both judge and exhibitor. He will check all the exhibits in and will hand out ring number cards. These identify the individual exhibits without disclosing the names of the dogs. The judge has to remain impartial and obviously is not expected to know anything about the dogs competing so that his opinion remains entirely unbiased. As a novice exhibitor you will undoubtedly be given advice by fellow competitors about particular judges. Sometimes they are verging on the slanderous, telling you that this particular judge is dishonest and that he gives prizes only to exhibitors who have used his dogs at stud. Another judge will be reputed to pay more attention to the person exhibiting than the actual exhibit and so on. It should be remembered that in any activity there are always people who are less scrupulously honest than they should be. However, the great majority of judges you will encounter are trying to do an honest job to the best of their ability. Obviously some are better at it than others and with experience you will soon discover which judges appear most popular. These are the people who the majority of exhibitors consider to give the most unbiased opinions. Remember, as has already been stated, you first obtain a schedule for any show and in that the names of the judges are displayed. It is then up to you to decide whether you want to exhibit under any particular judge. Nobody makes you pay your entry money, it is your choice.

Once you get bitten by the showing bug, it is very important that you never forget to record each and every placing you achieve with your dog. Previous descriptions of novice and undergraduate classes are but two of many classes scheduled at shows that are based on the dog's previous wins. If you really do get bitten and get into the show circuit you will find it difficult to remember previous placings, particularly after a hard summer season of showing, and if you do enter your dog in a class for which he is no longer eligible it is likely that you will be liable to disqualification.

Those of us who have had years of experience of the show ring will come to accept certain facts. One is that those who consistently have success over the years usually have the best dogs, irrespective of what people may say to the contrary. Equally important is the fact that the dog you take into the show ring is, and always will be, your dog, the original companion with whom you went into the ring for fun. Remember he is still your friend. If either of you, for any reason, cease to enjoy it, for goodness' sake stop. Please do not let the showing bug bite you so hard that you forget the bond that started it all. Whether you win or lose, remember it is only a hobby, and like all good hobbies it is there to be enjoyed, and that extends to both members of the team.

Good luck.

33

VETERINARY CERTIFICATION

In the eyes of the average dog owner, veterinary certification does not carry the importance that it does to the horse owner, but nevertheless as far as the issuing veterinary surgeon is concerned a certificate is a certificate no matter whether relating to a horse or a hamster. Written certification of any examination, treatment or necropsy carried out and signed by a veterinary surgeon is an important document, since it can act as the instrument upon which a law suit rests or compensation is decided. In some cases the reputation and standing of the veterinary surgeon may also be at stake. Obviously these thoughts are far from the average client's mind when a written statement is requested regarding the health status of a pet. It could be that the pet has been recently acquired and the written statement ends up as vital evidence in some form of litigation. Thus it is important that any certificate be prepared with care and accuracy after all the necessary steps have been taken to ensure that the matters to be certified are in fact true. Misleading, inaccurate or untrue certificates not only reflect adversely on the veterinary surgeon signing them but also affect the general reputation of the profession.

The Royal College of Veterinary Surgeons considers the issue of improper certificates an extremely serious offence and in some cases disciplinary proceedings have been taken against the offending veterinary surgeon.

When signing certificates in canine practice, one of the major problems is accurate identification of the animal. Remember that a vaccination certificate is still a certificate. How does the veterinary surgeon distinguish one male black Labrador puppy from another in a litter of, say, half a dozen males, all of the same age and same colour?

Perhaps more important is certification regarding some of the hereditary defects for which there are joint British Veterinary Association/Kennel Club schemes available, such as Progressive Retinal Atrophy affecting the eyes, or Hip Dysplasia. Despite every possible precaution being taken, at the moment such certification depends upon the co-operation and honesty of the owner to a large extent and it should be remembered that if the veterinarian is subjected to dishonest intentions by the owner, it is he and not the owner who is vulnerable.

IDENTIFICATION

Today there is much interest in the establishment of a national registration/ identification scheme and this would undoubtedly overcome many of the problems currently facing the certifying veterinary surgeon. Identification by tattooing may be permanent, but legibility tends to decline with time. The recently introduced microchip is perhaps less fallible, but does of course require the availability of expensive equipment in order to 'read' the code on the painlessly implanted chip. Perhaps we can now look forward to positive identification of our dogs in the future. At present the veterinary surgeon can only describe the animal presented as fully as possible, but in the case of a solid colour pedigree dog with no identifying marks this is less than ideal.

It is obvious that certificates are issued for a variety of purposes. Perhaps the commonest routine certificate is that handed to the owner when the course of primary vaccination has been completed. The Royal College of Veterinary Surgeons in Britain appreciates the difficulty of completing a vaccination certificate for a puppy in such a way to tie it without doubt to a particular animal, but emphasises that all parts of the certificate should be completed at the time of its issue. There can be no possible excuse for omitting relevant details concerning the sex of the animal, its known or approximate age, the name of the owner, the breed, a brief description of colour or any other matter with which the certificate should deal. Despite this, when inoculating a litter it is amazing the number of times that the breeder will ask for the name and address to be omitted because:

'I want to write in the name and address of the new owner and I don't have it. It will look messy if I have to cross out my name and address.' Another frequent comment when making out the certificate is:

'I'll fill that in for you when I get home, I'm in a bit of a hurry now, and it takes so long.'

On occasions I have had major confrontations with clients on these two simple issues. No doubt the client was in a hurry and I am appreciative of the fact that completion of a series of vaccination certificates often takes much longer than examination and vaccination of the puppies, but nevertheless there is a professional and legal aspect that may not be apparent to the client but which is very important for the certifying veterinary surgeon.

HEALTH CERTIFICATES

Less common, but even more important, are the certificates that are requested when examining a newly acquired animal. This may be a puppy from a local puppy farm or pet shop, or on occasions a rehomed animal from a less than reputable rescue organisation. The veterinary surgeon completes the examination and explains honestly to the owner that there are likely to be some problems. The owner then asks if he could have a note of the findings in writing. Frequently the client will be somewhat put out if asked to return at a later time for a correctly prepared certificate. There is also the question of cost. The cost of the vaccination certificate is included in the examination and vaccination fee, but this is not so in the case of the animal presented for examination with a later request for certification. A fee has to be levied because out of this very simple and honest request a situation may well arise where the veterinary surgeon's reputation is at stake. Litigation well may ensue if there is a dispute regarding the condition or suitability of the animal.

Unfortunately these are facts that are entirely unappreciated by the average owner, who presents the animal in all good faith. The examination is frequently considered a formality; he is hoping for the seal of approval from the veterinary surgeon followed by subsequent vaccination. To be told that it is a 'poor doer' or has some hereditary or behavioural problem which is causing anxiety is unexpected. Not surprisingly he wants this in writing and equally unsurprisingly can on occasion feel aggrieved if charged an additional fee for this written confirmation of findings.

I hope that this explanation of the implications will do something to explain the fee and to go some way to making its imposition a little more tenable.

Other certificates thankfully present less problems. Insurance companies will, on occasion, require certification regarding the health of a dog, as will airlines and other transit companies when animals have to be carried to far-flung destinations. Occasionally a certificate of health is required by an owner for his own purposes. For example, I have had such a request when an animal is about to be boarded. This can be at the instigation of the owner or the kennels in some circumstances. Similarly, injuries may require subsequent certification in some cases, e.g., if the animal is about to be exhibited.

Another common request for a health certificate is when a puppy is about to be sold and the breeder is asked for a certificate of health by the purchaser. Caring breeders will often provide these at their own expense, but I am of the opinion that it is not unreasonable for the purchaser to request from the breeder permission to take the puppy to a veterinary surgeon within a stated time, say 48 hours, and to bear the cost themselves. Unfortunately it is the cost of this certificate that can be a bone of contention. The veterinary surgeon carries out the examination, the cost of which is usually covered by the basic consultation examination fee. Certification is usually extra and can frequently amount to more than the basic consultation fees for the reasons already outlined. In view of the legal and professional implications this seems to me, as a veterinary surgeon, reasonable, but to the owner it is, after all, merely a piece of paper.

Vaccine certificates are not only issued for routine inoculations. Certain veterinary surgeons in Britain, authorised by the Ministry of Agriculture, Fisheries and Food and designated as Local Veterinary Inspectors (LVIs), are authorised to sign certificates following the administration of rabies vaccine for animals intended for export or for those in quarantine.

Another type of certificate which often has to be signed is the declaration of entirety of male dogs. In this case the issuing veterinary surgeon is certifying that both testes are descended and in the scrotum. These certificates can be for animals intended for export when often an LVI is involved, since he is already handling the export certification. On other occasions they may be requested either by purchaser or breeder for puppies that are intended ultimately for use at stud or for exhibition.

EXPORT CERTIFICATES

Health certificates for animals intended for export are commonly encountered in canine practice. Some countries, such as the USA, will accept a certificate from any qualified veterinary surgeon practising in Britain, whereas other countries require a certificate signed specifically by an LVI. The validity and terms of these certificates vary from country to country and their issue involves not only examination of the animal but also an appraisal of current regulations in respect of the importing country and often can involve special procedures, including blood sampling for Leptospirosis and Brucella canis, as well as certification that the animal has been sprayed with a parasiticide and, in some cases, has also been dewormed using specified drugs against tapeworm. Some countries require the veterinary surgeon to sign to the effect that the animal has been identified by the owner. LVIs are often involved also in the certification of imported animals.

RABIES CERTIFICATES

One certificate that causes confusion is the so-called 'Rabies Certificate,' for animals about to be exported. The Local Veterinary Inspector can obviously certify that in his opinion the examined animal is free from rabies, but he cannot certify that the area from which it is to be exported or for that matter the country (Britain) is free of the disease. This involves a special certificate issued by the Ministry of Agriculture and known as the Rabies Certificate.

AUTOPSY CERTIFICATES

Following a specific request for a post mortem examination many veterinary surgeons will issue a certificate. In many cases it completes the case in a much better way than a mere statement of autopsy findings, particularly if there is any suspicion of foul play. If this necropsy report is to assume the status of a certificate, great care is necessary in its precise wording and content. This is particularly important if owners are convinced that the death of their dog is due to malicious intent by some third party. It has been my experience in over 30 years of practice that in the majority of these unfortunate deaths suspected to be due to malicious intent, the actual facts are that common things are commonest and an accident or natural causes – heart or respiratory failure – are at the root of the problem.

CRUELTY CERTIFICATES

Finally we must consider the 'Cruelty Certificate'. Many veterinary surgeons today are involved in work with the leading charity organisations carrying out examinations and sometimes autopsies on cases of suspected cruelty. The carefully worded and often very comprehensive certificate which ensues is often used in subsequent litigation as a vital piece of professional evidence and often has to be substantiated by the veterinary surgeon in person. This is, of course, a prime example of the importance attached to veterinary certification.

It is hoped that this chapter has gone some way to clearing up the mystery attached to veterinary certification for dogs and to explain the reticence on the part of the majority of veterinary surgeons to put pen to paper without due thought and consideration of implications often unappreciated by owners requesting just a 'quick note of the diagnosis, treatment, or findings'.

34

PET INSURANCE IN THE UK

Over the last 40 years there has been a tremendous expansion in the scope and expertise of small animal practice. Conditions considered untreatable a few years ago can now be treated and repaired successfully thanks to major advances in veterinary anaesthesia together with the availability of excellent modern drugs and the increasing availability of specially designed equipment. Dogs with chronic disabling heart conditions can now be fitted with pacemakers and go on to enjoy many years of happy, active life. Cancer, one of the most common causes of death both in mongrels and pedigree dogs alike, is today routinely treated by the same methods as used with us: surgery, radiation therapy, cryotherapy, hyperthermia and chemotherapy are used on our pets just as they are on ourselves should the need arise. Bones shattered in road accidents can be plated and restored to normal function in a surprisingly short time. Hip replacement for our pets is now a practical consideration when we are presented with an animal with a crippling disability of the joint and no other signs of illness. Less obvious but equally important advances have been made in the treatment of chronic illness which inevitably involves maintenace of the animal on medication for long periods, often for life.

Unfortunately, however, accurate diagnosis and treatment costs money and with any complicated or chronic condition the bills soon mount up. Today for diagnosis alone the veterinary surgeon has at his disposal facilities unthought of a few years ago; X-rays, electrocardiographs (ECG) electroencephalographs (EEG) ultrasound techniques and endoscopic examination are all today available. In some cases they are unused solely because of the problems of finance.

Any veterinary surgeon in practice is well aware of the poignant and distressing situation where a dog owner is having to worry whether they can afford to have their badly injured or very sick pet treated without needing to deprive the family of essentials. The situation can be even more distressing if the pet happens to be elderly. The questions 'Can we afford it?' for the owner and, 'Am I right to suggest it and can I justify this course of treatment for an elderly dog?' on the part of the veterinary surgeon have to be answered and each can be equally agonising.

THE PHILOSOPHY OF PET HEALTH INSURANCE

Pet health insurance removes the need to confront decisions of this nature. It does not, however, provide an inexhaustible source of funding for every possible veterinary cost created by your dog. The philosophy is that the general maintenance of the dog can and should be budgeted for, unlike the traffic accident, poisoning episode or sudden onset of debilitating disease which causes unexpected expense and which insurance is there to cover. The essential feature of pet insurance is that it provides for the unexpected expense.

None of the pet insurance proposals covers preventative treatment such as primary vaccinations or annual boosters, and the elective neutering of either dogs or bitches, but if there is a disease condition present that makes such an operation a necessity then most companies will be prepared to cover the condition.

Hundreds of thousands of owners today realise that having insurance cover is the only practical way to ensure that their dog always has the veterinary care it may need, next week, next month, next year, right up to the end of its life so the pet will not have to suffer from any lack of ready cash at the time of crisis if ill or injured. Unfortunately fate seems to decree that adverse incidents always occur to coincide with other major expenses.

The Royal College of Veterinary Surgeons, the British Veterinary Association, the British Small Animal Veterinary Association, the Society of Practising Veterinary Surgeons, the British Veterinary Nursing Association and the Kennel Club all agree that having dogs insured is an important part of responsible ownership.

The pragmatist's view is that a puppy is a valuable asset. It is just as valuable in real terms as other valuable possessions. After all pet quality puppies in Britain today can cost up to £400–500 and this is only the beginning of getting the puppy 'on the road'. Primary vaccinations, check-ups, worming, leads and toys all add to the bill, and also do not forget that feeding in the first year or two is always the most expenseive. Thus it is soon evident that the family dog can be worth, in monetary terms, at least as much as a video, a hi-fi, a home computer or an engagement ring. All these articles we almost automatically insure because of their cost. Being purely practical, it does seem to make sense if one is making this rewarding investment of rearing and training a dog as a companion to protect one's investment if anything goes wrong. Letting the insurance company share the risks of dog ownership is thus a sensible way which many people are now beginning to realise.

SPECIALIST INSURANCE COMPANIES

Within recent years several specialist pet insurance companies have put forward practical proposals to cover unexpectedly heavy veterinary bills as well as providing a variety of other benefits to help dog owners in times of trouble. An example of some of the 1989 claims perhaps puts the whole question of veterinary treatment into perspective:

£150 for emergency treatment and hospitalisation over the weekend (treatment outside normal working hours inevitably costs more).

£600 for the repair of multiple road traffic accident injuries.

£252 for an exploratory operation which resulted in the removal of a pair of tights blocking the intestine of a young mongrel.

£194 for the treatment of a severe skin complaint in a West Highland White Terrier.

£347 for treatment by chemotherapy and in-patient care of a Golden Retriever with a form of leukaemia.

Figure 225   Irrespective of size, any dog from 8 weeks to 10 years of age can be initially insured and there is cover for cats too!

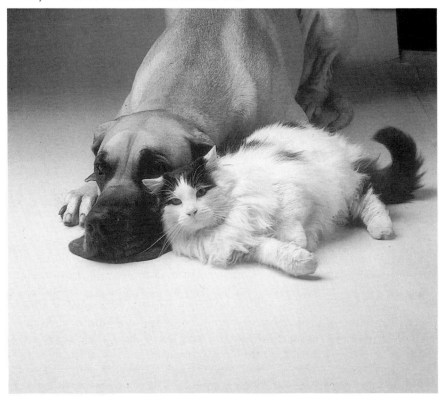

£245 to repair a sofa chewed by an Irish Setter left at a friend's house.

£250 for a puppy drowned in a swimming pool.

£297 for the removal of a malignant tumour from the leg of a Boxer bitch including follow-up consultations and dressings.

£139 for the renewal of regrowth of tumour on this bitch one year later.

£150 for advertising and reward for a straying Yorkshire Terrier.

Insured owners would only have to pay the first few pounds of the total veterinary bill in each case.

Cover for veterinary fees plus additional benefits is available according to the level of premium the owner chooses to pay. This varies from £400 up to a £1,000 for every individual illness and accident. Large dogs and giant dogs require higher levels of cover since treatment and medication will cost more due to the dog's size. A Labrador requires more anaesthetic and perhaps two or three times more medication than a small terrier and medication for, say, a Great Dane, will be even more costly. On the other hand very small or delicate animals like Italian Greyhounds, Papillons or Yorkshire Terriers will need very careful monitoring during surgery and special in-patient nursing so it may be wise to opt for higher levels of cover for these tiny dogs.

Most companies involved in pet insurance today offer these options but what are the advantages of insuring a dog with a specialist company rather than one of the larger 'household name' companies? Dogs with their ways and habits, their illnesses and their veterinary needs may be a relatively unknown area as far as the claims department of a multi-faceted company is concerned, whereas the specialist companies are very well acquainted with the canine race and their problems so that fewer queries and problems are likely to arise. All the leading pet insurance companies offer additional benefits as well as veterinary fees insurance and some offer a range of options so that owners may choose the benefit most suited to their own needs.

HOW UK PET INSURANCE WORKS

In Britain we are fortunate that pet insurance has been established for many years and has, with time, evolved so that it now has the confidence of the veterinary profession and the many hundreds of thousands of owners who already insure their pets. The procedure could not be simpler. Any dog can be insured from 8 weeks of age and initial insurance can be taken out for any animal until it is 10 years of age. Once accepted for insurance, cover should continue for the life of the dog. No initial veterinary examination is generally needed when the dog is enrolled although present or chronic illnesses must of course be declared. Premiums

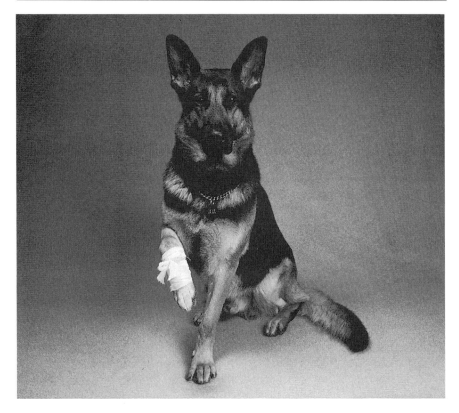

Figure 226 Insurance is there to cover the unexpected emergency

are the same irrespective of whether mongrel or pedigree. Hereditary conditions are generally not excluded.

Where to find dog insurance proposal forms

Proposals leaflets from one or more companies are to be found in practically all veterinary premises. Many dog breeders give information on insurance when they sell puppies and some actually have already insured the puppy before you purchase. One or two insurance companies usually have stands at championship dog shows and of course at Crufts. The Kennel Club will also give advice and some high street insurance brokers may be able to help. Thus the start on the road to insurance of your pet should not present too many difficulties.

Making a claim

Over the years the claims procedure has evolved along simple lines and today all the leading companies use a very similar, simple, straightforward system.

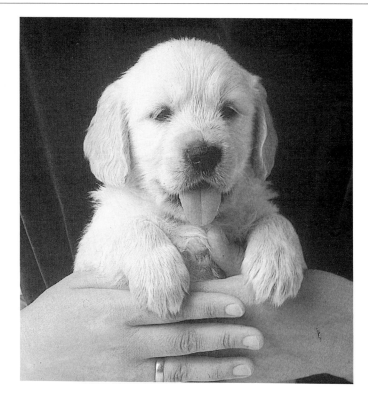

Figure 227 Puppies can be insured for life from 8 weeks of age

The owner takes the animal requiring treatment to the chosen veterinary surgeon. At this stage the insurance company need not be informed and there is no need to seek permission for the treatment to be started. Equally the veterinary surgeon has complete freedom to carry out whatever treatment is needed. At the end of the course of treatment the client pays the bill and the veterinary surgeon completes and signs the insurance claims form which has been obtained from the company. Provided the claim is legally acceptable a cheque for the amount less the statutory excess is then sent direct to the client within a very short time.

Package deals

Although the main benefit of pet health insurance is cover for veterinary fees, companies generally offer a collection of other benefits.

Third party cover is an absolute necessity to protect against claims from the victim of, say, a road traffic accident caused by a dog; or a farmer whose stock is attacked. Third party cover of up to one million pounds may seem extravagant but it can in some circumstances be necessary where an accident victim is incapacitated for life and makes a claim against the owner of the animal which caused the accident. Unfortunately the extent of third party cover is often misunderstood and therefore it is worthwhile explaining its scope.

It applies in incidents where the owner should be aware that the dog is likely to commit damage. The most common examples are traffic accidents caused by a dog running into the road and cars swerving to avoid it. Thousands of pounds worth of damages may be incurred if expensive cars have to be written off and the occupants are badly injured. Similarly the dog which trips someone up when dragging its lead can do a lot more damage than is at first obvious, for example if the person falls and hits the head on the kerb and suffers a long-term injury or sustains an incapacitating fracture. Third party cover can be worth literally its weight in gold in the case of dogs with farm animals. The mere sight of a dog may cause sheep to panic and kill themselves by running into field fencing, pregnant animals may abort solely due to fright and not because they are being actively chased. Claims in cases such as these can be heavy and it is then that the value of third party cover is fully realised.

There is another kind of cover which is available from only one insurance company at present. This gives protection against incidents when a dog damages other people's property even when under the control of the owner. An example will make this clearer. Recently a Bull Mastiff, on a lead, was startled by a collapsing tent while the owner was looking at an antique stall. The dog backed into a glass fronted display case which crashed to the ground breaking several pieces of valuable china. Under third party liability a claim would not be possible as the owner could not have been aware of what would have happened or how the dog would react. An accidental damage benefit would compensate for this incident as well as those embarrassing situations where the dog has spoiled furniture in a hotel or has chewed belongings on a visit to a friend's house.

Death benefit, usually equivalent to the purchase price of the dog, is paid by pet insurance companies in addition to veterinary fees if a dog should die from illness or accident before reaching 10 years of age. However it is important to check the small print of the policy carefully to see that the last veterinary bill will also be paid as well as the death benefit because this can vary according to the company.

Loss by theft or straying

The risk of losing a pedigree dog has accelerated in recent years. There have been many cases of dogs being stolen from cars or even from their own back gardens. A typical insurance package will include sums to pay for the cost of advertising for the missing dog as well as a reward for the finder. If the dog is not recovered the owner may claim a sum possibly equal to the death benefit but again, check the conditions of your particular policy very carefully.

Emergency boarding/caring

Many owners with sole responsibility for their pet or who live alone are often concerned about what will happen if an emergency should occur and they have to go into hospital or be otherwise away from home. Some companies actually pay boarding fees for the dog or pay for the dog to be looked after in its own home in such an emergency. If such a benefit interests you, be sure to enquire if the company offers these facilities.

HOW TO CHOOSE

It is worthwhile obtaining several prospectuses and reading them carefully. You must then decide which company offers the benefits you want with the premium you feel you can afford to pay. It may be that a simple veterinary fees cover, plus third party benefit, will fill your needs. If on the other hand you own a large dog or a delicate rare breed or a dog that tends to go off hunting you may find that you want more extensive cover and higher benefits. It is always necessary to read the small print when comparing one proposal with another. Your veterinary surgeon or the reception staff at the practice will willingly discuss any problems you have and may even be prepared to advise on the selection of a company. Do not be afraid to seek their advice, you will find they will be only too happy to help. Finally do not be afraid to clarify any particular points of cover with the company if you are in any doubt.

Special policies for exhibitors and dog breeders

The leading specialist pet insurance companies have realised for some time that people who keep a number of dogs and breed them, exhibit them or compete in obedience or agility trials have different, more specialised insurance needs from the general pet owner. Today at least two companies are offering policies in this field. For example, recognising that exhibitors often share cars with friends on the way to canine events, one company provides cover for dogs not belonging to the car owner which may be injured or go missing as the result of a motor accident. Breeding and whelping problems are often excluded from general pet health insurance policies but specialist policies are available which will cover breeders for many whelping risks and illnesses and even for the birth of puppies by Caesarean section if the veterinary surgeon considers the operation necessary. This is specialised cover however and a few of the Bull breeds such as Bulldogs and Boston Terriers are excluded since they have a notoriously high percentage of whelping problems. Therefore it is important to enquire from the insurance company if this is the type of policy which suits you.

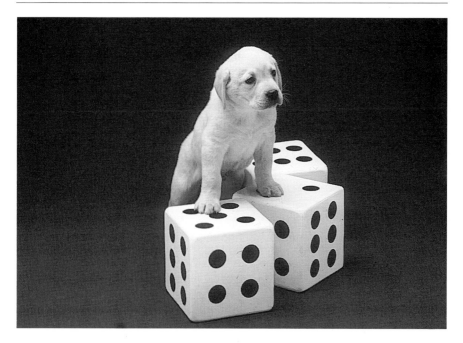

Figure 228 Breeders' puppy cover takes the gamble out of the first few critical weeks in a new home

Puppy cover

This is a short-term insurance which is sold only by breeders. It is intended to cover young puppies for the first few weeks in their new home. Costing only a few pounds, breeders generally include it in the selling price. The protection comes into operation directly the pup leaves the breeder so that accidents or illness which may occur even on the journey home will be covered. Market research has shown that new owners appreciate this type of insurance and associate it with a caring breeder concerned about the future welfare of the pups which are being sold.

Contact the following companies for information about aspects of canine insurance. Some also offer similar cover for cats and horses:

Pet Plan Ltd., Freepost, Pet Plan House, 10–13 Heathfield Terrace, London W4 4JE. Freephone 0800-282250.

Paws, c/o Jardine Insurance Brokers Ltd., Bristol & West House, 2 St. Philip's Place, Birmingham, B3 2QG. Telephone: 021-200-1010.

Pet Protect, 15 Knightsbridge Green, London SW1X 7QL. Telephone: 071-581 0187.

Dog Breeders' Insurance Co. Ltd., Freepost, Bournemouth, BH2 6BR. Telephone: 0202-295771.

35

VETERINARY MEDICINES
AND THEIR ADMINISTRATION

As the treatment of our pet dogs and cats has increased in importance since the beginning of this century, so the medicines used in their treatment have gradually evolved from the human counterpart. Many of the medicines used for the treatment of dogs are exactly the same as the human product but carry a veterinary label. In addition there are many human products used for the successful treatment of diseases in our dogs. For example, the treatment of chronic heart disease in the dog, which is becoming an increasingly important part of small animal practice, depends entirely upon the use of human cardiac drugs since there are no licensed veterinary counterparts.

All medicines in the United Kingdom are controlled by the Medicines Act 1968, be they intended for human or veterinary use. In addition certain drugs which can be the subject of abuse, e.g., morphine, heroin etc. are controlled by additional legislation under the Misuse of Drugs Act 1971. Further regulations under this legislation also came into force in 1985.

Under the Medicines Act, drugs intended for administration to animals are classed as veterinary drugs even though the same basic products may also be used for the treatment of humans. It should be appreciated that veterinary drugs are not only supplied to and by veterinary surgeons, but also include a large number of patent medicines sold for animal use in such places as supermarkets, pet shops and pharmacies. The safety, efficacy and quality of all medicinal products are controlled by a system of licences and certificates, issued by the Secretary of State for Health in the case of products intended for human consumption and by the Secretary of State for Agriculture in the case of veterinary drugs. Before a product licence is issued the manufacturer has to supply proof of quality, safety and efficacy; often involving extensive clinical trials. To obtain a product licence is therefore expensive and this is reflected in the cost of any new drugs on the market. However, one can at least rest assured that a drug carrying a licence for use in a particular species, for example a dog, has been thoroughly tested on that species and is safe and effective at the specifed dose rate.

Drugs on sale at the time of the introduction of the present legislation were granted 'licences of right' which are gradually being withdrawn to be replaced by a specific veterinary products licence. A similar and parallel procedure is occurring with human medicines. For drugs that are sold on the veterinary market in large quantities it obviously makes sound economic sense for the manufacturers to invest the not inconsiderable cost involved in obtaining a veterinary products licence. In the case of drugs with a limited use, for example those used in the treatment of fairly uncommon conditions, it is a different story. The cost of putting the drug through the test procedure is uneconomic and sadly these drugs are gradually being withdrawn as their licences of right expire.

The problem for veterinary surgeons is further complicated by the fact that veterinary products receive a licence for use only in particular species, the horse for example. Even though clinical experience shows that the drug is equally as effective when used for a similar condition affecting, say, the dog, because the product is not licensed for use in the dog, the manufacturer cannot be held responsible should anything go wrong. It is for this reason that some veterinary surgeons even go to the length of asking owners to sign a disclaimer if a non-licensed product has to be used upon their animal. An example of this is the use of a drug product called ivomectin which is licensed for use in the eradication of internal and external parasites in farm animals. This product is also known to be efficacious in some cases of demodectic mange in the dog. However, since its use is so limited, it is not and is unlikely ever to be, licensed for this condition. If you were unfortunate enough to own a dog with intractable demodectic mange, it is quite possible that your veterinary surgeon would advise you of the availability of this product, but would also explain that it is unlicensed for use in the dog and therefore neither he nor the manufacturer could be held responsible if any unexpected reactions occurred.

It should be remembered that many of the tranquillisers, sedatives, anticonvulsants, hormones and even cough medicines, in regular use in veterinary practice today do not carry veterinary product licences. They have been tested only for use in man but have established their worth in veterinary treatment. Insulin is an example of this. It is used in the treatment of diabetes which occurs frequently in the dog but for which there is no veterinary licensed product.

Both human and veterinary drugs are divided into three main categories.

1. General Sale Lists products (GSL)

These are the products that are considered safe enough to be sold freely in outlets ranging from petshops to supermarkets. The list of veterinary drugs on general sale is contained in an official order known as the Medicine (Veterinary Drugs) General Sales List Order 1984. Some of these veterinary drugs are on the general sales list only if they are intended for external use. There may be a limit on the maximum strength of the drug that can be supplied or on the total quantity in any pack. Veterinary drugs on the general sales list include medicated shampoos and parasiticides as well as certain anthelmintics (worm treatments), such as those containing piperazine which is a drug commonly used to treat roundworms.

2. Prescription Only Medicines (POM)

The second largest category of drugs are the Prescriptions Only Medicines (POMs). These are the drugs the average owner thinks of as 'veterinary medicines' although frequently they do not have a veterinary product licence and are actually 'human' drugs. These are the medicinal products which can generally be supplied by a qualified pharmacist upon receipt of a written prescription provided by a doctor, a dentist or a veterinary surgeon. There is a list of POMs which include all controlled drugs, (i.e., those listed under the Misuse of Drugs Act 1971,) antibiotiucs and sulphonamides, corticosteroids, barbiturates and tranquilisers as well as vaccines, antisera and many other categories of drugs. Apart from the drugs that are controlled under the Misuse of Drugs Act and which may be addictive, all the rest are controlled because specialist knowledge is needed for their administration or application and they should not be used indiscriminately.

3. Pharmacy (P) Medicines and Pharmacy Merchants Lists (PML) medicines

The third category of drugs falls between those on the General Sales List and the Prescription Only Medicines. These are the drugs that are designated Pharmacy or (P) Medicines. In general they can only be purchased by the public from a registered pharmacy but they do not require any prescription and can be freely bought. Many ointments and tablets used in the treatment of conditions in the dog fall into this category; for example, antihistamine creams as well as some of the non-antibiotic stomach remedies. In addition to these 'human' drugs there is also a specified range of veterinary drugs that are not General Sales List drugs and can be sold by agricultural merchants to farmers. These are drugs on the PML (Pharmacy Merchants List) and include preparations for sheep dips and worming. Mixed vitamin injections also come into this category and although intended for use by farmers in agricultural practice they are often used in canine practice, particularly the oil soluble vitamins A, D and E. (PML) medicines are thus the veterinary equivalent of (P) Medicines.

LABELLING

The labelling of veterinary medicines when dispensed by veterinary surgeons is as rigorously controlled as the labelling of similar drugs in human use. All medicines dispensed or sold by a veterinary surgeon are by definition 'dispensed medicines' and as such *must* be labelled in accordance with requirements. The container must carry the name and address of the owner, the name and address of the veterinary surgeon, the date dispensing took place, the words *For Animal Treatment Only* and the words *Keep Out of the Reach of Children.* Recent legislation discourages the use of pill envelopes and today containers must be of a more rigid nature and childproof. For the dispensing of tablets this usually means a plastic or glass tablet bottle with a childproof lid, but individually packed tablets in foil or bubble packs can be dispensed in envelopes. If the container is too small to allow labelling with all the mandatory information it is permissible to place the container in a larger envelope. These regulations frequently appear extremely irksome both to owners and to the veterinary surgeon but with the increasing number and complexity of veterinary products it is essential that mistakes are avoided and this can only be ensured if there is careful and meticulous packaging and labelling.

ADMINISTRATION

1. External applications

Having obtained your veterinary medicine there is then the problem of administration. Even the application of a cream or ointment is not always quite as easy as it would be in the case of humans. A frequent *crie de coeur* from worried owners supplied with an ointment to apply to an itchy spot, is that the dog licks it off as soon as it is applied. A good tip in this case is to apply the product just before the dog is fed or alternatively to distract him by taking him out for a walk. There are some dogs who are inveterate lickers and these simple ruses are doomed to failure. In such cases it may be necessary to resort to an 'Elizabethan' collar (Fig. 229). In the old days these used to be made of leather and were often unhygienic and certainly weighty. Today your veterinary surgeon will be able to supply you with a lightweight plastic collar which fits the bill admirably at little expense. Alternatively you may like to sacrifice a plastic bucket, break the handle off, cut a hole in the bottom and force it over the dog's head. Care is needed to adjust the correct size of hole to fit over the head and round the neck; if it is made too large, it will soon be removed. To prevent this, you can thread string through further small holes around the periphery of the 'neck hole' which can then be used to attach the bucket to his own collar, correctly adjusted in order that it cannot be removed. Although these

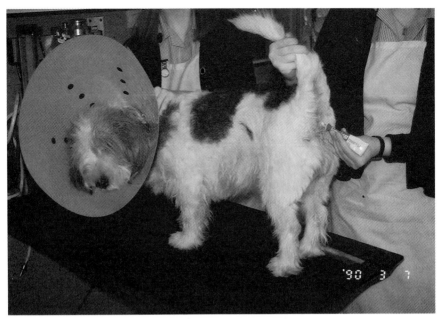

Figure 229   A lightweight plastic collar available from your veterinary surgeon
prevents self-inflicted trauma and unnecessary licking

devices are strongly resented by the majority at the beginning, it is amazing
how quickly most dogs will get used to them.

2. Administration of liquid medicines

Some medicines are reasonably palatable and can be given in the food,
although most veterinary surgeons are not keen on this method of
administration since it is imprecise. One is never quite sure if all the food
is going to be consumed! A much more precise method is to give measured
doses with the aid of a suitably sized plastic syringe. This is frequently
supplied by the veterinary surgeon at the time of dispensing the medicine.
The dose is measured into the syringe by sucking the medicine up by
withdrawing the plunger. The nozzle of the syringe can then be introduced
between the lips with the head tipped upwards (Fig. 230). The medicine
can then be gently dripped into the mouth rubbing the dog's throat at the
same time to encourage him to swallow. If the dog is very uncooperative
either a purpose-made muzzle or one fashioned from a piece of bandage
can be applied and the medicine gently dripped between the teeth
encouraging the dog to swallow at the same time (Fig. 231). It is important
that the medicine is not squirted down the throat. If a syringe is not
available a small plastic beaker can be used, which is preferable to
administering the medicine with a spoon since this is resented by the
majority of dogs. Today many specially formulated veterinary medicines

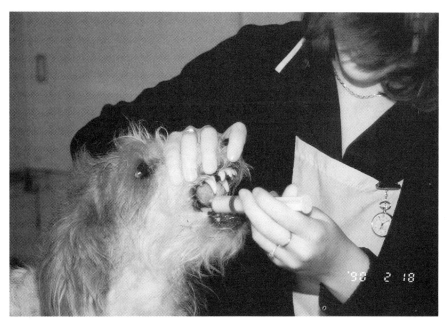

Figure 230   Using a plastic syringe the medicine can be dripped between the teeth

Figure 231   If the dog is uncooperative, a tape muzzle can be applied before administering medicine with a syringe

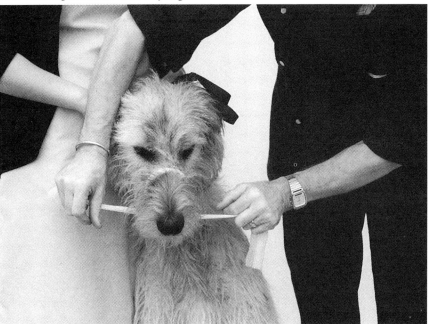

suitable for dogs are available in concentrated form requiring the administration of only a few drops. This is an advantage since the smaller the volume the greater the likelihood of success with the uncooperative patient.

3. Administration of tablets

As with the veterinary medicines mentioned above, manufacturers have also given thought to specially formulated veterinary tablets. These are made as palatable as possible. However if the dog is at all suspicious, he is unlikely to eat the tablet voluntarily, irrespective of how pleasant it tastes. Few owners have sufficient foresight to train a puppy to accept tablets pushed down the throat. This is a very useful technique to practise with the puppy, using innocuous vitamin tablets or even sweets. Make it a game and a lot of problems will be solved if solid medication is prescribed later on by the veterinary surgeon. It is a lucky dog that does not have to have tablets at some time during his life. If Fido really will not take the tablets, the technique is to try to take him by surprise without frightening him. Dogs quickly learn when it is 'tablet time' and will vanish from sight if given the opportunity. If a hand is placed across the muzzle and the forefinger and thumb gently inserted into the space between the jaws behind the canine teeth, the thumb can then be pressed on the roof of the dog's mouth. This will effectively prevent him from shutting his jaws on your hand provided you are dexterous enough to ensure that your thumb does not reduce pressure on the hard palate. With the tablet in the other hand it can then be pushed as far down the throat as possible and if the jaws are closed and the throat gently stroked, the tablet is usually swallowed (Fig. 232). Coated tablets are considerably easier to give than the rougher, uncoated type, but disguising these with butter or jam will often facilitate the operation. As little force as possible should be used to accomplish the task and this is why it is so much easier if the dog has been previously trained to accept solid medication. If you are not sure that the tablet has actually been swallowed, dripping a little water into the mouth with the aid of a syringe usually ensures that it is swallowed. Alternatively it is sometimes possible to disguise the tablet and mix it in the food, but if the tablet is divided or broken up, there is always the danger that the full dose is not taken.

4. Administration of drugs by injection

The only routine injections that have to be given by owners involve stabilisation of the diabetic dog using insulin. Most owners are extremely worried when diabetes is diagnosed in the dog, mainly because of the onerous responsibility involved in the administration of daily injections of insulin. Your veterinary surgeon will show you how to administer the drug. Since only very small quantities are necessary and the drug is administered

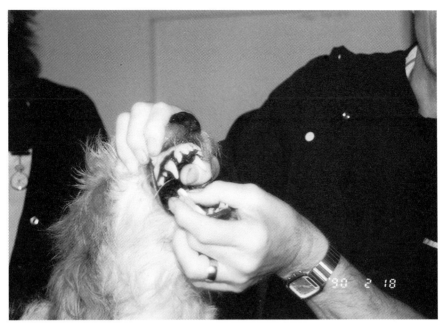

Figure 232 Pressing on the hard palate ensures the dog does not close its mouth on your hand when you are administering a tablet

Figure 233 Insulin injected on a daily basis is usually given by the owner

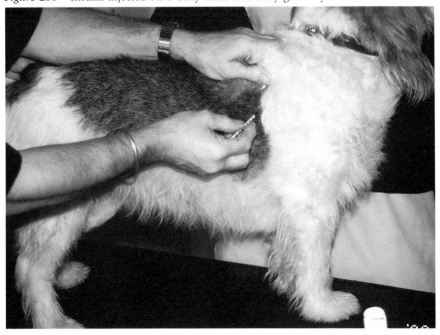

via a fine bore needle, little pain or discomfort is actually experienced by the dog. It is important that the whole dose is administered correctly and therefore it is worthwhile ensuring that the injection is given at the same time the dog is offered a small quantity of food. In this way at least the injection is associated with something pleasurable. Insulin injections are usually administered subcutaneously, which means that the injection is made into the tissue between the skin and the underlying muscle. The skin of the neck or upper part of the trunk is usually used. The skin must first be sterilised using surgical spirit or some other suitable skin cleanser on a swab and then a fold of skin is lightly held between thumb and forefinger and raised from the underlying tissue. The syringe should either be held like a pencil or dagger-like and the needle is then inserted swiftly into the fold of skin, keeping the syringe roughly parallel to the fold but with the needle angled downards. For insulin, 0.5 to 1.0 ml syringes are used and these are usually small enough to allow the plunger to be depressed with the palm of the hand once the needle has been positioned. Once the injection has been completed the needle is removed swiftly and the area thoroughly massaged.

36

YOU AND YOUR VET

The relationship between dog owners and their veterinary advisers should be as close or even closer than that between general practitioners and ourselves. In both cases there has to be complete mutual trust. If there is not neither side derives much benefit. Dog owners need their veterinarians and they need that bond of trust even more than we need it with our doctor. We can express what we feel is wrong when we enter the doctor's consulting room and can produce a fairly full and informative history of the problems we are experiencing. In the case of our dogs we need to be eternally vigilant to spot and record what is abnormal about them because we are probably the most important single factor in the vet's search for a diagnosis. If we are unable to give useful answers to the questions that are put to us it is unlikely that the vet is going to be able to do more than flounder in a vague half-light, handicapped by our lack of observation.

This bond of trust of course extends much further. If it is properly established we should not be afraid of tactfully suggesting to the veterinary surgeon in the puzzling case that perhaps we are barking up the wrong tree and perhaps the fault has been due to incorrect or incomplete history. Equally we should not take offence if the veterinary surgeon repeatedly cross examines us on the same topic.

Veterinary education in the UK

In Britain all practising veterinary surgeons have to be members of the Royal College of Veterinary Surgeons in order to be able to practise. They therefore display the letters MRCVS after their names. To gain membership of the Royal College they must study at one of the six university veterinary schools in the UK and complete a degree course which lasts at least five years. Present entry to the British veterinary schools is restricted to candidates who have obtained the highest standards in at least three subjects of their GCSE A-level examinations, and competition for places is very fierce.

The veterinary course is extremely complex and requires a great deal of concentrated application throughout the whole period. In addition to their academic work at university the students have, in their clinical years, to complete a minimum of 26 weeks 'seeing practice' with established veterinary surgeons in order to be able to sit for their final examination. Thus effectively they spend another academic year working 'in the field' before they qualify. Each veterinary school structures its particular course slightly differently, and at the end of it all a veterinary student receives a registrable degree that differs slightly from school to school. Cambridge graduates will end up with a BA and a Vet.MB degree, London graduates a B.VetMed, Glasgow, BVMS, etc. The mere fact that they are registrable degrees signifies that the basic course at all veterinary schools is similar and the degree is registrable by the Royal College of Veterinary Surgeons and allows membership for the recipient without having to sit further examinations.

Degrees offered by some of the veterinary schools within the Common Market and some Commonwealth countries are today also registrable, whereas other veterinary degrees, notably those from American universities, require the holder to sit a further examination set by the Royal College of Veterinary Surgeons before they can be admitted to membership and practise in Britain.

Figure 234   Veterinary Nurses provide a vital link between the worried client and the busy vet. Here a nurse helps an injured animal from car to examination room

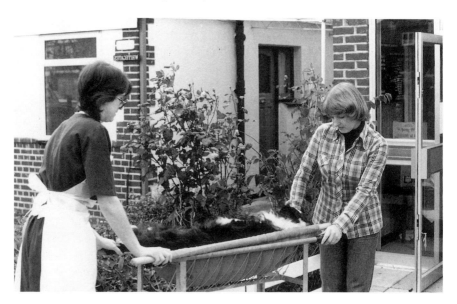

Once qualified, all veterinary surgeons in this country are supposed to be able to cope with all the problems which beset every possible animal from Retriever to racehorse, from walrus to Weimaraner. Quite obviously nobody can achieve omniscience of that order in a five-year degree course and, as in every other calling, learning continues throughout the whole of the lifetime career.

The Types of Practice

There are many veterinary practices which are run by only one vet and it is amazing the high standards that such solo vets attain. Other practices have anything from 2-20 vets all working within one group, but possibly covering a very large geographical area from several centres. Such a system enables individuals to concentrate on their own special interest, be it one particular animal, such as the horse, or one particular discipline, such as the heart or the eye. This specialist interest will be pursued right across the spectrum of patients.

Specialisation

Specialisation is being actively encouraged by the Royal College of Veterinary Surgeons and specific courses of postgraduate study are now available which can lead members to gain certificates or diplomas in subjects such as opthalmology, orthopaedics, radiography, dermatology and many other specialist realms.

Selection of Practice

It is not specialist services available at the practice which concern the ordinary dog owner in his initial selection of an appropriate practice. The prime consideration is, at that time, the availability and quality of the service offered. All veterinary surgeons in Britain are expected by the demands of their ethical code as laid down by the Royal College of Veterinary Surgeons to provide 'adequate cover' for 24 hours a day, every day of the year. This does not mean that any problem, large or small, will be dealt with at any hour of the day or night. Most routine illness can be attended to during normal consulting hours and do remember that these will involve the average practice and its staff in working considerably more than the normal 40-hour week. What is essential is that when a true emergency occurs, help can be obtained in a reasonably short period of time. Such help may come from within one's own veterinary practice or it may be from a neighbouring practice which is on emergency call. This is a normal arrangement that is frequently made between practitioners in an area so that all can be sure of some modicum of free time.

It will invariably happen on occasion that an owner will have to accept one of the other vets in a team, but most practices do try to provide their clients with regular cover from one individual in order that case continuity can be maintained and the bond of trust referred to earlier is not disrupted.

In recent times veterinary skills have advanced by leaps and bounds. Forty years ago the dog was considered, in many practices, to be the species which was dealt with once the more important horse and farm patients had been treated. Today the dog is the mainstay of more than half the practices in the country.

Most practices today run an appointment system, which usually means the minimum amount of waiting for both owner and patient and the immediate availability of patient records. However, it should be remembered that emergencies do happen and these can disrupt even the most well-run appointment system. In addition, in some areas traffic conditions are so horrendous that some practitioners are abandoning appointment systems and going back to the open clinics of 20 years ago, when you just walked in with your pet during clinic hours and took your turn. At least in this way there are no problems fitting in the person who arrives an hour late. This may be through no fault of their own, but solely due to delays due to traffic. On the other hand, some clients, having been late in the past, start off especially early only to arrive an hour early for the appointment. This is equally disruptive to a full appointment list.

Payment

Two or three decades ago it was considered unprofessional to ask for payment at the time of the treatment, whereas today most practices will expect payment on each and every occasion. This is in order that the cash flow of what is now a relatively sophisticated and labour-intensive business is adequate to pay the enormous expenses involved with drugs, equipment and staff.

Veterinary nurses

The trained veterinary nurse is now a familiar sight in most small animal practices. The days of the receptionist who doubled as nurse, anaesthetic assistant and general dog's body so graphically portrayed by James Herriot have long since gone. Veterinary nurses today spend a minimum of two years working in practices approved by the Royal College of Veterinary Surgeons as suitable training centres and have to undergo two stiff professional examinations, at the end of which time they are entitled to add the letters VN after their name. In the majority of approved training centres veterinary nurses can easily be spotted; trainees wear a green and white striped dress and white apron while VNs are usually dressed in a smart dark green uniform, often again with a white apron. They are a highly motivated, highly trained band of people who carry out crucial tasks in modern small animal practices. They are often the link between the worried owner and the veterinary surgeon and act as receptionist and counsellor as well as carrying out the many highly skilled jobs for which they are trained. These can range from the maintenance of anaesthesia, laboratory work and radiography to record keeping, in addition to routine nursing of the sick animal when hospitalised, together with all the monitoring necessary. Recently a further qualification has become available to nurses. This is a Diploma in Advanced Veterinary Nursing (Surgical) and will suitably acknowledge their undoubted skills in these fields.

Receptionists

In addition to veterinary surgeons and veterinary nurses many of the larger practices today employ trained receptionists. This training is designed to equip the receptionist with the necessary skills to deal with the emergency, and, let us face it, there are few jobs more tricky than calming the frantic owner whose dog has just been hit by a passing car. Naturally the owner wants immediate help, but is sometimes too distracted with grief that essential information such as the location, name of either owner or animal, or extent of the problem, is not relayed. An experienced receptionist is worth her weight in gold in a busy practice, especially as she is so often the first contact that the client has with the practice. Her projected image can either make or mar the relationship.

Premises and equipment

The days of the tiny, poorly equipped, lock-up consulting room are fast disappearing. Modern premises are smart, well equipped and with a great

Figure 235 Modern veterinary premises are smart, well equipped and with a lot of equipment never seen by clients

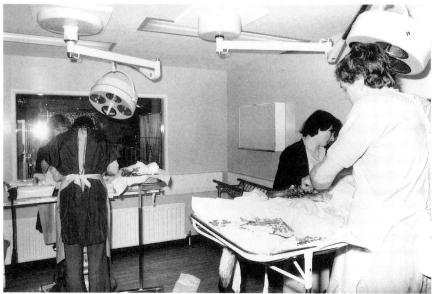

deal of vital and very expensive instrumentation, which regretfully the majority of clients never see.

The Royal College of Veterinary Surgeons which, in Britain, controls virtually every sphere of veterinary endeavour will, after inspection, allow the use of the protected title Veterinary Hospital to be applied to certain of these practices that have fulfilled the stringent requirements regarding equipment, facilities and staffing levels. However, there are many practices that do not carry the title of veterinary hospital but which are equally well equipped. It is entirely a decision of the principal whether or not application is made to the Royal College for inspection with a view to obtaining hospital status. Therefore, do not think that because any particular practice does not have hospital status the standard of diagnosis and specialised treatment, hospitalisation or intensive care is in any way inferior.

Most practices now run some form of practice laboratory. In some of these only very basic tests on urine or faeces may be carried out. More advanced laboratory work may be referred to specialised laboratory services. These are today offering ever more rapid and accurate results so that again one should not be concerned if the practice mentions that the samples urgently required for diagnosis have to be sent to a specialised laboratory. This can even happen in the most well-equipped veterinary hospital, since the range of diagnostic tests is becoming ever more sophisticated and some are conducted by only a very few specialised centres.

Computerisation has come to veterinary practice not only with computerised record-keeping, account administration, pricing, etc., but also in the sphere of laboratory services. Today there are many highly sophisticated microcomputer-controlled pieces of equipment that allow practices to conduct in-house investigations involving haematology and blood biochemistry, thus ensuring very rapid results. But, do remember the cost of such sophisticated apparatus runs into many thousands of pounds and one should not expect that because the result is available in sometimes a matter of seconds or minutes that it is any the less accurate or expensive than results from a source taking longer. Some practice laboratories carry out laboratory examinations on skin scrapings and biopsies, and antibiotic sensitivity testing of individual bacterial infections. This enables the clinician to prescribe with very much more accuracy than in times gone by.

This ever-expanding area of laboratory diagnosis increases the job satisfaction and depth of interest of those employed by the practice. Frequently it is a veterinary nurse who is trained to undertake this work.

Additional knowledge

It is not only in the practice laboratory that tremendous advances are being made; there are equal advances in anaesthetics, drugs and their administration as well as in surgical knowledge and skill. Thus treatment of injury, gastrointestinal blockage or cancer, as well as eye surgery, is now commonly carried out in many local practices with a success rate that would have confounded the veterinary surgeons of a few decades ago.

Preventive medicine

Preventive medicine is another area in which there have been great strides forward. Indeed, in some areas it has replaced the need for treatment of disease. Nowhere is this more obvious than in the routine vaccination against infections such as distemper, which were once dreaded and almost invariably fatal. Preventive medicine, however, does not only involve vaccination. Today regular treatment to control worm infestation using highly efficacious drugs which do not upset the animal is all part of the general health care programme.

Dental checks ensure the maintenance of good standards of oral hygiene and recently attention has been paid to the education of owners in home dental care involving brushing the teeth on a regular basis. This reduces the number of general anaesthetics and routine scalings and polishings that are required throughout the dog's life.

Many owners today have come to expect regular checks on heart, kidney and liver functioning, especially for geriatric animals, and these often involve sophisticated monitoring equipment, X-rays, ultrasonics and electrocardiograms as well as the supporting laboratory tests.

This catalogue of advance is heartening indeed for the caring modern dog-owning public, but it has one inevitable consequence; it costs money. The high standard of veterinary care today costs considerably more than the basic consultation and the packet of pills of our forefathers. Irrespective of the inflation factor the bill may reach quite large proportions in a relatively short time. Fortunately the veterinary world has mirrored the medical world and pet health insurance has become available from a number of companies. This does not cover routine vaccination, voluntary dental care or neutering, but it does mean that the severe injury sustained in a road traffic accident, the joint damage occasioned by an injudicious race after the neighbour's cat or the badly cut foot involving extensive tendon damage does not involve the owner in taking out a second mortgage to cope with the unbudgeted expense.

How do you select the practice?

The problems of selection of a veterinary practice is one that can often concern the new dog owner as well as those established owners who may be moving to a new area. The selection of the practice needs careful consideration. Personal recommendation from caring, dog-owning friends or neighbours is obviously one of the best guides, and for those moving into a new area a few minutes spent talking with other dog owners in local parks and public places is often time well spent. The *Yellow Pages* will often fill in other details of service and a prospective client should not be afraid of telephoning the practice to ascertain the extent of the services offered. The home or domiciliary visit is one area which worries many owners, since today an ever-dwindling number of practices offer this service on a routine basis. There are many reasons for this, time, cost and traffic delays being fairly high on the list as far as the veterinary surgeon is concerned. However, there are other factors to be considered. The well-equipped surgery is obviously the ideal place to examine a dog and in almost every situation it is best to transport the dog to that surgery. He will then not feel he has to defend his home territory against an invading stranger. In addition there will be a convenient table on which he can be handled; there will be adequate skilled help to hold him if that is needed and there will be effective light to examine him. All the other exotic hardware previously touched upon will be ready at hand. Even adequate light and handling facilities are rarely available in the home and polished tables or kitchen worktops do not make a very satisfactory or secure footing for the apprehensive, injured or ill pet. Thus it really is a good idea to take the dog to the vet as often as it is possible. It may also mean that he gets proper treatment very much more rapidly.

However, there are occasions when a home visit is required and it is worthwhile establishing what arrangements the practice can offer should such a service be needed. Many urban practices which today find it difficult to run an effective domiciliary visiting service will have ambulance services or a 'pet taxi' service that can be invoked in hours of need.

Some owners are particularly concerned about hospitalisation facilities or if the emergency service is in-house or whether telephones are transferred to sometimes far-flung practices. These are all questions which you should not be afraid of asking at the outset.

You will find, in the majority of cases, a caring veterinary nurse will be more than happy to answer all your queries on these points, patiently explaining routine procedures. Her training is such that you will be blissfully unaware that she may be endeavouring at the same time to change a drip on a critically ill dog just because the phone happened to ring at that moment.

Client loyalty

After you have satisfied yourself on all the questions that are important to you, choose your practice and then as far as possible remain with that practice. In that way the bond of mutual trust is soon established. There are no rules on the subject. No one can force an owner to go to the same practice all the time, but it is a fact that most practitioners like to build up a relationship with their clients and pets and that relationship does involve a modicum of loyalty on both sides. Remember that you, as the owner, are not bound by professional ethics, whereas they are stringent as far as the veterinary practitioner is concerned. It is for this reason that when you decide to visit a neighbouring practice, you will be subjected to what, on occasion, you may consider to be a quite improper 'third degree'. The practitioner is merely establishing to his own satisfaction that the animal is not currently under treatment.

Rapport with your veterinarian becomes even more important when emergency situations arise. Finding there is always a friendly voice at the end of the emergency line, even in the wee small hours, is vastly reassuring, particularly if you are about to invite that friendly voice to arise from a warm bed in order to attend to your bitch who happens to be in the middle of whelping and not making a very good job of it!

Second opinions

This relationship is even more called into question on those occasions when treatment does not seem to be going as well as the owner, the vet and assuredly the dog would like. It is in this situation that the possibility of another opinion, another view of the case, may be beneficial. The experienced veterinary surgeon knows that no one person can win every battle against every problem which is presented during a veterinary career. A good practitioner will know when another vet's examination, another colleague's line of therapy, may help towards a successful resolution of a worrying case. The suggestion for a second opinion should never be resented if it comes from your veterinary surgeon. It certainly does not mean that he is fed up either with you or the case but merely that he is caring and worried.

It may sometimes be necessary for an owner to express doubt about the progress of a dog's condition and there is absolutely no reason why an owner should be denied a second opinion. What is never a good idea is for an owner, however worried and distraught, to go and seek the second view behind the back of the regular adviser. This is not a matter of the oft-misused expression, 'professional ethics', it is a matter of what is best for the animal. To ask another veterinary surgeon to treat an animal that is already receiving professional attention, without making the existing situation quite clear, not only destroys your relationship with your veterinary surgeon but also risks the welfare of the animal. Treatment which has already been tried may be needlessly repeated, treatment which may be instituted by the second person may be incompatible with the therapy already employed. Tests and diagnostic aids may be invoked which have already been completed and this just involves a waste of time, money and further stress for the patient.

Embarrassing though it may be, it is far better to approach your veterinary surgeon and chat about the possibility of a second opinion.

The needs

It is sometimes helpful for veterinary surgeon and client alike if each is aware of the other's needs in their mutual relationship. Firstly, what are the client's needs?

1. Ease of contact, the ability to speak with the vet in person or over the telephone as and when appropriate.
2. A rapid reaction in an emergency situation.
3. Competent, sympathetic treatment. This extends to both client and animal in an emergency situation.
4. A true 24-hour service, again when such is necessary.
5. The availability of specialist advice when needed.
6. A genuine interest in your pet. This is especially important when breeding activity may be considered. Some practices encourage breeders to become clients, others do not, and it is better to know how breeding problems are handled within a practice before the need arises.
7. A scale of charges that is within your pocket, with the fixed tariff being available before treatment commences if this is required. Remember that few practitioners are in a position to give a quotation, but a rough estimate of costs should be available if required.
8. Mutually understood arrangements regarding domiciliary visits, pick-ups, etc. This is especially important in the case of large breeds of dog and whelpings.

The veterinary surgeon requires:

1. An acceptance of practice policy regarding consulting hours except in emergency or by special arrangement.
2. A readiness on the part of the client to provide an adequate history whenever a patient is presented for examination. This involves observation of the dog's general behaviour, appetite, production of urine and faeces and any obvious abnormality. These are essential to the veterinary surgeon if he is to attempt even a provisional diagnosis.
3. Ability to exercise reasonable control over any dog presented for treatment, while in the consulting room and in the reception area.
4. A readiness to accept advice and to act upon it. The course of treatment which is not carried out has little chance of influencing the condition for which it is prescribed and it is ridiculous complaining to the veterinary surgeon that 'the money spent on veterinary fees has been wasted because the condition is no better' if the treatment has not been carried out.
5. Client loyalty. Using one practice this week and a neighbouring one next week leads to inevitable loss of trust and interest.
6. Prompt settlement of accounts and a willingness to abide by practice policy in this respect.

I am sorry if these lists sound either dictatorial or perfectionist, they are not meant to. Hopefully they should be the basis of a lastingly satisfactory liaison between you and your vet.

INDEX